Effective Documentation for Physical Therapy Professionals

Second Edition

Eric Shamus, PT, DPT, PhD, CSCS
Associate Professor
College of Allied Health
Department of Physical Therapy & Human Performance
Florida Gulf Coast University
Fort Myers, Florida

Debra Feingold Stern, PT, DPT, MSM, DBA
Assistant Professor of Physical Therapy
College of Allied Health
Health Professions Division
Nova Southeastern University
Ft. Lauderdale, Florida

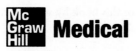 Medical

New York   Chicago   San Francisco   Lisbon   London   Madrid   Mexico City
Milan   New Delhi   San Juan   Seoul   Singapore   Sydney   Toronto

The McGraw-Hill Companies

Effective Documentation for Physical Therapy Professionals, Second Edition

2 3 4 5 6 7 8 9 0 QDB/QDB 15 14 13 12 11

ISBN 978-0-07-166404-2
MHID 0-07-166404-1

This book was set in Berling by Thomson Digital.
The editors were Joseph Morita and Regina Y. Brown.
The production supervisor was Catherine H. Saggese.
The index was prepared by Thomson Digital.
Quad/Graphics was the printer and binder.

This book is printed on acid-free paper.

Catalog-in-Publication Data is on file for this title at the Library of Congress.

Please tell the author and publisher what you think of this book by sending your comments to pt@mcgraw-hill.com. Please put the author and title of the book in the subject line.

McGraw-Hill books are available at special quantity discounts to use as premiums and sales promotions or for use in corporate training programs. To contact a representative, please e-mail us at bulksales@mcgraw-hill.com.

Effective Documentation for Physical Therapy Professionals

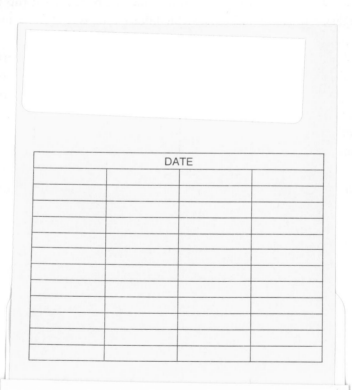

DATE			

Notice

Medicine is an ever-changing science. As new research and clinical experience broaden our knowledge, changes in treatment and drug therapy are required. The authors and the publisher of this work have checked with sources believed to be reliable in their efforts to provide information that is complete and generally in accord with the standards accepted at the time of publication. However, in view of the possibility of human error or changes in medical sciences, neither the authors nor the publishers nor any other party who has been involved in the preparation or publication of this work warrants that the information contained herein is in every respect accurate or complete, and they disclaim all responsibility for any errors or omissions or for the results obtained from use of information contained in this work. Readers are encouraged to confirm the information contained herein with other sources. For example and in particular, readers are advised to check the product information sheet included in the package of each drug they plan to administer to be certain that the information contained in this work is accurate and that changes have not been made in the recommended dose or in the contraindications for administration. This recommendation is of particular importance in connection with the new or infrequently used drugs.

This book is dedicated to our families;
Allan, Margot, and Darren
and
Jennifer, Grant, and Alexa
For their love, support and guidance.

CONTENTS

CONTRIBUTORS

Martha H. Bloyer, PT, PCS
Department of Physical Therapy
Florida International University
Miami, Florida
Pediatric Documentation

Nancy Campbell, PT
Orthonet
Fort Lauderdale, Florida
Utilization Review and Utilization Management

Keith E. Christianssen, PT, ATC
Impact Sports
Broomfield, Colorado
The Electronic Medical Record

Barbara Deering, PT
Director of URQA
Outreach Programs, Inc.
Ft. Lauderdale, Florida
Utilization Review and Utilization Management

Reuben Escorpizo, PT, DPT, MSc
Research Scientist of the ICF Research Branch of the
     World Health Organization
Collaborating Centre for the Family of International
     Classifications in German
Research Scientist of the Swiss
     Paraplegic Research
Nottwil, Switzerland
*WHO International Classification of Functioning
     Disability and Health (IFC) Model*

Helene M. Fearon, PT
Partner, *Fearon & Levine*
Phoenix, Arizona
The Electronic Medical Record

Gerard G. Fluet, DPT
Research Associate
Motor Control and Rehabilitation Laboratory
New Jersey Institute of Technology
Clinical Instructor
Department of Rehabilitation and Movement Science
University of Medicine and Dentistry of New Jersey
Newark, New Jersey
SNF, Medicare

Scott S. Harp, PT, PhD
Branch Director
Gentiva Home Health®
Orlando, Florida
Home Health Documentation

Stephen M. Levine, PT, DPT, MSHA
Partner, *Fearon & Levine*
Ft Lauderdale, Florida
The Electronic Medical Record

Rebecca S. Rosenthal, PT, JD
Physical Therapy Department
College of Allied Health
Nova Southeastern University
Ft. Lauderdale, Florida
Legal Issues in the Medical Record

Claudia Senesac, PT, PCS
Department of Physical Therapy
University of Florida
Gainesville, Florida
Pediatric Documentation

Jennifer Shamus, PT, PhD
Market Manager
Select Physical Therapy
Pembroke Pines, Florida
Documentation Content

Allan Stern, PT
Home Health Physical Therapist
Fort Lauderdale, Florida
Home Health

Kathy Swanick, DPT, MS
Department of Physical Therapy and
     Human Performance
Florida Gulf Coast University
Fort Myers, Florida
Documentation Content Exercise

Kay H. Tasso, PT, PhD, PCS
DLC Nurse & Learn
Jacksonville, Florida
Pediatric Documentation

Arie J. van Duijn, PT, EdD, OCS
Department of Physical Therapy and
  Human Performance
Florida Gulf Coast University
Fort Myers, Florida
Documentation Content Exercise

PREFACE

In a changing health care environment, physical therapists cannot afford third-party payer denial for medically necessary physical therapy services they provide. Common reasons for denials include:

- **Technical errors such as:**
  - identifier omission
  - incorrect form use
  - incorrect information
  - inadequate information

- **Non-technical errors such as:**
  - illegibility
  - good documentation in wrong place
  - bad documentation anyplace
  - billing information that does not match documentation of care
  - goals that do not match problems or diagnosis
  - outcomes or effectiveness of therapy services for patient's illness or injury (i.e., goals not achieved) are not documented
  - patient achieved their restorative potential and were provided repetitive, non-skilled exercises
  - patient did not require the care of a skilled therapist based on documentation
  - loss of function or functional limitation was not identified (problems were physiologically impairment based)
  - potential for significant improvement not identified (goals were not significant enough to justify care, or patient was too high level or too low level)
  - need for skilled therapist not identified (improvement would have been made without therapeutic intervention)
  - maintenance type therapies were being provided (rote, repetitive treatment to maintain same level of function)
  - lack of objective, measurable, or standardized evidence based tests and measures

Incorporating all of the general principles for documentation and health information management should help the therapist maintain records appropriately, organize the record, record appropriate information, and justify and receive reimbursement based on the documentation content. The therapist should seek to write only what is relevant and necessary in an objective manner, using verbiage that indicates skill, but is universally understood based on all purposes of the medical record. By appreciating why payment for skilled physical therapy services is denied, the therapist can reflect on documentation content guidelines and the importance of content adherence.

This textbook will help lay the foundation on What, How, and Why to document. Legal issues, coding, utilization review, and utilization management are just a few of the content areas covered.

ACKNOWLEDGMENTS

We would like to thank and acknowledge all the individuals who contributed to this book. Without their expertise and dedication, this book would not have been possible.

Special thanks Joseph Morita and the McGraw Hill staff for their never-ending help and encouragement.

Eric Shamus
Debra Feingold Stern

1 Introduction, Background, Purpose, and General Rules for Health Information Management (Medical Record Keeping)

I. INTRODUCTION, BACKGROUND, AND PURPOSES OF THE RECORD

Physical therapy (PT), although not known by name until modern times, has had a long history. Oral history, recorded information, documents, and archaeological discoveries enable tracing the history of medical practice, including physical medicine, through the ages. While some record keeping was important to previous generations, it is increasingly important for a variety of reasons, although modern standards did not appear until the 20th century. The Hospital Standardization Program established the first requirement for "complete and accurate reporting of the care and treatment provided during hospitalization" in 1918.[1] Before 1918, individual physicians haphazardly maintained records according to personal purpose and convenience, unless they were associated with research. With inadequate medical records, it was difficult to ascertain the results of treatment.[1] For physical therapists, the implementation of social security and Medicare in 1965 heralded the onset of record keeping or documentation as a component of the medical record.

In some respects, the purposes for documenting have remained constant. However, as the complexity of healthcare has grown, so has the management of medical or health information. Health information management (HIM) is replacing the term medical record keeping. As record keeping transitions increasingly from manual to electronic, the term is more appropriate. The American Health Information Management Association (AHIMA) is setting the standards for the overall science of HIM in an increasingly complex system. The patient chart/record itself is considered a legal document and is, therefore, subject to state and federal laws, as well as medical record laws, HIM laws, state licensure laws for healthcare practitioners, and federal regulation and acts, especially HIPAA (Health Insurance Portability and Accountability Act). HIPAA passed by Congress in 1996 and it was implemented in 2003. HIPAA set federal standards for accessing and handling medical information.

For physical therapy professionals, as with other health professionals, documentation is a required practice by federal, state, facility, and accreditation laws and guidelines. According to the American Physical Therapy Association (APTA) (*Guide to Physical Therapist Practice*),[2] documentation is "any entry into the medical record" and is required for all patient/client-related encounters. Although required in all settings with some differing requirements, effective, efficient appropriate documentation that complies with all purposes and regulations, and reflects skilled care, can be vexing to the practitioner. Fundamentals are traditionally taught in the academic setting, but the principles learned during one's education need to be practically adapted and applied in the working world. Additionally, as requirements and guidelines are frequently updated by the Centers for Medicare and Medicaid (CMS) for Medicare and Medicaid systems, it is the individual responsibility of each physical therapist or physical therapist assistant, to keep up with changing standards in all settings. As style and required content vary among facilities, organizations, agencies, and therapists, practical application is more challenging than theoretical application.

When the Medicare program was established with Title XVIII of the Social Security Act, physical therapy became a billable service. Under the Act, all practitioners are required to document patient care and ascertain and establish the medical necessity of care. At the time Medicare was implemented, most physical therapy was hospital based for both inpatient and outpatient, and payment did not depend on record content. Regulations existed for documentation in the Medicare program for all outpatient and skilled inpatient rehabilitation services as early as the 1970s (and remain in effect today, albeit much expanded). From a technical perspective, all delivered services initially required physician prescription or referral, ongoing physician visits, and justification of care as evidenced by documentation. Depending on the setting, hospital, skilled nursing, outpatient, or home health, reimbursement was on a fee-for-service or cost-based basis. In pure fee-for-service arrangements, increasingly rare in the 21st century, providers charged a fee and the third-party payer, including the designated Medicare intermediaries, paid. This was assuming the fees were reasonable and customary in the community. Medicare's cost-based reimbursement was derived from the costs incurred by the organization providing services to a Medicare beneficiary without regard for preset parameters. This was applicable to reimbursement in skilled nursing facilities, rehabilitation agencies, and comprehensive outpatient rehabilitation facilities (CORF).

The 1970s was a time of increasing medical malpractice claims, which continues today. Since the only evidence of care after patient discharge is the written or electronic medical record, the record content is critical in proving innocence (or potential guilt) of the healthcare provider. Although the number of malpractice suits against physical therapists was and continues to be small, it continues to be the documentation that supports innocence and protects or potentially contributes to convicting the provider. The cliché "if it wasn't written it wasn't done" aptly describes one aspect of the need for appropriate record content. Just having something written, however, is not adequate defense but rather having written information that is objective and complete, that justifies and describes skilled care provided.

With the APTA Vision 2020 of autonomous practice in an interprofessional environment, and the change in terminal PT educational degree to the doctor of physical therapy, PTs may see an increase in malpractice cases and therefore increasing need for thorough, accurate, complete, and skilled documentation.

Before healthcare costs began escalating in the 1970s and 1980s, documentation content was not used to any extent to deny reimbursement to the provider, as neither the federal government nor private industry had the technology to track claims in an efficient manner. However, with the advent of computerization in the 1980s, CMS/Medicare was able to track services for the first time. As this became possible, the Healthcare Finance Administration (HCFA, now CMS) embarked on a program to uncover fraud and abuse for all Medicare-provided services, including physical therapy. In the early 1990s, commercial payers determined that they could also track services and determine if documentation supported the care rendered, making appropriate and skilled physical therapy documentation increasingly important.

Tracking resulted in recovery of millions of dollars from fraudulent claims in the 1980s and 1990s, and continues today with expansion of Medicare and Medicaid fraud incorrect payment initiatives. According to the CMS, government website www.cms.gov, "In the Tax Relief and Health Care Act of 2006, Congress required a permanent and national Recovery Audit Contractor (RAC) program to be in place by January 1, 2010."[3] The RACs instituted a 3-year pilot test to "identify and correct past improper Medicare payments, reduce future improper payments, and improve the error rate (for all Medicare payments, not just physical therapy)." The RACs were implemented in 2009. During the RAC demonstration project alone, over $900 million in overpayments was identified based on audits of medical records/health information and billing records that did not support the care rendered with minimal underpayment discovered. It is in the best interest of the RACs to discover overpayment as they are paid based on discovery of overpayment and underpayment. Although this system is primarily Medicare based, similar types of audits are conducted by all third-party payers. In addition to the RACs, the federal Government Accountability Office (GAO) through the Office of the Inspector General (OIG), has historically conducted audits for the CMS and the Medicare and Medicaid programs. Physical therapy has regularly been identified as having documentation insufficient to support skilled care in a variety of domains.

There is a similar initiative in the private sector similar to the RACs which may be implemented in the near future as well, emphasizing the need for physical therapy professionals to document skillfully in all venues through the life span. CMS, relative to Medicare, does not include reimbursement in its list of purposes of medical records. Documentation and reimbursement is integrally related, however, as evidenced by the implementation of the RACs and GAO audits, which have historically required practitioners to "pay back" to the government any payments not supported by appropriate documentation.

In the last decades of the 20th century and the first decade of the 21st century, the healthcare delivery system has evolved into a managed care–oriented system. As the healthcare industry continues to undergo incremental reform, managed care—the initiative that seeks to deliver appropriate and cost-effective healthcare without sacrificing quality—demands an effective and efficient billing tracking process. Decreases in reimbursement by third-party payers within a managed care environment, whether by decreased dollars per visit, visit limitation, or capitation, have forced physical therapists to ensure reimbursement of all available funds through documentation. The documentation must justify care that reflects the need for skilled services, be concise and accurate (effective and efficient), and match all billing information with correct coding. According to Stewart and Abeln, 1993, "Carriers do not place a high value on physical therapy services as they relate to managed care concepts."[4] Therefore, the burden falls to the physical therapist (PT) to justify the value.

At the time this text is being written, the Senate and House have passed a national healthcare plan. It is unknown exactly how, it will impact physical therapy from delivery and record-keeping perspectives.[5] CMS, a division of Health and Human Services (HHS), is the largest payer of healthcare in the United States and dictates basic content for documentation for rehabilitation professionals, including physical therapists. Data gathered by the CMS are maintained in a national database where it is stored, analyzed and used to "make decisions related to healthcare reimbursement mechanisms, the effectiveness of healthcare services, and the general health of the Medicare population."[3] State governments (Medicaid) and other third-party payers maintain similar data for decision-making purposes. However, since a fiscal intermediary (FI) has historically contracted with CMS for payment to the care provider, the regulations are open to interpretation by the payer as well as the care provider. The one constant is that services must be skilled in nature and justified. It should be noted that as of 2010, MACs (Medicare administrative contractors) replaced the FIs. The intent was to "improve customer service … by offering a single

CMS point of contact and increasing provider education and training to improve claims accuracy." There are continued differences in interpretation of regulations regarding reimbursement with the MACs as there was previously with the FIs, by designated MAC coverage region.

Physical therapists (PTs) have historically been lax in making the connection in their documentation between the medical problem, the PT-related functional problem(s), treatment diagnosis or PT diagnosis, the PT initial examination and evaluation, treatment/intervention, and objective measures of findings and outcomes. PTs have also been challenged in relating treatment/intervention and goals to function, and providing evidence that PT is better than alternative patient management. Documentation content has long been impairment based, focusing on the physiology of a problem, with relatively little evidence-based, objective outcome measurement. As a result, PT has not been considered an essential medical service. With the current movement within the profession for evidenced-based practice, the future may be different. The APTA's *Guide to Physical Therapist Practice* stresses these relationships.[2]

Consistent terminology both in description and content is also a challenge for the physical therapist. AHIMA uses the general term health record to categorize what may be more commonly known, depending on the setting, as the patient records (acute care), medical records (physician offices, physical therapy practices/departments), resident records (skilled nursing facilities), or client records (ambulatory care, APTA). A health record contains all information about the patient/client, including the skilled documentation. The *Guide to Physical Therapist Practice*, 2nd edition refers to documentation as a role of the physical therapist.[2] Documentation is defined in the Guide as "any entry into the client record, such as consultation report, initial examination report, progress note, flow sheet/checklist that identifies the care/service provided, reexamination, or summation of care."[2] Colloquially, physical therapists are familiar with the term medical record, because the second Guide terminology was only developed in 2001 and neither APTA or non-APTA members may not be using the Guide regularly. Regardless of the terminology, the record is "the principal repository (storage place) for data and information about the healthcare services provided to an individual patient. It documents the who, what, when, where, what, and how of patient care."[2]

Historically, documentation has been by manual entry with maintenance of hard copy. Although costly and more commonly used by physicians, the practice of dictation and transcription was also adopted by physical therapists (primarily in the outpatient setting) for the same purpose. As we enter the 21st century, the future of recording and record keeping continues to evolve. The computer-based patient record (CPR) or electronic medical record (EMR) is gaining popularity, as are voice recognition systems and tablet-style laptop computers that translate handwriting into "typing." Whether an entry is made simply with a word processing program or through a custom-designed integrated record system, hard copy or paper records may soon become part of history.

"Under the American Recovery and Reinvestment Act of 2009 (ARRA), hospitals received payments from Medicare and Medicaid starting in October 2010 for the successful implementation and effective use of electronic health records (EHRs).... Hospitals that do not meet federal guidelines by 2015 face reductions in Medicare reimbursement."[6]

As the federal government mandates universal use of EHRs across all settings, regardless of whether a professional uses a pen, microphone or keyboard, narrative, SOAP format (subjective, objective, assessment, plan), or templates, the general principles, purposes, and content requirements remain the same.

II. FUNCTIONS AND USERS OF THE HEALTH RECORD

According to the AHIMA, the basic purposes of documentation are to serve as (1) a basis for planning and treatment; (2) a means of communication for attending health professionals; (3) legal entries describing the care the patient receives;

TABLE 1-1 · Primary Purposes of the Health Record

Patient Care Delivery (Patient)
- To document services received
- To constitute proof of identity
- To self-manage care
- To verify billing

Patient Care Delivery (Provider)
- To foster continuity of care (that is, to serve as a communication tool)
- To describe diseases and causes (that is, to support diagnostic work)
- To support decision making about diagnosis and treatment of patients
- To assess and manage risk for individual patients
- To facilitate care in accordance with clinical practice guidelines
- To document patient risk factors
- To assess and document patient expectations and patient satisfaction
- To generate care plans
- To determine preventive advice or health maintenance information
- To provide reminders to clinicians
- To support nursing care
- To document services provided

Patient Care Management
- To document case mix in institutions and practices
- To analyze severity of illness
- To formulate practice guidelines
- To manage risk
- To characterize the use of services
- To provide the basis for utilization review
- To perform quality assurance

Patient Care Support
- To allocate resources
- To analyze trends and develop forecasts
- To assess workload
- To communicate information among departments

Billing and Reimbursement
- To document services for payments
- To bill for services
- To submit insurance claims
- To adjudicate insurance claims
- To determine disabilities (for example, workman's compensation)
- To manage costs
- To report costs
- To perform actuarial analysis

SOURCE: Dick, Steen, and Detmer, p. 78.[7]

(4) verification of services for payers, and (5) basic data for health research and planning. The Institute of Medicine[7] divides the purposes into primary and secondary, where primary purposes directly relate to patient care (see Table 1-1) and secondary purposes indirectly relate to patient care (see Table 1-2).

The primary purposes identified by the institute are patient care delivery, patient care management, patient care support, and billing and reimbursement. *Patient care delivery* is the care provided by the professionals involved in a patient's care. This is used by providers to communicate what is being done and the outcome or patient response to treatment in order to ensure continuity of care. Therefore, it is imperative that the record be available to all providers and as appropriate, 24 hours a day. *Patient care management* refers to all of the activities related to a patient's management. *Patient care support* relates to facility management of resources, including trend identification for quality improvement and utilization review and management purposes. *Billing and reimbursement* is the use of the record to provide justification for reimbursement for the care rendered, by describing the care in skilled terms.

TABLE 1-2 · Secondary Purposes of the Health Record

Education
- To document the experience of healthcare professionals
- To prepare conferences and presentations
- To teach healthcare students

Regulation
- To serve as evidence in litigation
- To foster post-marketing surveillance
- To assess compliance with standards of care
- To accredit professionals and hospitals
- To compare healthcare organizations

Research
- To develop new products
- To conduct clinical research
- To assess technology
- To study patient outcomes
- To study effectiveness and cost-effectiveness of patient care
- To identify populations at risk
- To develop registries and databases
- To assess the cost-effectiveness of record systems

Policy Making
- To allocate resources
- To conduct strategic planning
- To monitor public health

Industry
- To conduct research and development
- To plan marketing strategy

SOURCE: Dick, Steen, and Detmer, p. 79.[7]

The secondary purposes are education, regulation (compliance and accreditation), research, policy making (allocating resources and planning), and industry (research and development).

Tables 1-3 and 1-4 list examples of the individual and institutional users of health records.[7] The patient identifiers are removed from all records used for purposes not directly related to patient care. In this way, the confidentiality of patient-identifiable information and the privacy of the individuals involved (both patients and providers) can be protected. However, HIPAA regulations require specific patient permission for most primary or secondary use of the medical record as of April 2003.

Based on the primary and secondary purposes of the record, a wide variety of individuals may require record access. With integrated EHRs, access through computers at convenient locations should facilitate optimal care through accessibility to all entries and integrated information. Although terminology must be sophisticated and skilled enough to justify care, it must also be clear and understood by other healthcare professionals, non-healthcare professionals, and others. Other users can be divided into individual and institutional. Each user may use and need the information from the record for a different purpose. A chaplain offering spiritual guidance and comfort uses information differently than a billing clerk, a third-party payer representative, physical therapist, or surveyor (i.e., Joint Commission on Accreditation of Healthcare Organizations [JCAHO] or Commission on Accreditation of Rehabilitation Facilities [CARF]). It is also becoming more common for patients or patient representatives, such as family, legal guardian, or healthcare surrogate, to take a greater interest in the care provided. With the exception of special regulations for psychiatric records, the Health Insurance Portability and Accountability Act (HIPAA), ensures a patient or designated representative the right to see the record. For more information on HIPAA, see Chapter 7, Legal Issues in the Medical Record. The security, confidentiality and privacy implications of HIPAA extend to current patients in any

TABLE 1-3 · Representative Individual Users of Healthcare Records

Patient Care Delivery (Providers)
Chaplains
Dental hygienists
Dentists dietitians
Laboratory technologists
Nurses
Occupational therapists
Optometrists
Pharmacists
Physical therapists
Physicians
Physician assistants
Podiatrists
Psychologists
Radiology technologists
Respiratory therapists
Social workers

Patient Care Delivery (Consumers)
Patients
Families

Patient Care Management and Support
Administrators
Financial managers and accountants
Quality managers
Records professionals
Risk managers
Unit clerks
Utilization review managers

Patient Care Reimbursement
Benefit managers
Insurers (federal, state, and private)

Other
Accreditors
Government policy makers and legislators
Lawyers
Healthcare researchers and clinical investigators
Health sciences journalists and editors

SOURCE: Dick, Steen, and Detmer, p. 76.[7]

practice and the maintenance of records as well. AHIMA recommends 10 years for retention of records, the JCAHO consistent with state law, CARF requires policies but specifies no time limits, and the National Committee on Quality Assurance (NCQA) does not specify.

Although the primary users of health records are patient care providers, many other individuals and organizations also use the information. Managed care organizations, integrated healthcare delivery systems, regulatory and accreditation organizations, licensing bodies, educational organizations, third-party payers, and research facilities all use information that was originally collected to document patient care.

The Institute of Medicine broadly defines the users of health records as "those individuals who enter, verify, correct, analyze, or obtain information from the record, either directly or indirectly through an intermediary."[7] All users of health records influence clinical care in some way, but use the information for various reasons and in different ways. Some users (e.g., nurses, physicians, and coding specialists) refer to the health records of specific patients as a part of their daily work. Many other users, however, never have direct access to the records of individual patients. Instead, they use clinical and demographic information.

TABLE 1-4 • Representative Institutional Users of Health Records

Healthcare Delivery (Inpatient and Outpatient)
Alliances, associations, networks, and systems of providers
Ambulatory surgery centers
Donor banks (blood, tissue, organs)
Health maintenance organizations (HMOs)
Home care agencies
Hospices
Hospitals (general and specialty)
Nursing homes
Preferred provider organizations (PPOs)
Physicians offices (large and small group practices, individual practitioners)
Psychiatrics facilities
Public health departments
Substance abuse programs

Management and Review of Care
Medicare peer review organizations
Quality management companies
Risk management companies
Utilization review and utilization management companies

Reimbursement of Care
Business healthcare coalitions
Employers
Insurers (federal, state, and private)

Research
Disease registries
Health data organizations
Healthcare technology developers and manufacturers (equipment and device firms, pharmaceutical firms, and computer hardware and software vendors for patient record systems)
Research centers

Education
Allied Health professional schools and programs
Schools of medicine
Schools of nursing
Schools of public health

Accreditation
Accreditation organizations
Institutional licensure agencies
Professional licensure agencies

Policy Making
Federal government agencies
Local government agencies
State government agencies

SOURCE: Dick, Steen, Detmer, p. 77.[7]

As already noted, many individuals depend on the information in health records to perform their jobs. The individuals who provide direct patient care services include physicians, nurses, nurse practitioners, allied health professionals, and other clinical personnel. Allied health professionals include physician's assistants, physical therapists, respiratory therapists, occupational therapists, radiology technicians, and medical laboratory technicians. Other medical professionals, such as pharmacists, social workers, dietitians, psychologists, podiatrists, and chiropractors, also provide clinical services.

The services directly administered by patient care providers are documented directly into the patient's health record. Other service providers (e.g., medical laboratory technicians) submit separate written reports that become part of individual health records, whether hardcopy or electronic.

III. SUMMARY

The medical or client record is a comprehensive set of information that chronicles an episode of medically related care rendered to an individual. Medical record keeping or the process of HIM is necessary in healthcare for a variety of reasons. It should include all information related to a patient, expressed in terminology understood by all record users, both primary and secondary. Primary users of the record include those primarily involved in the care itself. Secondary users include most others. Regardless of the purpose the record serves, the content should be the same. By following general rules of medical record keeping and content, the physical therapist in coordination with the Physical Therapist Assistant (PTA) should be able to create documentation or a complete record (depending on setting) that will be universally understood and withstand scrutiny by any reader, for any purpose.

REFERENCES

1. Affeldt JE. Proceedings of the Academy of Political Science. *Proc Acad Polit Sci.* 1980;33(4):182–191.

2. APTA. *Guide to Physical Therapist Practice*, 2nd ed. Alexandria, VA, American Physical Therapy Association, 2003.

3. CMS.gov: Monday, October 6, 2008. Details for: CMS Announces New Recovery Audit Contractors to Help Identify Improper Medicare Payments. Office of Public Affairs, 202-690-6145.

4. Stewart DL, Abeln SH. *Documenting Functional Outcomes in Physical Therapy*. St. Louis, MO. Mosby, 1993.

5. Healthcare Financial Management Association: Regulatory Alphabet Soup: Financial Implications of RACs. www.hfma.org/NR/exeres?A9a846FE-428D-4F1E-9F8F 0 167EC25E398.htm.

6. Federal Government Releases Electronic Health Record (HER) Requirements: CSC Survey Shows Hospitals are only 50% compliant. News Release- January 04, 2010. http://staging.csc.com/public_sector/press_releases/39178-federal_government_releases_electronic_health_record_ehr_requirements_csc_survey shows hospitals_are_only_50_compliant.

7. Dick R, Steen E, Detmer D. *The Computer-Based Patient Record: An Essential Technology for Health Care, Revised Edition* (Committee on Improving the Patient Record, Institute of Medicine). Washington, DC, National Academy of Sciences, 1997.

CHAPTER 1 REVIEW QUESTIONS

1. What is the relationship between health information management and medical record keeping?

2. Whose responsibility is it to determine medical necessity for physical therapy?

3. The advent of what technology facilitated the ability for Medicare and others to track services rendered to beneficiaries?

4. Relative to documentation, why has physical therapy not been considered an essential medical service?

5. What is documentation according to the APTA Guide to Physical Therapist Practice?

6. Are the principles for documenting by manual entry different than for the electronic medical record? Defend your answer.

7. According to AHIMA, what are the primary purposes of the medical record?

8. Describe five secondary purposes of the medical record.

9. What does "user" mean in the context of the medical record? Give five examples and the purpose each would need to record for.

10. What is HIPAA and how is it relevant to health information management?

11. How are the RACs impacting the relationship between documentation and reimbursement?

12. What is a MAC and what are the primary purposes of a MAC?

13. Why is it important for physical therapists to know what a RAC and a MAC are?

2 Record Organization and General Principles

I. GENERAL PRINCIPLES

The management of medical records, including content and organization, should be consistent throughout an organization and consistent within each discipline. Organizational policies and procedures should outline the general rules for the medical professional regarding documentation. Additionally, the records should be organized so that individual pieces of information are easy to locate within the record as a whole. Therefore, all records in the same facility should be organized the same way whether they are hard copy or electronic.

II. REFERRAL INFORMATION

Documentation should reflect how the patient/client arrived at your facility, for example self referred, physician referred or prescribed or physician extender. A non-physician practitioner (NPP) such as an advanced registered nurse practitioner (ARNP) or physician assistant (PA), or other—should be included in the patient's medical record. If the patient/client comes with a written order, that order becomes part of the record. If referred by telephone or verbal order, the person that took the order must transcribe it, consistent with state law and facility policy. The transcription of the referral should also be followed up by a signed written referral, preferably an original rather than a fax.

III. STORAGE

Records must be kept in locked, fireproof storage and must be accessible only to those directly involved with the patient/client. Electronic records must be password coded and screens must be shielded from public view. Security measures, such as firewalls, should also be in place.

IV. INDIVIDUAL CHARTS/FOLDERS

In facilities that use manual entry, there should be a single, hard copy "chart." If manila file folders are used, it is best practice to use a new folder for each new patient/client. If it is policy of the facility to reuse folders, all references on and in the folder to the prior patients/clients should be obliterated for privacy purposes. If records are maintained electronically, there should be separate electronic charts for each patient/client clearly identified.

A. Ink

For those organizations using manual entry, only ink should be used, preferably black or blue. In the recent past, black was generally expected and required. With the advent of improved copying systems, it can be difficult to discern an original from a copy. Therefore, from a legal perspective, some organizations have changed to blue ink. However, this is a decision for the organization or individual practitioner. There should be consistency in color within the practice as outlined in a policy. Generally, black ink is still the preferred color used for manual medical entries.

V. LEGIBILITY

All entries must be legible to anyone who may need record access. Illegibility may give the impression of carelessness and rushed efforts. For electronic records, consistent font style and size should be used. Some electronic systems allow manual entry. In these systems, entries must be legible. Legibility also refers to signatures. As most signatures are not legible, it is critical that all licensed professionals use their state license numbers following their names so they can be identified. In the case of students, following their designation of student physical therapist (SPT) or student physical therapist assistant (SPTA), they should also print their names for identification purposes.

VI. DATA TYPES

Although not applicable to individual entries, the record as a whole, regardless of the setting, consists of four types of data: (1) personal, (2) financial, (3) social, and (4) medical. This is true whether the record is manual or electronic.

VII. ERRORS IN THE RECORD

Entries cannot be physically removed, completely covered, or otherwise made illegible. If items that should have been entered are recalled at any time following the documentation for a specific encounter, an addendum can be added. It must be placed in the next available space in the record and should include the time and date of entry. It should then state "Addendum to entry of _____."

If an error in spelling, location, or other minor error is made, a single line should be put through the incorrect entry. The correction should be made above the incorrect entry with the date and the initials of the person correcting beside it. Neither correction fluid (White Out) nor correction tape should be used in a hard copy medical record (See Example 1).

■ Example 1

8/26/11 *ES*
18 y.o. male adm ~~8/25/11~~ with R femur fx.

Alterations to the medical record are considered fraudulent. Therefore, even if an incorrect entry is made on a new page and discovered, technically it should not be removed. Although this was the practice, the privacy and confidentiality components of HIPAA required a change in this practice, and it should be removed and noted. An example would be a note of a different patient written in someone else's chart. This note can be removed but some documentation of the removal needs to take place. The note should just not disappear.

Additionally, do not leave blanks or skip lines and always enter information chronologically. Blanks may give the impression that information was forgotten and may leave opportunity for record alteration. Single lines can be drawn through or across multiple blank lines or spaces. However, in a system in which there are running chronological entries, the space that follows the final signature on an entry is not considered blank space and should not be lined out.

In electronic records, corrections must be made consistent with laws and acceptable practice. Also in electronic records, errors should not just be deleted. It should be noted in an addendum that an entry is incorrect, and the addendum should then include the correction. As this is a relatively new phenomenon, facilities using electronic records, commonly referred to EMRs or CMRs, should have internal policies regarding entry error correction.

VIII. TIMELINESS OF ENTRY/TIME OF SESSION

Entries should be composed as close to the time of service delivery as possible, preferably at the time treatment is being rendered or immediately following. Entries can be manually written or typed. Dictated notes, either typed in or voice transcribed, need to be readily available. Timeliness of entry input saves time and ensures accuracy, as the PT/PTA does not have to "remember" what they did later. Additionally, if harm comes to the patient between PT visits, immediate documentation of patient status following treatment can protect the provider. If transcribed records cannot be obtained before the next patient visit, the provider should consider an alternate service that can deliver in a timely manner, or consider alternate forms of entry. This is especially relevant in the acute care setting with patients who are medically fragile or unstable. If another professional wanted to coordinate care, it could only be done if the records are entered in a timely manner. Discharge entries and summaries should also be completed in a timely manner for accuracy. Although good practice is to complete within 24 hours of discharge, it is up to the therapist to follow facility policies and procedures. There are regulations in place for some settings that do not require documentation for each visit; however, even if a full note is not required, the date and record of interventions performed should, at the minimum, be entered in some format. According to the American Physical Therapy Association (APTA), there should be an entry for every visit or encounter between patients and providers. Absence of an entry for any visit or encounter may result in denial of payment since there is no proof of the visit. Documentation for all patients treated or who did not receive treatment but were scheduled should be completed before a therapist or assistant leaves the facility for the day.

IX. SPELLING AND GRAMMAR

Although correct spelling and grammar would seem a given, carelessness does occur. The provider must correctly spell all words and write in a logical, coherent manner, as there are multiple uses for the record. Incorrect spelling and grammar may lead the reader to believe the care has been rendered with lack of skill. Professionals are expected to be able to spell. For electronic entry, some systems may have spell checks and grammar checks. If your system has these capabilities, it is recommended that they are used before finalizing entries. Spelling can also be checked easily with PDAs or cell phones with Internet capabilities or internal dictionaries.

X. ABBREVIATIONS

Only standard abbreviations and acronyms should be used. The dilemma in physical therapy is standardization. Refer to Appendix A for a list of some standard abbreviations. However, it is the organization's, facility's, or solo/independent practice PTs responsibility to have specific policies and procedures on using abbreviations. Individuals should not use self-developed abbreviations that are not universally understood. Abbreviations for specific PT treatments or interventions should only be used in conjunction with universally accepted Current Procedural Terminology codes

(CPT® codes, universally required for billing), to ensure categorical understanding. For example, other PTs or rehabilitation professionals may understand PNF for proprioceptive neuromuscular facilitation, but non-rehabilitation professionals would not know it is a form of therapeutic exercise. Additionally, if abbreviations have multiple meanings, such as WFL: within functional limits or within full limits, the PT should provide a key on the form being used. The latest Joint Commission regulations recommend elimination of the use of all abbreviations to minimize medical error and maximize effective interprofessional communication.

XI. ACCURACY

All documentation entries and intervention content should match billing dates, attendance grids, and appointment book entries. Each entry should match the appropriate billing date. The codes entered for billing purposes should match the codes and/or verbiage indicated in the record. CPT coding terminology should describe all interventions categorically.

The physical therapy diagnosis is not the same as the medical diagnosis, and is actually a determination of the primary problem for which the patient is receiving skilled care. For states in which PTs are not legally authorized to diagnose, the description would be the PT problem. The Medicare 700 series forms specifically require differentiation between the medical diagnosis and the physical therapy or treatment problem/diagnosis (see Appendix B).

In the content itself, the medical diagnosis should be the one established by the referring medical professional as appropriate. The PT diagnosis or treatment diagnosis should be established by the PT by description, matching The World Health Organization's (WHO) International Classification of Disease codes (ICD-9 code, see a sample of ICD-9 codes in Appendix D, soon to be the ICD-10 version). The PT diagnosis must match the patient complaints, objective findings and functional deficits. It will assist in establishing goals, therapeutic contents and determining frequency and duration of care. The PT diagnosis may be functionally oriented and, therefore, may differ or correspond with the medical diagnosis. The onset date of the PT problem should be clearly indicated and should be "recent", even if the medical problem is chronic in nature. Throughout the record, all information should match.

Careful attention should be paid to using the correct word for homonyms or words that sound the same but are spelled differently and have different meaning, such as gait and gate and their and there. Care should also be taken to avoid any other commonly confused terms or concepts, such as left and right.

Information should be presented in an organized manner and indicate functional goals attained by the patient/client in a linear progression. The appropriate forms, as determined by policy and procedure or external requirements such as third-party payers, should always be used.

XII. AUTHENTICATION AND COMPLETION

To ensure authenticity and to indicate completion, the medical record entry should be signed by the physical therapist or physical therapist assistant who writes it. With dictated entries, the individual who dictated should read the entry when it is returned, then follow the other applicable rules regarding error correction, and sign. Original signatures are required with manual entry or dictation. Electronic signatures have been deemed legally acceptable in electronic records and faxed documents. Signature stamps, however, are not acceptable.

A legible signature should appear with every entry. If the entry spans multiple pages, it should appear on each page with continuation indicated. The signature should be the provider's full name and appropriate professional designation (i.e., PT or PTA) and should be signed the same way each time. The individual's medical license number should accompany the signature to ensure identification and authentication of the provider of service. Educational degrees are not legal professional designations and do not replace PT (or RPT, LPT in some states). See Examples 2 and 3.

■ Example 2

Susan Smith, PT # 0001977

Depending on national, state, and local laws or accreditation requirements, SPTs and recent graduates with temporary licenses may require countersignature or co-signature for authentication by the supervising licensed physical therapist. According to Roach, "The purpose of countersignatures is to require a professional to review, and if appropriate, indicate approval of action taken by another practitioner. Usually, the person countersigning a record entry is more experienced or has received a higher level of training than the person who made the original entry. In any case, the person required to countersign should be the individual who has the authority to evaluate the entry."[1]

■ Example 3

Kevin Johnson, SPT Kevin Johnson

Susan Smith, PT # 0001977

John Doe, PT, DPT # 12340

XIII. COURTESY

The record is not the place for complaints, criticism, blame, anger, arguments, or expressions of frustration with other healthcare team members. The tone of the entries should be as neutral as possible. If multiple attempts have been made by the therapist to contact a physician or another professional and he or she has not responded, simply record the date and time the call was made. Let others pass judgment. Avoid underlining for emphasizing negatively toned entries, do not change from cursive to print or vice versa, and do not write larger in some parts of the entry than others or in capital letters in hard copy entries. In electronic records, or if manually printing, avoid using all capital letters as capitals indicate anger, bolding components, underlining, or series of symbols.

XIV. CONTENT INCLUSION

Document all telephone calls, missed appointments, instructions given to the patient/client or caregiver, discussion with families, verbal or telephone orders from physicians or other professionals (followed by signed written orders in as close to 24 hours as possible). It is also relevant to include instructions to other health professionals, all communication about the patient/client, and all session/encounter information, including identification of anyone who may have observed the therapy session.

All entries should be brief, meaningful, and as objective as possible, including primarily facts. Do not write just for the sake of writing. Avoid phrases and words that are meaningless or have multiple meanings. If tempted to use the adjective confused for example, it is better to describe the behaviors that led you to use the word (see Example 4).

Example 4

Instead of patient is confused, write:

- Although patient could not identify therapist nor where he was, he was able to actively participate in the therapy session.

Avoid phrases such as "tolerated treatment well," as it does not objectively describe any behavior or response to treatment.

- Describe, instead, what the patient or client accomplished in terms of time and aerobic capacity or endurance, or another choice of objective descriptions.

- Patient was able to complete 60 minutes of active therapeutic exercise and gait, with only brief rest periods in between, and stabilizing of blood pressure after 2 minutes of rest. This has improved as patient required up to 5 minutes for vital signs to return to normal previously.

Avoid PT jargon or terms and phrases only understood by PTs. What is written will influence the reader's impression of your care. Anyone who needs access to the record for any reason must be able to understand what is written. In the case of reimbursement, lack of understanding by the third-party payer representative may result in initial denial of a claim.

Terminology should be descriptive so that treatment can be duplicated or a clear picture of the patient/client is painted. Descriptive documentation should include impairments and functional limitations, justifying care based on functional improvement.

XV. HEADINGS OR TITLES

Preprinted forms or electronic templates usually include section headings or titles. In addition to section titles or headings, the whole entry itself should be titled (i.e., Physical Therapy Evaluation, Physical Therapy Notes, Physical Therapy Progress Report, etc.). In sections where narrative, paragraph, or "free-form" entries may be included, it is better to categorize information: e.g., interventions: gait training.... Even when using SOAP (subjective, objective, analysis/assessment, plan) format, subheadings can be used to clarify and better organize data than just the S, O, A, and P. If categories extend to more than one page, either the back of a page or a new page, there should be an indication that it is a continuation. All pages should be numbered and total number should be clear (i.e., 1/4, 2/4, 3/4, 4/4).

XVI. VERBAL, TELEPHONE, OR E-MAIL/ELECTRONIC ORDERS

The person taking the order should transcribe the verbal orders. State law may dictate who may take and transcribe it. In most cases it is the PT. The entry itself should include what the order is for, the time it was taken, how it was taken (i.e., phone, face-to-face, phone message, e-mail, fax, other), the prescribing individual's name, and the name of the person who entered it. Verbal, telephone, or e-mail electronic orders require authentication usually within 24–48 hours by the prescribing professional, based on organizational or accreditation guidelines or requirements. Electronic signature is considered acceptable in most cases.

XVII. ILLUSTRATIONS OR PICTURES

Pictures or illustrations can be effective tools for entering information into the record. They can be drawn with ink and must be clearly labeled, dated, and signed in addition to the body of the entry. Preprinted pictures must be clearly labeled

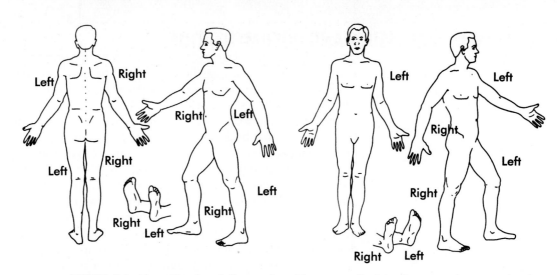

FIGURE 2-1. The pain chart.[2] (*Instructions: Please use all of the figures to show exactly where all your pains are, and where they radiate to. Please be as precise and detailed as possible. Shade or draw with blue marker for pain. Use yellow marker for numbness and tingling; red marker for burning or hot areas; and green marker for cramping. Only the patient is to fill out this sheet.*) (*Copyrighted by Ronald Melzack, 1970, 1984*)

as well (see Fig. 2-1 for an example of a body diagram that can be utilized for documentation purposes). Photographs or video/CD/digital recordings may also be included, but there must be signed permission and protection consistent with HIPAA rules and regulations.

XVIII. OBJECTIVITY

All entries should be as objective as possible, avoiding subjectivity and including facts. Personal opinion should be avoided. If patients come in smelling of alcohol, yelling obscenities, and staggering, avoid documenting that they are drunk by instead documenting your observations of their behavior. Drunkenness can only be established legally by blood alcohol levels. Indeed, other medical conditions such as ketoacidosis may mimic drunkenness or alcohol breath. Provide only the behaviors or signs that you have observed or assessed. When entering statements made by the patient/client, use quotation marks. When entering quotes, be careful when taking statements out of context.

Objective findings and progress over time can be established through the use of standardized test and measures with reliable and valid indicators.

XIX. ECONOMY OF VERBIAGE

All notes should be as efficient as possible, using only those words that are absolutely necessary. Nonessential words, such as pronouns and other modifiers, can be omitted. The reader will know, once the patient is identified, that entries are about the patient, unless otherwise stated. When selecting words, if there are short alternatives, employ them, as long as the issue of "skilling" the note or care is not compromised. The use of commonly used or facility-approved symbols is also acceptable as a means of economizing on words. Bulleting or numbering can be used to present items in series. Electronic entries may have a selection of phrases based on function or diagnosis (see Appendix A abbreviations). For patient goals, "Patient will be able to..." when written once, does not need to be repeated for every goal. It would only be necessary to clarify if a goal was for someone other than the patient. For example, the husband will be able to demonstrate safe and effective transfers with patient from the wheelchair (WC) to and from the bed.

XX. CLAIM DENIAL ISSUES AND DOCUMENTATION

Although communicating the care of the patient is probably the most important purpose of documentation, the record is also used for reimbursement purposes. There are APTA guidelines regarding pro bono care. However, a practice or practitioner cannot survive on sole provision of intentional pro bono services (unless supported by a grant or other sources of funding), nor can a practice or a practitioner survive if charged services are not reimbursed. It is the responsibility of the professional providing care to ensure that the contents of any entries in the patient/client record justify the intervention provided. The entries must, therefore, contain the information necessary to communicate with other practitioners involved in the care and ensure payment (as well as serve the other purposes of the medical record/documentation). When considering general principles of documentation and those specific to PT, discussion of the Office of the Inspector General (OIG)[3] reports and identification of reasons for physical therapy denials in the Medicare system are warranted. These reports are accessible to the public and are available on the OIG Web site (http://www.oig.dol.gov/), as well as the Centers for Medicare and Medicaid Services (CMS) Web site (http://cms.hhs.gov/medlearn/therapy/oigrpts.pdf).[4] The reasons include both technical errors and content errors that do not justify skilled PT intervention. Attention to the general principles of documentation can prevent denial for most of the elements cited and help the practitioner ensure appropriate content. The problems identified in the OIG audits, although performed on Medicare records, are universally applicable.

Common reasons for denials include:

- identifier omission;
- incorrect form use;
- incorrect information;
- inadequate/imprecise information/content;
- illegibility;
- good documentation in wrong place;
- bad documentation in any place;
- billing information that did not match documentation of care;
- goals that did not match problems or diagnosis;
- effectiveness of therapy services for patient's illness or injury (i.e., goals not achieved) not documented;
- patient had achieved their restorative potential and were provided repetitive, non-skilled exercises (care exceeded date of goal achievement);
- patient did not require the care of a skilled therapist (either care was not skilled, maintenance too general, or the documentation did not indicate skill);
- loss of function or functional limitation not identified (problems were physiological impairment based);
- potential for significant improvement not identified (goals were not significant enough to justify care, or patient was too high level or too low level);
- need for skilled therapy not identified (improvement would have been made without therapeutic intervention);
- no indication of medical necessity;
- maintenance type therapies being provided (rote, repetitive treatment to maintain same level of function).

There are other common reasons for denial that will be described for the general knowledge of the therapist. Since authorization is frequently required in a managed care system for PT services, the following reasons for denial deserve attention. Although not considered documentation of care, they are part of the medical/client record. Authorization or pre-authorization is the permission of the third-party payer or managed care organization (MCO) to provide a specified number of PT visits to a beneficiary. It usually includes the total number of visits to an approved provider, based on a specific diagnosis with treatment authorized for a specific diagnosis for a specific body area or body part. As large third-party payers such as Blue Cross Blue Shield (BCBS) provide multiple insurance products, having provider status with one type or division does not automatically mean the therapist has provider status with another. For example, if a PT has a Medicare provider number through BCBS, it does not give the individual provider status with the Health Maintenance Organization (HMO) or Preferred Provider Organization (PPO), unless the contract specifically stipulates otherwise. Pre-authorization or authorization does not necessarily ensure reimbursement. Documentation still has to support the necessity of skilled therapy services. For PTs providing Medicare Part B services, they must apply for individual Medicare identification numbers and ensure that a number is assigned and active.

Reasons for denials based on authorization include:

- unauthorized treatment (where pre-authorization is required);
- unapproved provider (practice is not an approved provider for the payer);
- exceeded approval limit (exceeded expiration date or pre-authorized number of visits in total, or goals were achieved in less than approved visits and treatment continued);
- treatment for other than "authorized" body area;
- part of care justified by documentation, but not all (partial denial, either patient reached goals and there was continued care or only some of the documentation was skilled in nature);
- documentation did not support the need for skilled PT (not medically necessary).

Millions of dollars in Medicare overpayments are identified annually. More than a third are a result of medical necessity identifiable in the documentation such as payments for skilled physical therapy for patients with *no functional* diagnosis requiring physical therapy. Incorrect coding was at the root of another percentage of the overpayments. Auditors check codes by comparing the code with the documentation in the medical record to support that level of code. Results such as these have led to increasingly aggressive efforts by the CMS to identify fraud and abuse in the Medicare system. All MACS and third-party payers are making the same efforts. With the advent of technology, audits and reviews can easily be performed to identify discrepancies. (Refer to Chapter 1 for information on Medicare RACs and MACs.)

XXI. NONCOVERED CONDITIONS AND SERVICES

It is also the service provider's responsibility to be aware of medical conditions and services not covered by the third-party payer. Regardless of the documentation, noncovered services will not be paid regardless of therapist efforts or goals. See Chapter 5, Coding and Documentation, for examples of Medicare noncovered services and conditions. Some payers may not pay for services rendered unless provided soley by a licensed physical therapist. This is also the responsibility of the physical therapist to know.

For Medicare purposes, if a service is covered, it is illegal to accept cash from a beneficiary. If a service is not covered, it is acceptable for the patient to agree to self pay and this must be documented.

XXII. SUMMARY

Incorporating all of the general principles for documentation should help organize the record, record appropriate information, and get services reimbursed based on the documentation. The therapist and/or assistant should seek to write only what is relevant and necessary, in an objective manner, using verbiage that indicates skill, but is universally understood by all potential users of the medical record. By appreciating why payment for physical therapy services is denied and why services are reimbursed, the therapy team can reflect on documentation content guidelines and the importance of content adherence.

REFERENCES

1. Roach William Jr. *Medical Records and the Law*, 4th ed. Chicago, IL, Aspen Publishers, 2006.

2. Melzack R. *Pain Measurement and Assessment*. New York, Raven Press, 1983.

3. OIG www.oig.hhs.gov

4. CMS www.cms.gov accessed Jan. 15, 2011

CHAPTER 2 REVIEW QUESTIONS

1. How should manual and electronic records be stored?

2. Why is legibility imperative in the medical record?

3. Describe the types of data found in the medical record.

4. Explain how errors in the record should be corrected. Give two examples in different domains.

5. Explain the risks involved if entries into the record are not timely.

6. Why is the use of abbreviations in the record a potential problem for physical therapists?

7. Explain the concept of accuracy in the record.

8. What is co-signature? Provide an example of application in physical therapy documentation.

9. What does objectivity in the medical record mean?

10. What is the relationship between reimbursement and documentation? Give six examples of denial based on the documentation.

11. What type of follow-up should there be for verbal, telephonic, or electronic referrals or orders?

12. A PT entry includes the statement "patient was uncooperative." Rewrite this statement using appropriate verbiage.

3 Application of Models for Organization and Guidelines for Content

I. RECORD FORMATS

There are a variety of record formats used by physical therapists and other professionals for manual entry or paper-based systems as well as electronic or computerized records. Categorically, they include source-oriented, problem-oriented, and integrated systems.

The *source-oriented medical record-keeping system (SOMR)* has been commonly used in hospitals and skilled nursing facilities (SNFs) for decades. Each record or "chart" is divided into sections by profession or service (i.e., physical therapy, nursing, medical, physician orders, laboratory, etc.). Patient problems are not separated and notes between caregivers are not integrated because they are "parallel" in nature. Entries in each section are usually in chronological order. It may be time consuming for the physical therapist to glean patient information from the SOMR because of this structure. Additionally, within each section, the methodology for recording information may be different for each discipline, but each discipline should be consistent with itself.

A component of the *problem-oriented medical record system (POMR)*, the SOAP (subjective, objective, assessment/analysis, plan) or SOAPIER (S, O, A, P, Implementation of plan, Evaluation of the implemented plan, Revision of the plan if necessary) note, is commonly used by physical therapists. Common use, however, should not be misunderstood to translate to the best or most effective or efficient for every situation. In an effort to improve patient record keeping, in 1958 Lawrence Weed, MD, of the University of Vermont began exploring alternative types of record entries. The POMR, developed in 1969, focuses on a patient's specific problems in an integrated and coordinated manner between professionals.[1,2] Weed's system includes the initial assessment, problem list, initial plan, progress notes, and discharge summary. All patient problems are included and numbered, active (current) and past, and all professionals involved in the patient's care contribute to the list. In the "pure" system, only one problem can be addressed on a SOAP progress note. Physician orders, not included in the initial plan, are cross-coded for relevance by number to the problems identified. Notes in the POMR are recorded in the SOAP or SOAPIER format. Dr. Weed offered categories to assist professionals in clarifying information.[1,2]

S   Subjective data (what the patient, family member, or significant other says the patient feels or is doing, *only as relevant to specific episode of care and problem*)

> **Author's Note:** Beware of inclusion of statements that are irrelevant to care or, out of context, may be misunderstood and result in denial of services.

O   Objective data (what the professional performs, observes, or inspects in a reproducible manner as relevant to function as possible and clearly presented)

A   Assessment or analytical (summary of S and O with interpretation and professional judgment in order to justify care including progress toward goals if using SOAP only vs. SOAPIER)

P   Plan (intervention plan)

I   Implementation of plan

E   Evaluation of the implemented plan

R   Revision of the plan if necessary

The SOAP or SOAPIER entries may be supplemented by flow sheets for ongoing and frequent interventions. For the discharge summary or summation of care, each problem identified needs a separate SOAP note by each professional providing intervention for the problem in the Weed format.

In order to adapt the SOAP note format to record-keeping regulations, an additional P for the patient problem may be added before the S, i.e., PSOAP. In a hospital setting or SNF, the record may be source oriented, but the physical entry may be in the POMR format, SOAP or PSOAP or SOAPIER. Another change in SOAP-type entries in the past decade is the introduction of functional outcomes reporting (FOR). In *Documenting Functional Outcomes*[3] furthered the concept of FOR, introduced by Swanson. This type of documenting stresses functions and goals related to the same problem, and can be presented in the SOAP format, the FOR format, or narrative.

Dr. Weed's contribution to health or medical record keeping has, to date, passed the test of time. He envisioned "a future in which every patient will have a birth to death problem list on record for use by any hospital. This list, available through a central computer bank, would provide healthcare professionals with a patient's complete data base, anytime, anywhere."[1,2] Although Dr. Weed's vision has been a long time in coming, it is interesting to note that it is being realized. The recent experimental advent of implantable data chips is the realization of Dr. Weed's vision.

The third category of record keeping is the *integrated health record format*. All entries and forms by each discipline are arranged in chronological order without separation.

II. INDIVIDUAL ENTRY FORMATS

There are a variety of formats for individual entries, in addition to SOAP, including problem, status, and plan (PSP); problem, status, plan, and functional goals (PSPG); data, evaluation, and performance goals (DEP); functional outcomes report (FOR); narrative; patient/client management format; use of clinical tools; flow sheets/checklists; and illustrations. The latter three should be used more as supplements to the others than as stand-alone entries. In the past decade, documentation by exception and critical pathway documentation have also been introduced.

A. Problem Status Plan

P   Patient problems and or medical diagnosis

S   Patient/family/caretaker input as relevant and objective data

P   Treatment plan/treatment rendered

B. Problem Status Plan and Functional Goals

P   Patient problems and or medical diagnosis

S   Patient/family/caretaker input as relevant and objective data

	P	Treatment plan/treatment rendered
	G	Functional goals/progress toward goals

C. Data Evaluation Performance Goals

D	Patient/family/caretaker input as relevant and objective data
E	Identification of patient problems, interpretation of data, treatment plan/ treatment rendered
P	Functional goals/progress toward goals

D. Functional Outcome Report (FOR)

The FOR includes the reason for referral, functional limitations (these differ some from the American Physical Therapy Association [APTA] Nagi Model), physical therapy assessment, physical therapy problems, functional outcome goals/progress toward goals, treatment plan/treatment rendered, and rationale.

E. Narrative

Entries are made by the category of intervention but should be consistent with terminology from the Current Procedural Terminology (CPT) coding, in that prior to listing individual interventions they should be preceded by the CPT code verbiage (i.e., gait training, therapeutic exercise, therapeutic activities) in a paragraph-style format, objective intervention and patient response, progress toward goals, and plan or modifications to plan. There may be conclusions or assessments drawn, depending on the purpose of the entry (i.e., treatment vs. progress over time). Headings should be differentiated so that information can be readily identified.

F. Templates

Templates may be hard copy of electronic and actual format may vary. They usually include preset of predetermined categories. The categories may include blanks to be filled in or boxes to be checked off. Electronic templates often include "drop down menus" as fill-in selections.

III. PATIENT/CLIENT MANAGEMENT

This method is related to the patient/client management process in the *Guide to Physical Therapist Practice*. In it, appropriate categories are used as headings in which information can be included, consistent with Guide categories of the systems and subcategories such as aerobic capacity, assistive and adaptive devices, sensory integrity, etc.

IV. CLINICAL TOOLS

A variety of scales, indexes, tests, and measures are commonly used in physical therapy. However, the use of tests and measures must be coordinated with the diagnosis (if there is a disease-specific tool), interventions and results external to the assessments or data gathered and entered onto the tool form. The information contained in the tool should always be summarized in supporting entries in a functional, objective manner in order to be meaningful to other professionals involved in care and any reader. Examples of commonly used evidenced based, reliable and valid and clinical tools are the Berg Balance, Timed Get Up and Go, and the Folstein Mini Mental. If PT intervention is addressing the deficits identified by a tool, the tool should be repeated at minimum at discharge. The OPTIMAL,[4] developed in coordination with the APTA, is an example of a survey-style tool that can be used both at initial exam and evaluation that focuses on function. The OPTIMAL is one of the tools recommended by the Centers for Medicare and Medicaid (CMS) for Medicare Part B outpatients.[4]

V. FUNCTIONAL INDEPENDENCE MEASURE (FIM)™

The Functional Independence Measure (FIM)™ (Guide for the Uniform Data Set for Medical Rehabilitation, 1996) is used to determine the severity of disability on a scale of 1–7. Developed by the University of Buffalo, the FIM scores are used to measure progress as a result of intervention and are commonly used for inpatient rehabilitation. The Uniform Data Set administers the system.[5] Fees are charged for participation in the system and analysis of the data for one organization compared to similar organizations in the system. The FIM is functionally oriented, using variables such as transfer, toileting, and gait. It is an 18-item ordinal scale. The WeeFIM is the version of the FIM used for pediatric application. All professionals using the FIM are specially FIM trained and certified for consistency with scoring. There is also a Spinal Cord Independence Measure (SCIM) for use with individuals with spinal cord injuries. The information provided by the FIM data can be used by a facility to benchmark its outcomes.

VI. FOCUS ON THERAPEUTIC OUTCOMES, INC. (FOTO)™

The Focus on Therapeutic Outcomes, Inc. (FOTO)™ system is designed to measure outcomes of care in the outpatient setting. Like the FIM system, fees are charged for participation in the system and analysis of the data for your organization compared to similar organizations in the system.[6] The information provided from participation in FOTO can facilitate or reinforce effective and efficient outpatient PT.

VII. FLOW SHEETS AND CHECKLISTS

Flow sheets and checklists may contain dates, treatments, attendance, or a variety of other activities. Generally, a check mark is used to mark a specific box for the care provided. Initials of the person who provided the care are preferable to discourage others from entering on the record. Flow sheet or checklist entries should be accompanied by notes to clarify entries and "skill" or rate the effectiveness of the intervention. Although functional, they should not be used as stand-alone forms. See Table 3-1 for a flow sheet example. The downside of using these types of entries is that treatment sessions may appear unskilled if there are no clarifying entries addressing the skill needed, and the same interventions are included with changes limited to repetitions or weight.

TABLE 3-1 • Flow Sheet Example

TX:	8/26/10	8/27/10	8/28/10
Therapeutic procedures	JLS		
Gait training	JLS		
Therapeutic activities		JLS	
Self-management		JLS	

Supplemental entries by date:
8/26/10 "Pain at 3/10 during activity after last session." Able to inc. resistance from 5 to 8#'s for quad ext/flex, 30 reps. Demonstrated ability to ascend and descend 5 steps without use of handrails, no knee buckling. Requires tactile facilitation during LE ther ex to fully engage the L quadriceps and control contractions. Steady improvement noted toward goals. *Jon L. Smith, PT,* #1234

Note: Other data entries should also include supplemental information.

VIII. CRITICAL PATHWAYS/CLINICAL PATHWAYS

Within each patient's therapy plan, target processes and sequences of care, known as critical or clinical pathways, are determined upon the initial visit or diagnosis and generally follow a precise timeline. The pathways are generally experiential or evidence based, and may be used to replace traditional forms of documentation since they require only a signature and date when a goal is achieved on a preprinted pathway form. The term critical pathway relates to the original pathways developed in acute care for "critically ill" patients. Clinical pathways are more applicable in rehabilitation for patients not "critically" ill. See Table 3-2 for a clinical pathway example.

TABLE 3-2 • Clinical Pathway Example

Medical Diagnosis: _____

PT Diagnosis: _____

Weight Bearing Status: _____ RLE _____ LLE

PT Name: Print: _____ Signature: _____ Initials: _____

PT Name: Print: _____ Signature: _____ Initials: _____

PT Name: Print: _____ Signature: _____ Initials: _____

PT Name: Print: _____ Signature: _____ Initials: _____

PT Name: Print: _____ Signature: _____ Initials: _____

Post-op day achieved	IEP: Quad sets, ankle pumps	Able to recall precautions	LTD Asst bed mob	I bed mobility	I sit <> supine	Min Asst Sit <> stand	Min Asst Gait with walker, 25'	Sup standing with device	Pain level with movement
1	JLS	JLS							10/10
2			JLS						9/10
3				JLS	JLS	JLS			7/10
4							JLS	JLS	6/10
5	Discharge status:								

Indicate if status different from that above:

_____

Supplemental entries as indicated:

_____

_____

_____

IX. DOCUMENTATION BY EXCEPTION

The documentation by exception style of record keeping consists of using anticipated or typical treatments and goals that are preestablished and available on preprinted forms in manual entry systems. The only entries required would be variations from the established "norms." In electronic or computerized systems, the user enters the initial diagnosis and the treatment information appears in a retrievable file in a data bank. This method is not recommended because it does not allow for entry of specific patient information and is often too generalized.

X. PRINCIPLES SPECIFIC TO PHYSICAL THERAPY

Documentation content can be organized and simplified with the use of conceptual models or frameworks. Models are frequently used in industry and theoretical sciences to make categorization of information easier to study, organize, apply, and discuss. The APTA provides models in the *Guide to Physical Therapist Practice*.[7] The information in the current edition (as of this writing) of the Guide is presented using a Nagi-based disablement model and the Clinical Decision-Making Model (CDMM) (see Fig. 3-1). Using the disablement model and the CDMM can help therapists organize their examination (tests and measures), evaluation, interventions, and all record-keeping documentation.

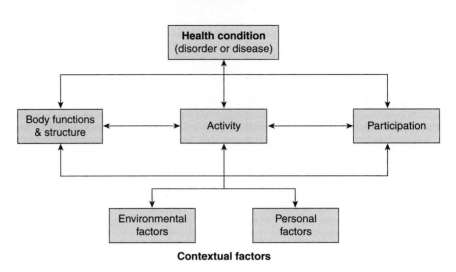

FIGURE 3-1. The WHO - ICF model.

In May 2001, the advent of the International Classification of Functioning, Disability and Health (ICF) began with its approval by the 191 member states of the World Health Organization (WHO)[8] during the 54th World Health Assembly (WHA). The ICF is a conceptual framework and classification system that provides a universal understanding of health using a broad consideration of functioning-related factors and contextual factors to include personal and environmental factors. The ICF was intended for use in research, surveillance, and reporting per the WHA resolution. The World Confederation for Physical Therapy endorsed the ICF in June 2003, and the APTA followed with its endorsement of the ICF in June 2008. According to the APTA, the model will be presented in the next edition of the *Guide to Physical Therapist Practice*.

Exclusive of the models, guidelines for documentation were first established for Medicare by the Healthcare Finance Administration (HCFA, now CMS). Initially, they were used by the Medicare fiscal intermediaries (FIs) or carriers to verify provision of services to beneficiaries by physicians. The guidelines were not, however, used extensively until the 1970s. By the 1970s, computers could track adherence and costs to the system, which began to grow exponentially. When non-Medicare providers (also known as carriers or third-party payers) gained access to technology and the revelation that they too could track provision of care, documentation for non-Medicare beneficiaries had to undergo the same scrutiny. Although somewhat general in nature, there is standard information required by Medicare. Many of the guidelines were written into Medicare manuals in the 1970s and 1980s, but it was not until a decade later that Medicare attempted to standardize forms or formats for reimbursement.

The information required in Medicare documentation is very similar to that recommended in the APTA *Guidelines for Physical Therapy Documentation*. The Medicare documentation guidelines can be obtained on the Internet by accessing Medicare provider manuals at www.cms.gov.

XI. THE DISABLEMENT MODEL

As early as the 1970s, disablement models were developed with the following help of sociologist Saad Nagi to categorize the impact of medical conditions on function for the WHO.[8] The WHO, part of a component organization of the United Nations, which also developed the International Statistical Classification of Diseases and Related Heath Problems or commonly known as ICD (i.e., ICD-9), developed an alternative model in 1980, the International Classification of Diseases, Impairments, Disabilities, and Handicaps (ICDIDH). The National Center for Rehabilitation and Research developed a similar model in 1992. See Table 3-3 for the disablement models.

TABLE 3-3 • Disablement Models

	Nagi	WHO	National Center for Rehabilitation and Research	ICF
Categorization of condition	Active pathology: interruption or interference with normal processes and efforts of the organism to regain normal state	Disease: the intrinsic pathology or disorder	Pathophysiology: interruption with normal physiological developmental processes or structures	Health condition: diseases, disorders, and injuries
Impairment	Anatomical, physiological, mental, emotional abnormalities, or loss	Loss or abnormality of psychological, physiological, or anatomical structure or function at organ level	Loss or abnormality of cognitive, emotional, physiological, or anatomical structure or function	Impairments are problems in body function or body structure such as a significant deviation or loss.
Activities	Functional limitation: limitation in performance at the level of the whole person	Disability: restriction or lack of ability to perform an activity in normal manner	Functional limitation: restriction or lack of ability to perform in action in the manner or range consistent with the purpose of an organ system	Activity limitations are difficulties an individual may have in executing activities. Participation restrictions are problems an individual may experience in involvement in life situations.
End state	Disability: limitation in performance of socially defined roles and tasks within a social, cultural, and physical environment	Handicap: disadvantage as a result of impairment or disability that limits or prevents fulfillment of a normal role depending on age, gender, or sociocultural factors for the person	Societal limitation: restriction attributable to social policy or barriers that limit fulfillment of roles	
Other factors				Environmental factors as facilitators or barriers to functioning Personal factors as positive or negative influence at the individual level

In its current version, the *Guide to Physical Therapist Practice*[7] uses the Nagi framework as the theoretical basis for its terminology. Familiarity with the model should help the PT in conceptualizing and actualizing documentation of care, as all components should be addressed in the medical or client record. There are four categories in the model: pathology or pathophysiology, impairment, functional limitation, and disability. Pathology or pathophysiology is the state caused by a disorder, condition, or disease. Impairment is the physiologic or system problem itself (i.e., integument, cardiopulmonary or neuromuscular, psychological, or anatomical problem). Functional limitation is activity limitation that occurs as a result of the impact of the impairments on a physical "action, task, or activity in an efficient, typically expected, or competent manner."[7] Disability is the inability to perform expected self-care, leisure, work, community, and social roles.

With the endorsement of the ICF by the APTA, plans are being undertaken to facilitate the integration of the ICF in the Guide. This development makes the awareness and understanding of physical therapists of the ICF a necessary tool in order to document a comprehensive picture of their patients' health, functioning, and disability. The ICF (see Fig. 3-1) is made up of different interactive components—health condition, functioning variables (body functions and body structures, activity, and participation), and contextual factors (environmental and personal). Within the ICF, functioning (or disability) as it relates to the patient's health condition does not only provide information at the individual (intrinsic)

Health condition: diseases, disorders, and injuries

Functioning Components:
1. Body Structures: anatomical parts of the body such as organs, limbs and their components
2. Body Functions: physiological functions of body systems (including psychological functions)
3. Activity: execution of a task or action by an individual
4. Participation: involvement in a life situation

Contextual Factors:
5. Environmental Factors: make up the physical, social and attitudinal environment in which people live and conduct their lives.
6. Personal Factors: include gender, age, coping styles, social background, education, profession, past and current experience, overall behavior pattern, character and other factors that influence how disability is experienced by the individual.

FIGURE 3-2. Definition of the ICF components.

level but also at the societal (extrinsic) level. This makes the ICF framework essential in the whole process of documentation because of its inclusiveness. See Fig. 3-2 for the definition of the different components included within the ICF.

The ICF is part of the Family of International Classifications (FIC) by the WHO. The 9th edition of ICD {{1345 World Health Organization 2007}} or ICD-9 is also part of the FIC. ICD-9 classifies health conditions while the ICF classifies functioning and disability. Therefore, both the ICF and the ICD-9 could complement each other. In some cases, both could also overlap, i.e., impairment of body parts and/or body function. Both the ICF and the ICD-9 are under the auspice of the WHO Collaborating Centre for the Family of International Classifications. In future versions of the ICD, the integration of the ICF is being planned to enable complementary role of each system. In physical therapy practice, comprehensive description of functioning regardless of the etiology is vital in addressing problems of the patient that are common to more than one health conditions.

Author's Note: Although the ICD-9 edition is being used in the U.S., the WHO has completed the ICD-10 version.

Other related roadmap developments in the implementation of the ICF include the following:

- Consolidated Health Informatics (CHI) recommended the use of ICF as the "vocabulary," November 2006.
- National Committee on Vital and Health Statistics, an advisory to the Secretary of Department of Health and Human Services in the United States, agreed with the recommendation of CHI regarding the use of ICF Initiative 2006 Recommendations on the Functioning and Disability Domain (accepted by DHHS secretary in 2007).
- Integration of the ICF in the Unified Medical Language Systems (UMLS).

The prevailing trend in the evolution of disablement (or enablement) models is toward functioning-based rather than the pure medical/diagnostic model. This trend reflects consideration of society and the environment (macro-level) in addition to capturing information at the individual level (micro-level). As we go further into the realm of an ICF-based system of healthcare documentation, physical therapists must be ready to deal with reimbursement and payer requirement system—a system that would eventually reflect the ICF.

Figure 3-3 illustrates the application of the ICF in a case format. The main purpose of this figure is simply to convey to the documenting clinician a framework by which the ICF can operate to define "what" needs to be documented in order to

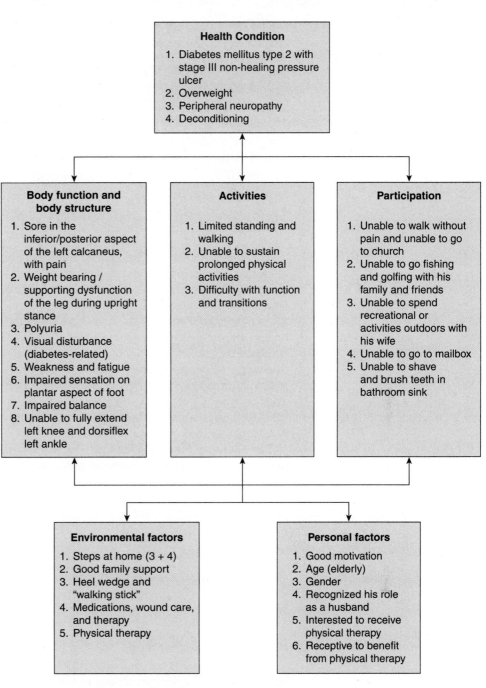

FIGURE 3-3. Case illustration based on the ICF components.

generate informed clinical management. Having said that, the clinician can modify "how" the ICF could be applied depending on the documentation and reimbursement requirement of the payor. Because the WHO's ICF is universal, specific adaptations should not be a problem but would rather create a positive impression to the payors of the clinicians' effort to document a patient's level of functioning.

By addressing all four elements of the disablement model, the PT should be able to appropriately address patient/client needs and problems, regardless of the format the PT selects to enter the information (i.e., SOAP or narrative). The functional goals of the episode of care should be based on resolution or management of the impairments as they relate to function, decrease or eliminate functional limitations, and decrease or eliminate disabilities. The record should not, however, ever reflect concentration on physiologic impairment or resolution of impairments, unless a clear relationship is established between the impairment and its impact on functional improvement. Patient problems can be summarized in the Initial Examination/Evaluation by using the classification headings, which better articulate the treatment goal. *If specifics have already been stated in the body of the document,* deficits can be summarized in Example 1 as follows:

Example 1

Impairments	Functional limitations	Disabilities
• Limited bilateral knee flexion limited 30°/135°	• Unable to climb stairs in home • Unable to sit at table or desk • Unable to squat	• Unable to work as a truck driver

The above is characteristic of the functional reporting model. With an appropriate form of development and organization, goals and anticipated dates can be added as columns to clearly relate impairments to functional limitations and disabilities, as well as specific categories of interventions.

Another application of the disablement model as a tool to facilitate thinking and organization of record content is the CDMM (Fig. 3-1). The CDMM helps the therapist organize the patient/client management process from initial visit through discharge, using the same documentation process throughout. Recording of the information gained by history and interview and various tests and measures should assist in filtering the data for relevance to PT management. Clearly documenting problem summaries and setting realistic functional goals should result in a well-constructed initial evaluation document.

The *Guide to Physical Therapist Practice* suggests five elements for patient/client management that lead to "optimal outcomes":

Examination

↕

Evaluation

↕

Diagnosis

↕

Prognosis

↕

Intervention

The five elements can be correlated to the categories of information that should be included in the written record as follows.

A. Diagnosis

Based on the examination results and clinical judgment, the therapist determines the PT diagnosis or problem and correlates it with the appropriate functional ICD-9 code or ICD-10 (if in use at time). The initial examination/evaluation should also include the physician's or appropriate professional's referring diagnosis. However, the therapist should beware of medical diagnoses that absolutely do not match actual treatment diagnoses, as they will interfere with reimbursement as in Example 2.

Example 2

Medical Diagnosis: fractured humerus

PT Diagnosis: fractured humerus

ICD-9: 812.12 (closed, unspecified), 812.30 (open)

This may be sufficient if the referral was for treatment of the healing humerus or the individual had become dependent in self-care. However, if the referral was because the patient/client had lost functional gait because of prior walker use, then the PT diagnosis or problem should be different as in Example 3.

Example 3

Medical Diagnosis: fractured humerus

PT diagnosis: gait abnormality   ICD-9: 781.2

Followed by an explanation in the history and reason for referral.

A diagnosis that does not match the problems, interventions, or goals identified will result in denial of the claim.

Generally, an acute medical event such as the onset of a cerebrovascular accident (CVA), fracture, multiple trauma or multisystem illness, or presence of comorbidities or complex medical condition will justify, with appropriate documentation, skilled physical therapy. However, the additional of functionally oriented diagnoses such as cerebellar, cerebellar ataxia, and gait abnormality, paralysis or ataxia will better support the need for therapy intervention.

B. Examination

Information and data obtained during the examination process (tests and measures) lead the therapist to clinical judgments, including appropriate systems, screening, and more specific tests and measures to determine the patient/client needs. The specific tests and measures are usually categorized on a "form" entitled PT Evaluation with varying formats. For certain Medicare venues such as a SNF or a Certified Outpatient Rehabilitation Facility (CORF), the results of the initial examination and evaluation are entered into the CMS 700 form (see Appendix B), or a self-designed form that includes the same information. It is critical that the examination be objective, using standardized, evidence based tests and measures whenever possible.

C. Evaluation

Based on information and data collected in the initial examination, the therapist makes clinical judgments regarding patient care, including identification of the PT problems or diagnosis(es) and potential need for consultation or referral. According to the APTA *Guidelines for Documentation*, this stage is called the Initial Examination and Evaluation/Consultation. In total, this entry should answer the following questions:

1. Who is the patient?

   Demographics, medical history, social history, prior or concurrent services (avoid duplication), onset

2. Where is the patient functionally?

   Causative impairments, functional limitations, disabilities

3. What is/are the primary problems the patient has?

   System tests and measures, impairments, medical/social/psych problems that may impact care

4. What is the applicable PT diagnosis?

   The primary problems that will be addressed correlated to the appropriate ICD-9 code

5. Can the problems be impacted by PT intervention?

   Identification of effective and efficient intervention for the problem(s) as determined by the PT and consistent with patient/client family perceptions and needs

6. If yes, which will be addressed during this episode of care?

   Identification of the problem(s) that will be addressed in the plan of care and goals established by the PT in cooperation with the patient/family/responsible party

7. If no, what will the disposition be?

   If not accepting the individual for care, identify reason: lack of expertise in area of problem, has other problems that need referral in addition to those for PT, problems identified are not within scope of PT

D. Prognosis

According to the *Guide to Physical Therapy Practice*,[7] the prognosis is included in the Initial Examination/Evaluation document, including the plan of care (interventions), goals or level of function anticipated as a result of the therapeutic intervention, and frequency and duration of treatment. Contents for the plan of care are outlined by the CMS for Medicare beneficiaries. However, they can be applied to all settings and carriers. The prognosis also includes the individual's rehabilitation potential, which is relevant to the PT goals and prior level of function. If an individual is accepted for care, the rehabilitation potential should be at minimum good as it is based on the goals established Excellent may appear to indicate to the reader that the individual may not need services. If the PT chooses fair, it may be acceptable assuming the patient is too ill to make any other determination at the time and the documentation reflects this.

E. Intervention

These are the specific skilled PT treatments and methods used to impact the patient's problems and achieve goals established by the PT in conjunction with the patient/client. The treatments should be described with terminology that matches Current Procedural Terminology (CPT), the AMA billing codes, or HCPCS (refer to Chapter 5). All interventions must match specific problems identified in the initial examination or reexamination (with goals modified as indicated) and specific goals.

F. Outcomes

This phase of treatment occurs when the results of the interventions or treatments are evaluated. The *Guide to Physical Therapy Practice*[7] includes the reexamination of the patient/client with intervention to determine if changes or modifications are needed in the interventions. If the patient is not demonstrating progress toward the desired outcomes or achieving the anticipated results from the physical therapy at any point in time, reevaluation of treatment options is necessary. Possible adjustments include changing intervention and determination of change in medical status necessitating referral back to the physician or initial referral in states with direct access. The outcome or progress level during care must be clearly indicated in the documentation. If some or all of the goals are not achieved, the reasons for lack of accomplishment must be included. These outcomes must also reflect back to the initial goals and modifications during the episode of care. By administering standardized tests and measures at initial examination and throughout treatment, progress can be measured objectively.

XII. SUMMARY

There are three basic formats for medical/client record organization: the SOMR, POMR, and integrated systems. Of the three, the SOMR, the system that divides the record by service or discipline, is the most common. Each service, however, may choose within the SOMR to make their entries in the "model" of their choice. The most common entry formats for PT are a SOAP and narrative, for ongoing entries, with flow sheets and checklists for intervention parameters. A variety of customized formats, often self-designed, are used for initial examination/evaluation and discharge summaries and disposition/discharge plan.

In the *Guide to Physical Therapist Practice*, 2e[7] the APTA purports using the Nagi Disablement Model to help organize patient/client care and the documentation. In the model, information is divided into pathology, impairment, functional limitation, and disability. The Guide identifies six elements that must be included in the record: the PT diagnosis or problem (as well as the medical as applicable), examination, evaluation, prognosis, intervention (continuation of care), and outcomes assessment (summation of episode of care). Application of the concepts presented in the *Guide to Physical Therapist Practice* and the CDMM can assist the PT is completing appropriate documentation.

With the APTA's recent endorsement of the WHO/ICF, it is expected that the Guide and documentation in physical therapy will reflect the ICF language in the coming years. As the ICF shares a common interface with the Guide and the CDMM; it was meant to be complementary. While the ICF defines "what" to measure, the Guide could provide ways and means on "how" to operationalize the ICF components in practice.

The recognition and understanding of enablement models, particularly the ICF, is helpful in daily documentation within the context of CMS guidelines and private insurers. They facilitate more standard formats for documentation and resultant reimbursement. The enablement models also facilitate standardization of documentation content, enhancing the ability of the clinician to track treatment outcomes.

Links to ICF-related Web sites:

- http://www.icf-research-branch.org/
- http://www.icf-casestudies.org/
- http://www.who.int/en/
- http://www.rehabnet.ch/index.php?page=30&lang=0
- http://www.paranet.ch/en/pub/pan.cfm

REFERENCES

1. Weed L. Medical records that guide and teach. *The New England Journal of Medicine*. 1968;278:11, 593–599, 652–657.

2. Weed L. *Medical records, medical education, and patient core: The problem oriented medical record as o basic tool.* Cleveland, Ohio, Case Western Reserve Press, 1969.

3. Abeln S, Stewart D. *Documenting Functional Outcomes in Physical Therapy*, 1st ed. St. Louis, MO, Mosby-Year Book, 1993.

4. APTA's Outpatient Physical Therapy Improvement in Movement Assessment Log (OPTIMAL). http://www.apta.org/OPTIMAL/. Accessed April 15, 2011.

5. Uniform Data System for Medical Rehabilitation. http://www.udsmr.org.

6. Focus on Therapeutic Outcomes. Inc. www.fotoinc.com. Accessed April 12, 2011.

7. APTA. *Guide to Physical Therapist Practice*, 2nd ed. Alexandria, VA, American Physical Therapy Association, 2003.

8. World Health Organization. www.who.int/en. Accessed April 16, 2011.

CHAPTER 3 REVIEW QUESTIONS

1. What are the basic types of medical record organization? Compare and contrast these types.

2. Explain what goes in each section of the SOAP formatted note. What is the difference between the SOAP and the SOAPIER?

3. Give examples of three types of individual entry formats. Compare and contrast each format.

4. What is your opinion regarding the popularity of the SOAP format?

5. What is a clinical tool and its relevance to documentation? Give two examples.

6. Why is it not prudent to use a checklist or flow sheet without additional narrative or written entries?

7. What are the different models that are being used in physical therapy practice?

8. Explain what a disablement model is. Which model is used by the APTA in the *Guide to Physical Therapist Practice?*

9. What is the ICF? What are the different components of the ICF?

10. Give your own example entry for each of the ICF components?

11. Explain the categories in the disablement model employed in the *Guide to Physical Therapist Practice*. Include examples for each category.

12. Give an example of an impairment, the resulting functional problem, and possible disability.

13. Compare and contrast the medical diagnosis and the physical therapy diagnosis (physical therapy problem).

14. What is the difference between the initial examination and the evaluation?

15. How can the ICF help in patient evaluation and tracking patient progress?

4 Content Standardization/ Component Requirements

I. GENERAL DOCUMENTATION REQUIREMENTS

The Centers for Medicare and Medicaid Services (CMS), formerly HCFA, was the first to delineate documentation requirements for physical therapists (PTs) by a payer. Although there are some differences depending on setting and type of organization, there are basic requirements for all PT services: physician/appropriate referral (except for direct consumer access, although it may be required for third party reimbursement), initial examination/evaluation, plan of care (POC), certification of the POC (dependent on setting), ongoing documentation of care/continuum of care, reevaluation, and discharge summary or summation of care. There are also states, such as Florida, that include documentation requirements in the state practice act, although they are similar to those required for Medicare. In the past two decades, the American Physical Therapy Association (APTA) has developed guidelines for documentation that are similar to the Medicare guidelines (see Table 4-1). It is interesting to note that the Medicare program does not require providers to abide by the same requirements for Medicare and non-Medicare patients. However, in the states in which documentation requirements are included in the laws, and for those therapists that follow APTA guidelines, the requirements are similar and represent best practice standards.

The use of standardized forms for documentation and billing purposes aids in maintaining consistency within an organization and between therapy personnel. Blank forms or pages lead to inconsistency and omission of information that may be crucial in supporting medical necessity for skilled physical therapy (PT) services. Although pre-designed or keyed forms (or formats in the electronic medical record) do not guarantee the quality of content, if keys or legends are provided in each category, the information is more likely to be included. The APTA's *Guide to Documentation* includes sample forms (see Appendix E).[1] The forms in the guide are not detailed (with exception of the history) and therefore should be used only as a guide to develop forms that best suit a facility's or organization's needs. This is applicable to manual entry forms as well as electronically generated forms or formats.

Because APTA documentation elements are generic and widely used, therapists should attempt to use them consistently, regardless of the third-party payer or payment system. The only documentation differences between patients should be age and activity appropriate goal (i.e., pediatrics vs. geriatrics) or form requirements for billing and documentation (i.e., CMS 1500 vs. CMS 700 or 701). Durable medical equipment, such as orthotics or wheelchairs, may require not only the standard documentation to identify need, but additional supporting letters from the therapist and/or physician, or state-specific forms, such as for Florida Medicaid wheelchairs.

There are varieties of forms or formats required or strongly recommended for billing of services or to accompany billing forms (if requested) depending on the payer. Examples include Medicare's 700 series forms (see Appendix B), the CMS 1450 (UB 92) which has been revised to include the NPI (National Provider Identification) number, and the CMS 1500 form modified in 2005 (see Appendix C). The forms come with the instructions pre-printed on them. Adherence to the instructions will

TABLE 4-1 • Medicare (CMS) and APTA Guidelines for Documentation

Medicare (requires some forms or similar format and content)	APTA: Guide for Documentation (provider choice of format)
Physician's referral or approval/signature on initial POC	Referral or referral mechanism (prescription)
Developed by PT	
Evaluation	Initial Examination/Evaluation
	History
Identification of objective losses by system	Systems review
	Tests & measures
	Evaluation: judgment
	PT diagnosis
Prognosis	Prognosis
	Patient/client involvement in goals
	Measurable goals related to impairment, functional
Plan of care	Limitations, disabilities
	Plan of care
	Authentication
Ongoing documentation of interventions	Progress report at least every ten days
	Continuation of care
	Every visit or encounter
Reevaluation/Recertification	Reexamination
Discharge	Summation of episode of care

help to ensure that they are completed appropriately. Although the billing may not be completed by the treating professional, there should be familiarity with information required. There should also be agreement with the billing and coding personnel regarding who will be providing what information (see Example 1).

Example 1

Coding for billing and documentation content

The treating PT or PTA documents the treatment preceding all descriptions with CPT verbiage:

Therapeutic procedure: passive stretching; × reps × 15 sec of the hamstrings, reciprocal inhibition quadriceps/hamstrings to facilitate hamstring lengthening, manual resistive exercise with progressive resistance knee extension/flexion.

Since this is a timed code, either the billing department or the treating PT/PTA would need to ensure that the time was included:

1 unit 97110/15 minutes: Therapeutic procedure: passive stretching; × reps × 15 sec of the hamstrings, reciprocal inhibition quadriceps/hamstrings to facilitate hamstring lengthening, manual resistive exercise with progressive resistance knee extension/flexion.

The 700 series forms are used to document initial examination and evaluation, interim monthly reports, and discharges in skilled nursing facilities (SNFs), comprehensive outpatient rehabilitation facilities (CORFs), and outpatient rehabilitation agencies (ORFs). These accompany, if requested, the billing forms that are submitted to the MAC. The CMS 1500 form is used for all other outpatient or Part B services rendered in other settings. The 700 series forms are available and were developed by the CMS in an attempt to standardize documentation to complement billing. Although the forms themselves are not required, the information requested on the 700 series forms is required. The authors of this text recommend that the forms be used with minor adaptations that provide all of the information required in a skilled manner. If a facility decides that the form is too limiting because of space, the form that is "self or facility" designed should include all of the information required on the 700 series forms. It is recommended that the PT contact the fiscal intermediary (FI), now called MAC, to get approval for use of a self-designed form. Regardless of the form used, the goal of the provider should be to submit a clean—error free—claim that matches the information both in the initial forms/reports and subsequent. If information is requested to support the bill, it should be self-explanatory and reinforce the information and charges on the claim form. It is essential that the instructions that come with each form be followed. In some cases, as in the use of the CMS 1500 form, omission of a modifier, such as -59 if interventions are provided during the same session and can only be so with clarification by a modifier, will result in a denial that cannot be appealed in the Medicare system. Most non-Medicare payers have begun to follow the same coding and documentation initiatives as Medicare, the CCI (Correct Coding Initiative). It is the responsibility of individual therapists to be familiar with CCI edits.

> **Author's Note:** The -59 modifier needs to be used for other CPT codes if manual therapy is being billed. Manual therapy is considered as a bundled code for other techniques like therapeutic exercise. If the therapist performed 15 minutes of manual therapy and then separately did 15 minutes of therapeutic procedures, the therapeutic exercise would need a -59 modifier code next to it. If not included, the payor will reject, stating that the therapeutic exercise is part of the manual therapy and cannot be billed separately unless using the modifier. Documentation would also have to delineate this in the treatment.

It is the responsibility of the treating PT/PTA to know, for the sake of documentation and billing, if a payer has adopted the -59 modifier.

In addition to the use of forms, the terminology used in the documentation must be universally understood by all possible record "readers," yet sophisticated enough to justify the skilled care rendered. In this context, there are terms that can and should be used and terms that should be avoided. Terms that may be used by the therapist in conversation, should not necessarily appear in the documentation. According to Baetan, Philippi, and Moran, "Functional phrase alternatives are terms or phrases that convey to the reviewer the skilled nature of the service provided.... the concept of using functional phrase alternatives can be expanded to all practice setting."[2]

Appropriate identification of patient/client problems with relevant goals is another key to successful documentation. Although goals should be functionally oriented, impairment-based goals should be included as they relate to function. The goals of the patient/client or caregiver(s) need to be addressed in these. However, they must be achievable and appropriate for the episode of care. The therapist should provide goals for the episode in which they are providing care only. If a continuum is expected (i.e., acute care to inpatient rehabilitation to home health to outpatient), each therapist establishes the goals for the setting and length of stay (LOS)/time period for which the patient/client is under their care. In the discharge or summation of care, the therapist should address the need for the patient/client to receive continuing services in the next setting. A therapist in one setting should never establish goals for therapy rendered in another setting at another time. At the time of patient/client discharge, the PT should avoid stating that the "patient has reached maximal potential." This may limit an individual's ability to obtain services in another setting. It is best to simply state the patient has reached the goals established for the episode of care. If additional services are needed, the discharging therapist should simply state "the patient will benefit from continued PT in the _____ setting."

II. CATEGORIES AND APPROPRIATsE TERMINOLOGY

A. What to Avoid

There are words and verbiage that are considered "red flags" in professional documentation and may result in an automatic denial from some payers, but not necessarily others.

Avoid using the terms "walking" when referring to gait training and "maintain" (unless used in the context of balance ability). The word walking should only be used in the context of quoting a patient, as in the patient stated: "he wants to walk." Also avoid repeated statements that indicate a patient is not progressing, noncompliant, or uncooperative, still unable, unless the intention is to discontinue the PT. If any nonspecific words such as these are used, they should be clarified (Example 2).

■ Example 2

Patient is demonstrating noncompliance with his home exercise regime; stated: "I hate doing those exercises, so I'm not."

Patient was uncooperative during therapy today; he shouted to therapist "Go to hell," then picked up the walker and threw it toward the therapist.

This should also be avoided when describing the training or education a caregiver is receiving. For most skills that involve caregivers, a reasonable time must be established similar to that for a specific patient goal (see Example 3).

■ Example 3

An initial established goal on a POC is:

Husband will be able to safely and consistently transfer patient (his wife) from the WC to and from the bed by _____ (indicate date or number of sessions)

- Avoid, in treatment or progress reports comments such as "husband is still unable to safely transfer wife" in spite of multiple training sessions.
- Instead: Husband is now able to transfer his wife from the WC to the bed with minimal verbal instructions.
- If it appears that the husband will not be able to execute a stand pivot or sliding board transfer, the goal needs to be terminated or modified, e.g., the husband will be able to safely and consistently transfer patient from the WC to bed using a mechanical lift.

Avoid using nondescriptive terms such as patient is "the same," "not improving," or "still not compliant." It is better to identify some aspect of the treatment that the patient is able to perform and demonstrate progress in such as "The patient is now able to…"

Avoid terms without clear meaning, such as "uncooperative, confused, agitated," unless the plan is to discharge (DC) or unless there is specific clarification that follows. Use of the word "Maintain" should be used with caution. Other terms without clear meaning include tolerated well; general increase in; general improvement, strengthening, or supervision; poor carry through; declined in function; not responding to treatment; improved (unless objective data follows); and increased or decreased pain without reference to a scale that can be measured and related to function.

B. What to Include

Descriptive, Objective Terminology and Data/Measures. Examples of descriptive, objective terminology and data/measures include functionally oriented goals; distances, deficits with progress toward goals, and functional limitations and disabilities that can be impacted during the episode of care by resolving impairments.

For Medicare purposes, focus on essential function versus nonessential function, especially in inpatient and home health. Essential functions are those that an individual has to do versus wants to do. Any type of leisure activity for example, is not an essential function. The ability to achieve in one's home the functionality to move from room to room, self-care, or to get to the bathroom for toileting in functional times are essential. Once a patient/client has progressed to outpatient (OP), community safety and function must also be addressed. Use comparisons that illustrate progress and provide instruction in precautions, independent exercise, and caregiver training. Use skilled terminology that matches CPT code verbiage for interventions (i.e., therapeutic exercise, gait training) so that the documentation content truly matches the billing codes. Terminology as indicated in the *Guide to Physical Therapist Practice*[2] is also acceptable and should include application of practice patterns for goals, interventions and progress.

Whenever possible, numbers, assuming they are universally understood or a key is provided, should be used to communicate in the medical record. Range of motion (ROM) should be expressed as fractions, indicating total "normal" range based on a standard, i.e., 120°/180° for shoulder flexion/extension, 45°/135° for knee flexion, and so on. ROM goals should be written to indicate the goal ROM and the reason it is necessary or the "in order to…" component. Percentages should be avoided as they lack the same clarity (see Example 4).

■ Example 4

Increase AROM L shoulder flexion from 95°/180° to 180°/180° in order to maximally flex L shoulder and return to job as house painter.

Muscle performance or strength should be expressed in fractions based on a standardized scale such as the 0/5 to 5/5 scale (using + or − as indicated). Strength goals should be written to indicate the goal strength and the reason it is necessary. Stating in a goal that "muscle strength will be increased by 1 grade" does not include a frame of reference for anyone reading the record (see Example 5).

■ Example 5

Increase strength of L shoulder flexion from 3/5–5/5 in order to return to job as house painter, and sustain full flexion of the shoulder up to 6 hours/day.

However, if a patient, such as a geriatric client, can only perform maximal resistance with a single repetition or only early in the day, caution should be used when using a standard strength scale to describe muscle performance. In this case, the therapist may prefer to use verbiage that more accurately describes the reality of what the patient can do or describe strength relative to functional activities performed.

Author's Note: For example, able to tolerate single repetition of L hip flexion moderate resistance only, with inability to repeat flexion in sit or stand against gravity.

Records should also include numeric expression of assistance with component for which help is needed (i.e., minimal or limited assistance of 25%, moderate or extensive assistance of 50%, maximal or extensive assistance of 75%, or total assistance 100%), applied for transfers, transitional movements, gait, wheelchair mobility, balance, or other objective measures of gait with use of consistent terminology. Since the CPT code is gait training, consistently use gait throughout the entry, avoiding introduction of the term ambulation (although the CMS accepts the use of the term ambulation) Walking is not a skilled term. It should also be noted that when using percentages to describe patient/client ability or dependence, the part of the activity that the patient/client needs assistance with should be included in the daily or weekly documentation, although it is not needed in the initial goal setting (see Example 6).

> ### ■ Example 6
>
> O: Gait Training: fixed front wheeled rolling walker, even surface, no directional changes, 3-point discontinuous pattern; PWB LLE, minimal assist to keep walker from veering L/R, verbal instructions for consistent pattern and for intermittent facilitation of PWB on LLE.

Refer to Chapter 5 for additional information on content. The initial examination is presented again as an overview, because its importance cannot be stressed enough. If the appropriate content is in the initial examination/evaluation, including objective measures, reliable and valid tests and measures that are functionally oriented and or disease specific, identified physical therapy problems, clear delineation of the patient's deficits/problems that can be impacted in a reasonable amount of time (frequency and duration), with appropriate goals and interventions, the appropriate baseline will be established for the total episode of care or length of stay.

III. INITIAL EXAMINATION OR EVALUATION

The APTA includes four categories of content: general guidelines, initial examination and evaluation/consultation, continuation of care, and summation of the episode of care. Practitioners may be more familiar with the colloquial terms of initial evaluation, daily/weekly notes, progress notes/reports, and discharge reports or summaries.

What is important for each, regardless of the name, is the content. The initial report sets the tone for the record and should clearly establish the need for skilled therapy. Many of the elements included should be repeated in the discharge summary to determine if the care rendered matched the initial problems and plan; especially standardized tests and measures. All data should be communicated as objectively as possible to allow for objective goal setting and justification of care. The therapist will have to make decisions regarding which baseline tests and measures should be included based on the patient/client primary complaint(s) and if disease-specific measurement tools are indicated and available. Medicare Part B outpatient regulations require measurement tools and recommend four, one of which is the APTA/Cedaron developed OPTIMAL instrument.

A. Initial Visit

For record authenticity purposes, it is preferable to include as much information as possible in the record at the initial visit. In some situations, some of the tests and measures may have to be completed on subsequent visit(s), although as much as possible should be completed so an initial plan can be developed. All initial patient/client visits should also include patient/client or caretaker completion of an intake form with demographic information, payer/insurance information, reason for PT, other treatment for current condition, and medical history form that has information that can be easily checked off. Medications, including prescription, over the counter and supplements should also be included for the PT to review.

Content of Initial Visit Documentation

Referral information. The types of referrals in PT are self-referred and physician or physician extender (NPP, non-physician provider), or other appropriate health professional depending on state law and from whom a payer will accept referral or approval of a POC. If the patient is physician referred, the diagnosis(es) and treatment requested must be included on the referral, i.e., S/P R patella fracture, evaluate and treat.

To become a patient of an outpatient facility, a Medicare beneficiary must be under the care of a physician who certifies that the beneficiary needs skilled rehabilitation services. However, the physician who approves the POC need not have seen the patient immediately preceding the referral. (It does not have to be the same physician that approves and signs subsequent POC for recertification). He or she must advise the PT of the beneficiary's medical history, current diagnosis and medical findings. The desired rehabilitation goals should be established by the PT, with the POC approved by the physician within the first month of care. This should include any precautions or contraindications to specific activity or indicate intensity of rehabilitation services.

The referral process may also include specific authorization if the patient is a member of a managed care plan or Medicare Advantage plan.

HIPAA acknowledgement. Signed acknowledgement of organization HIPAA policies is required for all patients.

Signed consent. Consent to treat by patient/client, legal guardian, or parent is required. There should also be signed consent to treat once treatment and effects are explained or the therapist should state that treatment was discussed and patient/client or appropriate representative has agreed to treatment.

Patient/Client identification information. Full name, gender, date of birth, and language spoken: primary and secondary, health insurance claim or identification number.

Start of care date (SOC). Date of the initial examination/evaluation for the episode of care.

Medical diagnosis. If physician referred or referred by other health professional or if known by patient.

Physical therapy diagnosis. PT diagnosis or primary PT problem. If an injury, list the mechanism of it. This is established by the PT based on the initial examination.

Onset date. Should be recent, if a chronic condition, list date of acute or recent exacerbation. Recent is usually no more than 3–6 months prior to start of care.

Medical history. Include co-morbidities (may be summarized if on separate intake form completed by patient/client with only relevant information summarized in the evaluation) and all medications prescription and over-the counter (OTC), as they may impact physical therapy, recent hospitalizations, circumstances regarding onset, general medical history including surgeries and any prior treatment for same problem by PTs or other practitioners. Information should also be obtained to ensure the patient is receiving any simultaneous services that could be considered duplicative.

Related medical testing results. As available to PT.

Patient/Client/Family therapy goals. Goals are determined based on examination results and needs of patient/client/family that are relevant and appropriate for the episode of care. This is a critical component consistent with the WHO's ICF model. Acknowledgment of patient/client/family/caregiver input or inclusion is also required.

Prior functional level. This should include mobility (home and community); work, school, leisure, and self-care (ADL [activities of daily living], IADL [instrumental activities of daily living]); family care responsibilities/child care/elder care, in the recent past.

Social history/support. Handedness: right/left; employment income source, school, leisure; family status; living arrangements (type of dwelling, presence or absence of stairs, location of bedrooms and bath); support system, caretaking responsibilities, ability to drive or dependence on public transportation.

Precautions/contraindications/barriers. Precautions may relate to medical conditions as with cardiac precautions, seizures, diabetes, oxygen dependency, surgical as in total hip precautions for posterolateral approach, weight bearing, or other.

Contraindications would indicate that some procedure should not be performed for a specific reason (i.e., electrical stimulation to a body area close to a non-shielded pacemaker), or ultrasound use over a non-healed fracture site. Barriers may include such things as physical barriers in a living environment, illiteracy, language, financial limitations or lack of regular transportation.

Baseline data from tests and measures. (Examples are not all inclusive)

- Activities of daily living (instrumental and functional, compare to prior level of function). Instrument examples: Bethel Index, Katz
- Aerobic capacity; activity tolerance/endurance. Examples: Borg RPE, Dyspnea scale, vital signs
- Balance BERG, Timed get up & go, Tinnetti, Functional Reach, Dynamic Gait, Romberg
- Cardiovascular/pulmonary HR, BP, P, RR & quality, pallor
- Cognition - Folstein Mini-Mental Status Examination
- Coordination - reciprocal activity R/L, speed
- Gait ability or non-gait mobility - observational using Rancho Los Amigos or traditional terms.
- General integrity - speed, balance with directional change, ability to maneuver wheelchair manual or power.
- Hearing - finger rub, whisper test
- Joint integrity
- Bed mobility (wheelchair) - Ability, assist time required
- Motor control/movement patterns (gross and fine motor skills)
- Muscle performance/strength 0/5 to 5/5 scale and or verbiage if scale inappropriate
- Musculoskeletal status/findings special tests
- Neuromuscular/neuromotor development
- Pain (measurable scale of 0/10 to 10/10, specifying body part and pain at rest and activity)
- Posture - sitting and standing
- Range of motion: active vs. passive; vs. active assistive; joint contracture in fractions and numbers
- Reflexes - DTRs, abnormal presence of primitive reflexes
- Sensory/proprioception - light touch/monofilaments, pain (sharp/dull)
- Systems review (as relevant to problem for specific episode of care)
- Tone - Modified Ashworth
- Transfers/transitional movement; sit to/from stand, bed-chair, supine to/from sit
- Vascular: capillary refill, skin temperature/condition, edema, extremity hair patterns, nails
- Vision - pocket snellen chart for general ability, tracking, peripheral
- Vital signs: radial pulse (other peripheral as applicable, blood pressure, respiration rate, breathing pattern) before, during, and after
- Anthropometrics - height, weight, abdominal girth, waist to hip ratio, body type, BMI
- Integument integrity: wounds/ulcerations/any abnormalities or potential areas of concern
- Functional deficits/abilities

Whenever possible, standardized tests and measures functionally based or disease specific, should be used. These can then be repeated throughout the patient/client length of stay as intervention and measure of progress and at discharge to measure progress based compared to initial results. Medicare Part B requires that standard tests and measures be used at initial exam/evaluation. The APTA OPTIMAL is one of the recommended. However, the clinician can determine which test or measure is most appropriate. Examples are provided in the categories above.

Device use. Protective or adaptive; orthotics (including splints and supports); prosthetics; assistive gait devices; communication devices (i.e., augmentative communication devices, communication boards, speech, hearing aids, contact lenses, glasses, electrolarynx [external].

Note: Passy–Muir valves have replaced the need for electrolarynx in most cases in recent years.

Results of any special tests. If any special tests are conducted, they should be documented by name with the results.

Architectural/safety considerations. The physical considerations of the home, work, school, and other environments/buildings including access, presence of stairs, elevators, ramps, bathrooms, door widths, bathroom accessibility, indoor/outdoor surfaces, type of transportation and access to the same and so on. Safety relates to the patient/client's ability to function safely in an environment based on their abilities.

Prior level of function (PLOF). This is a general description of what the patient was able to do functionally prior to the "current episode" of illness, pathology, surgery, etc. (see Example 7).

■ Example 7

PLOF
Patient was independent in gait without an assistive device, able to drive, perform all self-care, work, and participate in leisure activities.

Reason for skilled care, referral or need for therapy services, assessment/professional judgment (see Example 8).

■ Example 8

Patient is now dependent for gait, transfers, bed mobility and self-care.

Problem Summary. The PT medical record should also include a summary of deficits identified in baseline data, preferably delineating the relationship between impairments and the functional limitations and disabilities, but avoiding physiological impairment focus. The ICF model includes a "list of body functions and structure, and a list of domains of activity and participation. Since an individual's functioning and disability occurs in a context, the ICF also includes a list of environmental factors." (WHO). There is a difference in functional outcome reporting versus the *Guide to Physical Therapist Practice* regarding impairment and functional limitation. In the Nagi disablement model, which is used in the second edition of the Guide, gait is considered an impairment. Gait in different environments and levels of quality, speed, and functional purposes are considered functional limitations. For Medicare purposes, concentration should be on essential functional activities (EFA) as much as possible, based on the setting in which the patient/client is being treated. For example, home health would concentrate on EFA in the home. Once the progression is made to outpatient, essential activities would expand into the environment outside the home and appropriate safe function. The concept of EFA is usually not as limiting in non-Medicare reimbursed therapy.

Plan of care (POC). The PT POC should include specific planned interventions using CPT or the related CMS/Medicare HCPCS terminology, including patient/caregiver instruction and a statement regarding patient/family involvement in goal setting. The POC should list the frequency and duration of the treatment and include all short- and long-term goals (time defined, functionally oriented). Rehabilitation potential for achievement of goals/prognosis should also be included along with a statement of the medical necessity or need for skilled PT.

> **Author's Note:** If the LOS is only several days, i.e. acute care, delineator of short vs. long terms is not necessary.

> **Author's Note:** Medicare providers may have a separate document entitled POC since physician/nonphysician provider (NPP) signature is required.

Authentication. Authentication consists of the signature of the both the PT and the referring physician (for a Medicare POC) with attestation of the need for skilled PT and agreement with the POC.

According to the Medicare Carrier manual, the following must be included:

a. Identification of the physician's agreement with the POC for physical therapy

b. Indication that the patient is under the care of a physician for the presenting diagnosis

c. Indication of the potential prognosis for restoration of functions in a reasonable and generally predictable period of time

d. Patient identification information

e. Precautions/contraindications/barriers

All providers billing for physical therapy services are required to maintain an established plan of treatment as a permanent part of the patient's clinical record. The plan must be established as soon as possible relative to the start of care or within 30 days. The re-certification does not need to be by the same physician or non-physician provider (NPP), as long as it is the person responsible for the patient oversight at the time of the recertification.

> **Author's Note:** This is applicable for Part B in outpatient venues such as skilled nursing facilities (SNFs), long-term residents (ORFs), home health, and independent practitioners. For Certified Outpatient Facilities (CORFs) it is 60 days for the initial POC (plan of care), then every 30 days is recommended. For other outpatient settings it can be for 90 days, then every 30. However, It is recommended that in all settings for adults, recertification for the POC should be every 30 days. In the SNF, it is 30 days for residents receiving Part B services.

The plan must be kept on file and available for carrier review if requested.

A physical therapy plan of treatment must include the type, amount, frequency, and duration of the services that are to be furnished and indicate the treatment diagnosis and anticipated goals. Any changes in the treatment plan must be made in writing and signed by the physician/NPP. The frequency and duration must be specific especially for Medicare, and not given in ranges (see Example 9).

■ Example 9

Frequency and duration: 5×/week for 2 weeks, then 3×/week for 2 weeks

3×/week for 6 weeks

Medical record documentation maintained by the physical therapist with referring physician/NPP signature, must clearly indicate the medical necessity of each physical therapy modality covered by the Medicare program or appropriate payer.

The physician/NPP or therapist *must document the patient's functional limitations in terms that are objective and measurable.* Documentation must show objective loss of joint motion, strength, or mobility (i.e., degrees of motion, strength grades, levels of assistance), related to function.

All claims submitted with an unlisted service or procedure must be accompanied by documentation that describes the service, supports medical necessity, and the rationale for using the treatment modality.

The Medicare guidelines, available at www.cms.gov in the provider manuals and on the First Coast of Florida Web site for Florida, emphasize the following:

Services must be furnished under a plan of treatment that has been written and developed by physical therapist is cooperation with the physician/NPP. The plan must be established within 30 days of the initiation of treatment, must be signed by the physician, and must be incorporated into the physician's permanent record for the patient. The services provided must relate directly to the written treatment regimen.

The POC must contain the following information (see Example 10):

1. Patient's diagnoses that require physical therapy

2. The patient's significant past history

3. Related physician orders if there are any

4. Therapy goals and potential for achievement

5. Any contraindications/precautions

6. Patient's awareness and understanding of diagnoses, prognosis, treatment goals

7. When appropriate, the summary of treatment provided and results achieved during previous periods of physical therapy services

The plan relates the type, amount, frequency, and duration of the physical therapy that are to be furnished to the patient and indicates the diagnosis and anticipated goals. Changes are made in writing and signed by the physician, a qualified physical therapist (in the case of physical therapy), a qualified speech pathologist (in the case of speech pathology services), a registered professional nurse, or physician on the staff of the clinic pursuant to the attending physician's oral orders.

Outpatient physical therapy may be furnished under a written plan of treatment established by the qualified physical therapist providing such physical therapy services as long as the physician periodically reviews the plan. The physician no longer needs to see the patient in order to sign or approve the POC.

Physical therapy services are to be furnished in accordance with the POC established by the physical therapist and approved by the physician responsible for the patient's care and may not be altered in type, amount, or duration by the therapist (except in the case of an adverse reaction to a specific treatment).

2206.1 Physician's Certification and Recertification

A. *Content of Physician's Certification*—Medicare does not pay for outpatient physical therapy unless a physician certifies that:

• The services are or were required by the patient.

• A plan for furnishing such services is or was established and periodically reviewed by the physician.... A plan of treatment for outpatient physical therapy services is established by either the physician or the qualified physical therapist providing such services. However, a plan established by a physical therapist must be periodically reviewed by the physician ... (See §2206.3.)

The outpatient physical therapy services are or were furnished while the patient was under the care of a physician. (See §2206.2.)

Since the certification is closely associated with the plan of treatment, the same physician who established or reviews the plan of treatment should certify the necessity for services but it may be a different physician. Obtain certification at the time the plan of treatment is established or as soon thereafter as possible.

> **Author's Note:** For non-Medicare patients, the referral requirements, including pre-authorization, may be different for each provider and must be verified before treatment is initiated.

■ Example 10

EXAMPLE FOR BEGINNING HISTORY: initial visit record; SOC 4/9/10

Medicare: 81 year old English speaking female referred to outpatient PT with acute onset of R shoulder bursitis 4/1/10. Referred by physician for evaluation and treatment after taking NSAIDs for a week without significant relief.

Past Medical History: CABG x 10 years, HTN, osteoarthritis B shoulders and knees, occasional distal LE edema, hyperlipidemia, TAH

Medications: atenolol, lasix, ramipril, simvastatin, baby aspirin

Social: Patient is a widow, lives alone in a condo on the first floor of a multistory building, drives, is independent in gait without an assistive device, and eats meals out frequently. Two daughters live several hundred miles away. Plays cards several times a week, and swims, weather permitting. At this time, is unable to participate in these activities.

Patient Client Goals: "Get rid of shoulder pain so she can move her shoulder again and take care of herself," as she is having difficulty dressing herself, with personal hygiene, and sleeping, as she awakens every time she turns onto the RUE.

Precautions: Cardiac; s/p CABG, HTN

Prognosis and Rehab Potential: Good for goals and to return to pre-bursitis functional status

IV. CERTIFICATION AND RECERTIFICATION INCLUDING PLAN OF TREATMENT (PLAN OF CARE)

Depending on the payer source, initial certification of the POC, may be a physician or NPP. In the case of self referral the POC is internal to the provider, but may be requested by a payer. The following POC content information:

1. The plan of treatment must contain the diagnosis (referring medical diagnosis and the established PT diagnosis or PT problem established by the PT and preferably functionally oriented) type (interventions stated in CPT or HCPCS verbiage), amount (parameters), frequency (× per day, week, etc.), and duration of services (total length of time for episode of care or length of stay [LOS]) to be performed and the anticipated rehabilitation goals, emphasizing function that can be achieved in a reasonable time (preferably 30 days or less, unless acute co-morbidities or devastating condition such as acute CVA or multiple trauma).

2. Indicate services are or were required because the patient needed skilled rehabilitation services (for an acute condition or recent exacerbation resulting in functional decline from a chronic condition, or an improvement in condition or cognition allowing participation in PT not previously possible).

3. Be sufficiently detailed to permit an independent evaluation of the patient's specific need for the indicated skilled PT services and of the likelihood that he/

she will derive meaningful benefit from them (goals must be significant from a functional perspective).

4. Indicate the services are or were reasonable and necessary to the treatment of the patient's condition and not harmful (identifying all precautions and any contraindications).

5. Be reviewed by the physician at least once every 30 days or initial 60 days for a CORF. Following the review, the physician must certify that the plan of treatment is being followed and that the patient is making progress in attaining the established rehabilitation goals (established by the PT in conjunction with the physician). When the patient has reached a point where no further progress is being made toward one or more of the goals, Medicare coverage ends for that aspect of the plan of treatment.

6. Since the certification is closely associated with the plan of treatment, the same physician who establishes or reviews the plan must certify the necessity for the services. Obtain the certification at the time the plan of treatment is established or as soon thereafter as possible.

7. Obtain the recertification at the time the plan of treatment is reviewed since the same interval (at least once every 30 or 60 days depending on outpatient setting) is required for the review of the plan. Recertifications are signed by the physician who reviews the plan of treatment and has examined the patient/client in the recertification period. The PT may choose the form and manner of obtaining timely recertification, i.e., electronic, mail, and fax.

> **Author's Note:** Sending recertifications out a few days prior to the due date with a note of explanation and a return addressed envelope with an arrow "sticky" indicating where the signature goes, or faxing and then sending it out to be signed, may prevent undue delay.

Any changes to this plan must be made in writing and must be signed by the physician and therapist. Changes to the plan may also be made pursuant to oral orders given by the attending physician to a qualified physical therapist.

Changes to such plans may also be made pursuant to verbal/oral orders, telephone orders, email, fax or electronic orders by the physical therapist to another qualified physical therapist, or by the therapist to a registered professional nurse on staff. Such changes must be immediately recorded in the patient's record, preferably by the individual who received them and must be signed by the individual receiving the orders. While the physician may change a plan of treatment established by the therapist providing such services, the therapist may or may not alter a plan of treatment established by a physician unless the PT established plan is expressly signed off on by the physician. Each facility should have a policy on how to obtain an original signature on orders or referrals taken verbally, fax or other means if not in writing by the physician.

> **Author's Note:** The patient's plan normally need not be forwarded with the claim, but is retained in the provider's file. The provider must certify on the billing form that the plan is on file. The plan and other documentation must be submitted upon request.

Make sure the plan is established or reduced to writing either by the person who established the plan or by the PT when the PT makes a written record of that person's verbal/oral, electronic, email or faxed orders, before treatment begins. The plan must be promptly signed by the ordering physician, and therapist, and incorporated into the patient's clinical record.

A. Types of Entries Beyond the Initial Exam/Evaluation

APTA: Continuum of Care. Daily Note/Treatment Note (format of choice)

For daily treatment notes or progress notes:

- Title of entry if not provided on form e.g. PT treatment note, PT progress note
- Date
- Patient's legal name: first and last
- Number of units for each intervention or time

> **Author's Note:** Most timed codes with the exception of Medicare which is 8–22 minutes, are in 15 minute intervals.

- Where treatment rendered and how patient arrived (if it is not standard for all patients)
- Specific interventions where applied, i.e., lower extremity, with parameters including patient position
- Equipment issued, if any
- Response to intervention at that visit (+ or –)
- Instructions given/communication and if patient was accompanied and who it was.
- Patient/client statement of response to treatment for that session
- Statement regarding plan for next visit (in SOAP note of progress note)
- Authentication (signature of PT or PTA)

Note: Medicare: Treatment or Encounter Notes

The purpose of the encounter note is not to document medical necessity, but to create a record of all encounters and skilled interventions. Tips to keep in mind with encounter notes are as follows:

- Documentation is required for every treatment day, and every therapy service.
- The encounter note must record the name of the treatment, intervention or activity provided.
- Total treatment time must be documented.
- The signature of the professional delivering the service must be included.

If the entry is a progress note (narrative or SOAP format), the following is also needed:

- Brief statement of overall functional progress, not necessarily addressing all goals (as in progress reports) In a SOAP format, this would be the "A" or assessment/ analysis section.
- Additions/deletions of treatments

Medicare: progress notes.

The Progress Report provides justification for the medical necessity of treatment. For Medicare payment purposes, information required in Progress Reports should be provided at least once every 10 treatment days, or once during the treatment interval of 1-month or 30-calendar days, whichever is less. Objective measures of progress should be included when available. A treatment note justifies the billing for each treatment day. It may also (at the clinician's option) include information required for the Progress Report. Note: Documentation requirements apply to all outpatient therapy services regardless of therapy caps.

If the Treatment Notes completed during the Progress Report period have sufficient information to fulfill the requirements of the Progress Report, information does not have to be re-written into a Progress Report at the end of the reporting period. www.hhs.gov[4]

- Date of the beginning of the treatment interval
- Date the report was written

- Signature of the qualified professional
- Objective reports of the patient's progress
- Objective measurements of changes in status relative to current goals
- Plans for continuing treatment
- Changes to long and short-term treatment goals (time defined)

> **Author's Note:** A progress note would include the same information as a treatment note in addition to a statement of progress relative to the initial or interim goals established. It is usually longer as it relates to a longer period of time, i.e., a week, multiple weeks.

APTA Continuum of Care, Forms/Checklists.

Forms include space for consecutive days/sessions, modalities/interventions requiring a check or initials to indicate care. As necessary, forms should be supplemented by brief daily notes to avoid appearing unskilled. In some settings allowed weekly entries by regulation, checklists may be used on daily basis. However, if anything unexpected happens, such as issuance of equipment, communication with family, or other unplanned event, a supplemental daily note is written for that day. Authentication is required for all changes in care and supplemental or supporting entries.

APTA Reexamination, Progress Notes/Reports.

Periodic entries—weekly, biweekly, or monthly—are compiled based on the daily entries. According to Baeten, Moran, and Phillippi, "The focus of the progress report is on the problems identified in the initial evaluation or any new problems that have developed since the last formal reevaluation [*or initial examination/evaluation*]. Documentation describing the skilled intervention provided, complicating factors that may have affected the duration of skilled care, and comparative data."[2]

Significant progress toward functional goals, modification of goals, and completion of goals should be evident. If progress is not demonstrated, justification of this lack of progress as well as justification for continued care with modified goals and plans as indicated must be included. Authentication of any change in care is required.

> **Author's Note:** Refer to Initial Examination/Evaluation for content categories. For Medicare beneficiaries, recertification for care and payment is based on 30-day (or 60 as applicable) progress reports. However, unless there has been devastating injury or neurological problem (i.e., stroke) most episodes of care should average 30 days. Treatment beyond 30 days may result in higher possibility of review of care by the carrier.

Discharge Summary: APTA Summation of Episode of Care, Discharge Report/Discharge Evaluation.

At the end of the episode of care, patient status, summarized from initial examination/evaluation through the final visit, is required. This summary should address all initial or modified goals and progress or achievement of them. If goals were not achieved, indicate why.

The summation should also include a description of interventions rendered during care, including total number of sessions and the duration (dates) and frequency of the sessions. If specific tests and measures were administered at the initial visit, they should be repeated to show objective change and improvement.

The discharge report should also include the patient's discharge disposition, plan for next level of care with recommendations as applicable (including home with home instructions), and any other instructions or training, equipment dispensed, and safety concerns. Authentication is required.

Author's Note: In circumstances where timely discharge reports are not completed, a summary may be the best way to close out a record, based on the information included in the daily entries. If a patient self-terminates care, a discharge summary indicating such with a summary of care determined by the daily entries should be completed when it has been established that the patient is not returning. A discharge report or evaluation that includes analysis and plans for further care requires completion by a PT. According to the APTA, all summations of care should be completed by the PT. Medicare requires that a PT see a Medicare patient pre-discharge and complete the discharge summary.

When doing internal utilization review, peer review, or quality assessment, the evaluation and discharge should contain the information necessary to determine if the services were skilled, appropriate, effective, and efficient. If the format is similar, it is easier for the reader to make a determination. In facilities that use outcome assessment measures such as the FIM (Functional Independence Measure) used in rehabilitation hospitals or units or FOTO (Focus on Therapeutic Outcomes), used in outpatient, values at initial examination and final reexamination should be included. The same concept is applicable to any standardized measure used during initial examination or throughout care. Participation in outcome systems allows a facility or organization to benchmark their care against other facilities for quality and to easily identify patient progress.

V. RECERTIFICATION DOCUMENTATION: MEDICARE SPECIFIC BUT APLLICABLE TO ALL

When outpatient physical therapy services are continued under the same plan of treatment for a period of time, the physician must recertify at intervals of at least once every 30 days that there is a continuing need for such services and estimate how long services are needed. Obtain the recertification at the time the plan of treatment is reviewed since the same interval (at least once every 30 days) is required for the review of the plan. The physician who reviews the plan of treatment signs the recertifications. The form of the recertification and the manner of obtaining timely recertification is the responsibility of the individual clinic.

Author's Note: For Certified Outpatient Rehabilitation Facilities (CORFs), the requirement for recertification is every 60 days for the initial 60. It is then every 30 days. All other outpatient physical therapy, skilled nursing, and home health requires 30 days. The requirements for outpatient coverage by Medicare are essentially the same for all settings. For non-Medicare, the Medicare guidelines can be applied by provider choice.

A. Coverage and Limitations

Medicare Guidelines, Section 2206.2 B: Method and Disposition of Certifications. There is no requirement that the certification or recertification be entered on any specific form or handled in any specific way as long as you can determine, where necessary, that the certification and recertification requirements are met. The certification by the physician is retained by the clinic, and the clinic certifies on the billing form that the requisite certifications and recertifications have been made by the physician and are on file in the clinic when it forwards the request for payment to you.

Medicare Guidelines, Section 2206.2 C: Delayed Certification. The clinic must obtain certifications and recertifications as promptly as possible. Payment is not made unless the necessary certifications are secured. In addition to complying with the usual content requirements, delayed certifications and recertifications are to include an explanation for the delay and any other evidence the clinic considers necessary in the case. The format of delayed certifications and recertifications and the method by which they are obtained is left to the clinic.

Medicare guidelines further state that it is expected that therapy services be performed as indicated by current medical literature and/or standards of practice. When services are performed in excess of established parameters, they may be subject to review for medical necessity. This concept should guide the therapist in all entries and treatments.

VI. DOCUMENTATION OF CONTINUATION OF CARE

According to the Medicare regulations, "The office/progress note must contain necessary and sufficient information, which indicates the services were actually provided and were reasonable and necessary to treat the patient's condition." The categories described in the APTA guidelines include "documentation of intervention or services provided and current patient/client status, and documentation of reexamination."[1] It is the therapist's or organization's responsibility to determine the format in which the information should be included.

The APTA guidelines do not describe types of entries, but rather content. However, as PTs and PTAs tend to describe types of entries, following are descriptions of entry types, but not descriptions of format. Again, that is the decision of the therapist.

A. Medicare

271.1. Physical Therapy Services: Conditions of Coverage. To be covered, physical therapy services must relate directly and specifically to the plan of treatment described in §270.3, and be reasonable and necessary to the treatment of the individual's illness or injury. Services related to activities for the general well being and welfare of patients (i.e., general exercises to promote overall fitness and flexibility and activities to provide diversion or general motivation) do not constitute physical therapy services for Medicare purposes.

> **Author's Note:** According to the *Guide to Physical Therapist Practice* there are five elements of patient care: Examination, Evaluation, Diagnosis, Prognosis, and Intervention.

Evaluation. The evaluation is an integral component of physical therapy services. It is the clinical judgments of the PT based on the synthesis of data/information/ findings to establish the diagnosis, prognosis, and POC. It establishes the baseline data (including identified functional problems and related impairments that can be impacted by skilled PT intervention) necessary for assessing expected rehabilitation potential, setting realistic (functionally oriented) goals, and measuring progress. The evaluation of the patient's condition must form the basis for the physical therapy treatment goals. A physical therapy initial evaluation (excluding routine screening) is covered when it is reasonable and necessary for the qualified physical therapist to determine if there is an expectation that either restorative or maintenance services are appropriate for the patient's condition. When a patient exhibits a demonstrable change in physical functional ability, reevaluations are covered to reestablish appropriate treatment goals (Reevaluations are also covered for ongoing assessment of the patient's rehabilitation needs). Initial evaluations or reevaluations that are determined reasonable and necessary are covered even though the expectations are not realized or when the evaluation determines that skilled rehabilitation is not needed.

> **Author's Note:** Evaluations only, without justification for intervention may not be reimbursed.

Reasonable and necessary. In order for services to be considered reasonable and necessary, the services must be considered under accepted standards of medical practice to be a specific and effective treatment for the patient's condition.

The services must be of such a level of complexity and sophistication or the condition of the patient must be such that the services required can be safely and effectively performed only by or under the supervision of a qualified physical therapist. Services that do not require the performance or supervision of a physical therapist are not considered reasonable or necessary physical therapy services even if they are performed or supervised by a physical therapist.

There must be an expectation that the condition will improve significantly in a reasonable (and generally predictable) period of time based on the assessment made by the physician of the patient's restoration potential after any needed consultation with the qualified physical therapist. Alternatively, the services must be necessary to establish a safe and effective maintenance program required in connection with a specific disease state. The amount, frequency, and duration of the services must be reasonable.

> **Author's Note:** When the intermediary determines the services furnished were of a type that could have been safely or effectively performed only by or under the supervision of a qualified physical therapist, it presumes that such services were properly supervised. However, this assumption may be rebutted. If, in the course of processing claims, the intermediary finds that physical therapy services are not being furnished under proper supervision, the intermediary denies the claim and brings this matter to the attention of the Division of Health Standards and Quality of the CMS RO.
>
> Medicare will not reimburse for PT student-rendered care. However, the student may assist the PT if the PT is directly supervising and not engaged in treating other patients at the same time.
>
> Claims for physical therapy services denied because the services are not considered reasonable and necessary are excluded from coverage and are thus subject to consideration under the waiver of liability provision in §1879 of the Act.

B. Types of Continuing Care

Restorative Therapy. To constitute physical therapy, a service must be reasonable and necessary to the treatment of the individual's illness. If an individual's expected restoration potential is insignificant in relation to the extent and duration of physical therapy services required to achieve such potential, the services are not considered reasonable and necessary. In addition, there must be an expectation that the patient's condition will improve significantly in a reasonable (and generally predictable) period of time. If at any point in the treatment of an illness it is determined that the expectations will not materialize, the services are no longer considered reasonable and necessary and are excluded from coverage.

Maintenance Program. The repetitive services required to maintain function generally do not involve complex and sophisticated physical therapy procedures and do not require the judgment and skill of a qualified physical therapist for safety and effectiveness. However, in certain instances, the specialized knowledge and judgment of a qualified physical therapist may be required to establish a maintenance program. For example, a patient with Parkinson's disease who has not been under a restorative physical therapy program may require the services of a physical therapist to determine the most effective type of exercise to maintain the patient's present functional level.

In such situations, the following services constitute physical therapy:

• The initial evaluation of the patient's needs

• The design by the qualified physical therapist of a maintenance program appropriate to the capacity and tolerance of the patient and the treatment objectives of the physician

- The instruction of the patient or supportive personnel, i.e., aides, nursing personnel or family members, if furnished on an outpatient basis, in carrying out the program; and reevaluations as required

If a patient has been under a restorative physical therapy program, the physical therapist regularly reevaluates the condition and adjusts the exercise program. The physical therapist should have already designed the required maintenance program and instructed the patient, supportive personnel, or family members, if the services have been furnished on an outpatient basis, in implementing the program before it is determined that no further restoration is possible. Therefore, when the therapist does not establish a maintenance program until after the restorative physical therapy program has been completed, no further physical therapy services are reasonable and necessary. Therefore, establishing such a program is not reasonable and necessary to the treatment of the patient's condition and is not covered.

VII. 271.2 APPLICATION OF GUIDELINES (FROM CMS MEDICARE CARRIERS MANUAL)

Coding should generally apply to "more common modalities in which the reasonableness and necessity of physical therapy services is a significant issue."

Medicare Considerations

Hot Pack, Hydrocollator, Infra-Red Treatments, Paraffin Baths, and Whirlpool Baths. Heat treatments of this type and whirlpool baths do not ordinarily require the skills of a qualified physical therapist. However, in a particular case, the skills, knowledge, and judgment of a qualified physical therapist might be required in such treatments or baths, e.g., when the patient's condition is complicated by circulatory deficiency, areas of desensitization, open wounds, or other complications. Also, if such treatments are given prior to but as an integral part of a skilled physical therapy procedure, they are part of the physical therapy service and must be documented.

> **Author's Note:** However, hot pack treatments and other modalities may be bundled for payment (see Chapter 5) and not be individually reimbursed.

Gait Training. Gait evaluation and training furnished to a patient whose ability to walk has been impaired by neuromuscular, musculoskeletal, cardiopulmonary, integumentary, or medical pathology abnormality requires the skills of a qualified physical therapist. However, if gait evaluation and training cannot reasonably be expected to significantly improve the patient's ability to walk, such services are not considered reasonable and necessary. Repetitious exercises to improve gait or maintain strength and endurance and assisted walking are appropriately provided by supportive personnel (i.e., aides or nursing personnel) and do not require the skills of a qualified physical therapist.

It is necessary to include skilled terminology when evaluating gait, describing dependence versus independence, all gait deviations, and need for assistive devices or adaptive equipment.

Ultrasound, Shortwave Diathermy (SWD). These modalities must always be performed by or under the supervision of a qualified physical therapist. Therefore, such treatments constitute physical therapy.

> **Author's Note:** Ultrasound requires constant attendance from a coding perspective, but SWD does not. Microwave is no longer covered by Medicare.

Range of Motion Tests. Only the qualified physical therapist may perform range of motion tests, and such tests constitute physical therapy.

> **Author's Note:** Objective measurements must be provided indicating available active or passive ROM measured over normal ranges for the joint. They should be stated in fractions, and ultimately relate to lack of function as the reason for care.

Therapeutic Procedures. Therapeutic exercises that must be performed by or under the supervision of the qualified physical therapist because of either the type of exercise employed or the condition of the patient constitute physical therapy.

Range of motion exercises require the skills of a qualified physical therapist only if:

1. They are part of the active treatment of a specific disease which has resulted in a loss or restriction of mobility (as evidenced by physical therapy notes showing the degree of motion lost and the degree to be restored).

2. Such exercises, either because of their nature or the condition of the patient, may only be performed safely and effectively by or under the supervision of a qualified physical therapist.

Generally, range of motion exercises that are not related to the restoration of a specific loss of function but rather are related to the maintenance of function (see §271.1D2) do not require the skills of a qualified physical therapist.

The following conditions must be met: The services must be considered under accepted standards of practice to be a specific and effective treatment for the patient's condition.

Co-Treatment

503.3 Occupational Therapy Availability. There may be instances where two or more disciplines are providing therapy services to the same patient. There may also be occasions where these services are duplicative. The MAC uses the documentation to determine if duplication exists. The following are some examples where there is not a duplication of services:

Transfers. Physical therapy instructs the patient in transfers to ascertain the level of safety with the techniques. Occupational therapy instructs and utilizes transfers as they relate to the performance of daily living skills, e.g., transfer from wheelchair to bathtub for bathing.

Pulmonary. Physical therapy teaches the patient an adapted breathing program. Occupational therapy carries the breathing retraining program into activities of daily living training.

Hip Fractures/Arthroplasties. Physical therapy instructs the patient in hip precautions and gait training. Occupational therapy carries out and reinforces the precautions when training the patient in activities of daily living, e.g., lower extremity dressing, toileting, and bathing.

CVA. Physical therapy utilizes upper extremity neurodevelopmental treatment (NDT) techniques to assist the patient in positioning the upper extremities on a walker and in gait training. Occupational therapy utilizes upper extremity NDT techniques to increase the functional use of upper extremities for dressing, bathing, grooming, and so on.

As with all rehabilitation services, your documentation must indicate a reasonable expectation that the patient will make material improvement within a reasonable period of time.

Professional Services. Services are sometimes performed by speech–language pathologists, occupational therapists, and physical therapists in concert with other health professionals. Services may be documented as performed by a team with each member performing unique roles. Do not document duplicate services. Clearly delineate roles. Services may include, but are not limited to the following example. (See example 11)

■ Example 11

One professional assisting with positioning, adaptive self-help devices, inhibiting abnormal oromotor and/or postural reflexes while another professional is addressing specific exercises to improve oromotor control, determining appropriate food consistency form, assisting the patient in difficulty with muscular movements necessary to close the buccal cavity or shape food in the mouth in preparation for swallowing. Another professional might address a different role, such as increasing muscle strength, sitting balance, and head control.

Relate the documentation to either loss of function or potential for change. As with other conditions/disorders, the reasonableness and necessity of services must be evident in your documentation.

Include:

- changes in condition or functional status;
- history and outcome of previous treatment for the same condition; or
- any other information that would justify the start of care.

Even where a patient's full or partial recovery is not possible, a skilled service still could be needed to prevent deterioration or to maintain current capabilities.

When rehabilitation services are the primary services, the key issue is whether the skills of a therapist are needed. The deciding factor is not the patient's potential for recovery, but whether the services needed require the skills of a therapist or whether they can be carried out by non-skilled personnel (see §214.3.A).

A service that is ordinarily considered non-skilled could be considered a skilled service in cases in which, because of special medical complications, skilled nursing or skilled rehabilitation personnel are required to perform or supervise it or to observe the patient. In these cases, the complications and special services involved must be documented by physicians' orders and nursing or therapy notes.

The existence of a plaster cast on an extremity generally does not indicate a need for skilled care. However, a patient with a preexisting acute skin problem, preexisting peripheral vascular disease, or a need for special traction of the injured extremity might need skilled nursing or skilled rehabilitation personnel to observe for complications or to adjust traction.

Whirlpool baths do not ordinarily require the skills of a qualified physical therapist. However, the skills, knowledge, and judgment of a qualified physical therapist might be required where the patient's condition is complicated by circulatory deficiency, areas of desensitization, or open wounds.

The importance of a particular service to an individual patient, or the frequency with which it must be performed, does not, by itself, make it a skilled service.

Author's Note: If there are complicating co-morbidities or the potential for decline, skilled services may be indicated on an inpatient, home health, or outpatient basis (see Examples 12-16).

Example 12

A primary need of a non-ambulatory patient may be frequent changes of position in order to avoid development of decubitus ulcers. However, since such changing of position does not ordinarily require skilled nursing or skilled rehabilitation personnel, it would not constitute a skilled service, even though such services are obviously necessary. However, if instruction to caretakers is needed for positioning and transfer training, the short-term skilled instruction, with appropriate documentation should be covered.

Example 13

A patient has undergone peripheral vascular disease treatment including revascularization procedures (bypass) with open or necrotic areas of skin on the involved extremity. Skilled observation and monitoring of the vascular supply of the legs is required, especially during functional training activity.

Example 14

A patient has undergone hip surgery and has been transferred to an SNF. Skilled observation and monitoring of the patient for possible adverse reaction to the operative procedure, development of phlebitis, skin breakdown, or need for the administration of subcutaneous heparin, is both reasonable and necessary, as well as rehabilitation services to regain function.

Example 15

A patient has been hospitalized following a heart attack and, following treatment but before mobilization, is transferred to the SNF. Because it is unknown whether exertion will exacerbate the heart disease, skilled observation is reasonable and necessary as skilled mobilization and rehabilitation is initiated, until the patient's treatment regimen is essentially stabilized.

Example 16

A frail 85-year-old man was hospitalized for pneumonia. The infection was resolved, but the patient, who had previously maintained adequate nutrition, will not eat or eats poorly. The patient is transferred to an SNF for monitoring of fluid and nutrient intake, assessment of the need for tube feeding and forced feeding if required. Observation and monitoring by skilled nursing personnel of the patient's oral intake is required to prevent dehydration. In order to remobilize the patient, skilled rehabilitation services to regain function are needed.

If a patient was admitted for skilled observation but did not develop a further acute episode or complication, the skilled observation services still are covered so long as there is a reasonable probability for such a complication or further acute episode. "Reasonable probability" means that a potential complication or further acute episode was a likely possibility.

VIII. TEACHING AND TRAINING ACTIVITIES

Teaching and training activities that require skilled nursing or skilled rehabilitation personnel to teach a patient how to manage his treatment regimen would constitute skilled services. Some examples are: gait training and teaching of prosthesis care for a patient who has had a recent leg amputation; teaching patients the use and care of braces, splints, and orthotics, and any associated skin care; and teaching patients the proper care of any specialized dressings or skin treatments.

According to the SNF Carriers Manual, available at www.cms.gov, the following are relevant to physical therapy. Please note that they are not distinctly different than in any other setting, and are therefore, included. They are also applicable for patients of any age and payer source.

A. Direct Skilled Rehabilitation Services to Patients

Skilled Physical Therapy.

General. Skilled physical therapy services must meet all of the following conditions:

- The services must be directly and specifically related to an active written treatment plan designed by the physician after any needed consultation with a qualified physical therapist.

- The services must be of a level of complexity and sophistication, or the condition of the patient must be of a nature that requires the judgment, knowledge, and skills of a qualified physical therapist.

- The services must be provided with the expectation, based on the assessment made by the physician of the patient's restoration potential, that the condition of the patient will improve materially in a reasonable and generally predictable period of time, or the services must be necessary for the establishment of a safe and effective maintenance program.

- The services must be considered under accepted standards of medical practice to be specific and effective treatment for the patient's condition.

- The services must be reasonable and necessary for the treatment of the patient's condition; this includes the requirement that the amount, frequency, and duration of the services must be reasonable (see Example 17 and 18).

■ Example 17

An 80-year-old, previously ambulatory, post-surgical patient has been bedbound for one week and, as a result, has developed muscle atrophy, orthostatic hypotension, joint stiffness, and lower extremity edema. To the extent that the patient requires a brief period of daily skilled physical therapy services to restore lost functions, these services are reasonable and necessary.

Author's Note: Based on progress, this patient would probably qualify for continued services on a home health and possibly on an outpatient basis to return to independence.

■ Example 18

A patient with congestive heart failure also has diabetes and previously had both legs amputated above the knees. Consequently, the patient does not have a reasonable potential to achieve ambulation, but still requires daily skilled physical therapy to learn bed mobility and transferring skills, as well as functional activities at the wheelchair level.

Author's Note: If the patient has a reasonable potential for achieving those functions in a reasonable period of time in view of the patient's total condition, the physical therapy services are reasonable and necessary.

If the expected results are insignificant in relation to the extent and duration of physical therapy services required to achieve those results, the physical therapy would not be reasonable and necessary, and thus would not be covered under skilled physical therapy services.

Author's Note: The following are also excerpted from the Carrier Manual at www.cms.gov. They are found in the SNF guidelines, but are consistent for coverage for Medicare beneficiaries in other settings as well.

Application of guidelines. Some of the more common physical therapy modalities and procedures are:

a. Assessment (examination)
   The skills of a physical therapist are required for the ongoing assessment of a patient's rehabilitation needs and potential. Skilled rehabilitation services concurrent with the management of a patient's care plan include tests and measurements of range of motion, strength, balance, coordination, endurance, and functional ability.

b. Therapeutic procedures
   Therapeutic exercises that must be performed by or under the supervision of the qualified physical therapist, due either to the type of exercise employed or to the condition of the patient, constitute skilled physical therapy.

c. Gait training
   Gait evaluation and training furnished to a patient whose ability to walk has been impaired by neurological, muscular, or skeletal abnormality require the skills of a qualified physical therapist and constitute skilled physical therapy if they reasonably can be expected to improve significantly the patient's ability to walk.

   Repetitious exercises to improve gait or to maintain strength, endurance, and assistive walking are appropriately provided by supportive personnel, i.e., aides or nursing personnel, and do not require the skills of a physical therapist. Thus, such services are not skilled physical therapy.

d. Range of motion
   Only the qualified physical therapist may perform range of motion tests and, therefore, such tests are skilled physical therapy. Range of motion exercises constitute skilled physical therapy only if they are part of active treatment for a specific disease state which has resulted in a loss or restriction of mobility (as evidenced by physical therapy notes showing the degree of motion lost and the degree to be restored).

   Range of motion exercises, which are not related to the restoration of a specific loss of function may often be provided safely by supportive personnel, such as aides or nursing personnel, and may not require the skills of a physical therapist. Passive exercises to maintain range of motion in paralyzed extremities that can be carried out by aides or nursing personnel would not be considered skilled care.

e. Maintenance therapy
   The repetitive services required to maintain function sometimes involve the use of complex and sophisticated therapy procedures and, consequently, the judgment and skill of a physical therapist might be required for the safe and effective rendition of such services (see §214.1.B). The specialized knowledge and judgment of a qualified physical therapist may be required to establish a maintenance program intended to prevent or minimize deterioration caused by a medical condition, if the program is to be safely carried out and the treatment

aims of the physician are to be achieved. Establishing such a program is a skilled service (see Example 19).

> ### ■ Example 19
>
> An individual with Parkinson's Disease who has not been under a restorative physical therapy program may require the services of a physical therapist to determine what type of exercises are required for the maintenance of his present level of function. The initial evaluation of the patient's needs, the designing of a maintenance program which is appropriate to the capacity and tolerance of the patient and the treatment objectives of the physician, the instruction of the patient or supportive personnel (i.e., aides or nursing personnel) in the carrying out of the program, and such infrequent reevaluations as may be required, would constitute skilled physical therapy.
>
> While a patient is under a restorative physical therapy program, the physical therapist should regularly reevaluate his condition and adjust any exercise program the patient is expected to carry out alone or with the aid of supportive personnel to maintain the function being restored. Consequently, by the time it is determined that no further restoration is possible (i.e., by the end of the last restorative session), the physical therapist will have already designed the maintenance program required and instructed the patient or supportive personnel in the carrying out of the program.

f. Ultrasound, shortwave, and microwave diathermy treatments
These modalities must always be performed by or under the supervision of a qualified physical therapist and are skilled physical therapy.

g. Hot packs, infra-red treatments, paraffin baths, and whirlpool baths
Heat treatments and baths of this type ordinarily do not require the skills of a qualified physical therapist. However, the skills, knowledge, and judgment of a qualified physical therapist might be required in the giving of such treatments or baths in a particular case, i.e., where the patient's condition is complicated by circulatory deficiency, areas of desensitization, open wounds, fractures, or other complications.

IX. SUMMARY

According to the APTA and AHIMA, medical records should be maintained for all patient/client care, regardless of the payer source, including self-pay or pro bono. In some states, record keeping is mandated by statute. All therapy professionals must be aware of their practice act and accompanying rule requirements as well as other applicable state and federal regulations. The CMS mandates specific documentation requirements for all Medicare beneficiaries in all venues. The CMS requirements for all settings include the same elements as the APTA Guide to Documentation. All third-party payers require documentation that accurately reflects the PT care rendered and justifies medical necessity, although they may not dictate format or content, even though many are now mandating provider compliance to the Medicare Correct Coding Initiative (CCI Edits). The guide categories are Initial Examination and Evaluation/ Consultation, Documentation of Continuation of Care, and Documentation of Summation of Episode of Care. The Medicare requirements fit into these categories. Adherence to the APTA and CMS/Medicare guidelines will assist in producing effective documentation that will withstand scrutiny by any reader.

All payers of physical therapy require that billing be completed on specific forms. However, most payers use a standard CMS 1500 form (some use UB forms) that includes only demographic information, with diagnosis codes, and CPT codes relating to the diagnosis, with the date(s) of service. If records are requested to support the claims, copies of all patient/client records for the dates of treatment are required in whatever format the provider PT uses at their facility. The CMS, however, for Medicare beneficiaries, requires the CMS 1500 form (see Appendix C) be used for most billing with the 700 series (see Appendix B) forms or facsimiles for the initial evaluation, monthly progress and discharge. For Medicare billing, there are specific documentation requirements that must be followed. Reimbursement can be denied for lack of compliance to the documentation regulations by any payer. The billing forms should also include the appropriate modifiers as needed, e.g., the -59 or KX. Medicare may not allow appeal if a modifier is missing from the initial billing.

Regardless of the format for billing, attention must be paid to consistent terminology and the matching of all elements; billing dates, treatment dates and times, diagnostic codes (IDC-9), procedural codes (CPT), identified patient problems, established goals, interventions, initial examination results, all visit entries, and discharge information. All entries must indicate the necessity for skilled PT. If progress plateaus or stops at any point in the care, consideration must be made to discharge the patient. All care must be reasonable and necessary. The documentation content is the only supporting evidence of medical necessity and the justification of reasonable and necessary care.

REFERENCES

1. Baeten AM, Moran ML, Phillippi LM. *Documenting Physical Therapy: The Reviewer Perspective*. Wo burn, Butterworth-Heinemann, 1999, 215 pp.

2. *Guide to Physical Therapist Practice*, 2nd ed. American Physical Therapy Association, 2003.

3. ICF: International Classification of Functioning, Disability and Health. World Health Organization, Geneva, 2001.

4. HHS.gov. Centers for Medicare and Medicaid http://questions.cms.hhs.gov/app/answers/detail/a_id/7100

CHAPTER 4 REVIEW QUESTIONS

1. What are the basic requirements for Medicare documentation?

2. Identify ten content elements required in the initial examination and evaluation.

3. Provide five categories of systems review with two examples of content for each.

4. What is the relationship between the patient/client's prior level of function and physical therapy?

5. What are the basic content requirements for a plan of care?

6. From a Medicare perspective, what is recertification and what is the relationship to continuing physical therapy?

7. What does the APTA describe as the Continuum of Care? Provide examples.

8. What is authentication and describe its relationship to documentation?

9. What is the APTA recommended frequency of documentation?

10. What is a problem summary?

11. What are the advantages of using pre-made forms for documentation and billing purposes?

12. Provide four examples of terms that should be avoided in documentation.

13. Can Medicare be billed by the PT for restorative services? Defend your answer.

14. In order for PT services to be considered reasonable and necessary, what criteria have to be met?

15. What is co-treatment? Can more than one service bill for co-treatments? Explain your answer.

16. Compare and contrast certification and recertification in the Medicare context.

17. Under what circumstances is gait training skilled versus unskilled?

18. What constitutes an evaluation?

19. What is the difference between a CMS 1500 form and a CMS 700 form?

20. What are duplicate services? Provide examples of a procedure that might be considered duplicative unless the documentation indicates otherwise.

5 Coding and Documentation

Correct coding on the medical/client record is required for all reimbursement. Current Procedural Terminology (CPT) codes, developed and owned by the American Medical Association (AMA), are numeric codes for medical procedures. They are required for billing of all medical services including physical therapy. As of 2010, the most recent CPT-4 edition contains over 10,000 codes. The Centers for Medicare & Medicaid Services (CMS) Healthcare Common Procedure Coding System (HCPCS), Levels I and II, identify specific codes that may be used for billing services delivered to Medicare beneficiaries. Level I codes are most similar to the CPT codes; Level II codes are not found in the CPT codes. As reimbursement is integrally linked to documentation, the knowledge and inclusion of CPT code verbiage when entering into the medical record is key to third party payers, internal organization billing and coding personnel for correct coding and billing for services.

Also required for documentation are International Classification of Disease codes (ICD-CM, which will be referred to as ICD in this text), which are numeric codes for diseases and pathologies, medical procedures including surgeries, and functionally oriented deficits or conditions. As of fall 2002, ICD-9 (9th revision, Clinical Modifications, 1993, with annual updates in the fall of each calendar year) code versions are in use for physical medicine and physical therapy procedures. Although the ICD-10 was published in 2001, there is now an ICD-11 version. As of the middle of 2010 the transition to ICD-10 use has not been made in the United States. CMS is replacing ICD-9 with ICD-10 for diagnosis and procedural coding by 2013. The ICD codes were developed by the World Health Organization (WHO) as a way to standardize classification of diseases worldwide (see a sample of ICD-9 codes in Appendix D).[1]

As the CPT codes that describe physical therapy–related procedures have historically been categorized as physical medicine codes, it has been difficult for physical therapists to distinguish themselves from others licensed to administer some of the same procedures. Although recent changes have resulted in evaluation and reevaluation codes unique to physical therapy, it remains incumbent on the physical therapist to prove medical necessity of the service based on consistent matching of CPT codes, ICD-9 codes, and appropriate documentation of what classifies the intervention as skilled.

Another category of code the physical therapist must be familiar with is the Relative Value Resource Based Systems (RVRBS). The RVRBS is a standard system developed by the federal government that assigns a dollar value to medical treatments in order to standardize reimbursement to physicians, with slight adjustments for geographic area. The values are derived from the time and skill (work) required for administration, the related practice cost, and professional liability costs. RVRBS values have been established for reimbursement by the federal government for physical therapy (PT) services rendered by physical therapists in private practice (PTPP, formerly referred to as physical therapists in independent practice, PTIPs) for outpatients that are Medicare beneficiaries. However, the use of RVRBS is not limited to the Medicare system. RVRBS is used in some states for Medicaid, by managed care organizations (MCOs), and other payers. Medicare calculates the RVRBS payment for PT and other rehabilitation services using the following formula:

$$RVU \times GPCI = ARVU$$

where RVU is the relative value unit or component (work, practice, professional liability cost), GPCI is the geographic practice cost index, and ARVU is the adjusted relative value unit.

I. PRINCIPLES OF CODE USE

One of the challenges of including coding information as a component of documentation is the constant modification of the codes themselves. However, since correct coding is required in order to effect reimbursement, it cannot be ignored. By following the principles and knowing where to obtain the updated information, the physical therapist can ensure that the latest principles and guidelines are consistently applied. Depending on the facility, it may or may not be the PT's responsibility to identify the code numbers. However, in order for a third party such as a billing clerk to correctly code a record, the verbiage that precedes specific intervention components must be correct. Based on the size of the CPT and ICD-9-CM books, learning the verbiage may seem a daunting task. However, many facilities use the same categories for their patients/clients on a regular basis. Therefore, it is common for facilities to establish a list of frequently used CPT and ICD-9 codes or to include in electronic systems in drop down menus. Lists save time and ensures better consistency throughout facilities. They also eliminate errors if interpretation is left to another party. Most CPT codes with the exception of the evaluation and reevaluation codes are billed and documented in 15-minute units/increments. Refer to the 8–22 minutes as one unit for Medicare later in the chapter.

II. INDIVIDUAL CODES

A. New Codes/Correct Coding Initiatives

It is the PT's responsibility to keep up with the most current coding. Members of the American Physical Therapy Association (APTA) can refer to the APTA Web site for updates.[2]

CPT and HCPCS. The verbiage in the documentation should match the code that will be used in the billing. Always precede specific types of interventions identified colloquially with abbreviations, with the code terminology. The PT is responsible and should record and enter the specific codes for the patients they are treating.

> ### ■ Example 1
>
> Incorrect: CPT 97110: General strengthening, PNF
> *Correct*:   CPT 97110: Therapeutic procedure: isotonic strengthening, PNF
>
> Incorrect: CPT 97116: Ambulated patient with straight cane L hand
> *Correct*:   CPT 97116: Gait Training: straight cane in L hand

ICD-9. The therapist must always include the medical diagnosis established by the physician as the referral diagnosis. However, the PT's diagnosis or problem for which the therapy is being rendered must be established by the PT, since the physician's diagnosis is not always the same as the physical therapist's diagnosis. Regardless, all diagnoses must have verbiage that specifically matches an ICD-9 (or relevant version) code. When appropriate, the PT diagnosis should be functionally oriented and should establish the relevance between the treatment diagnosis, the interventions selected, and the goals established. Do not create "new" diagnoses and always refer to the ICD-9 book for guidance. The ICD code should be carried to at least four number places when available (see examples 2 and 3).

■ Example 2

Same:
Medical diagnosis: 727.71: tendinitis, Achilles
PT diagnosis: 727.71: tendinitis, Achilles
Note, however, that there should also be additional PT treatment diagnosis for gait deficits, motor performance deficits, that are consistent with findings on initial examination.

Different:
Medical diagnosis: 812.40: closed fracture of humerus, lower end, unspecified
PT diagnosis: 781.2: abnormality of gait
Referred to PT for gait training with quad cane, as can no longer use walker secondary to humerus fracture.

ICD-9 Diagnosis Order. List the code for the primary treatment diagnosis first, followed by the others. Comorbidities may help justify the need for skilled services.

Author's Note: The *Guide to Physical Therapist Practice* includes medical diagnoses and functional diagnoses commonly used in physical therapy. The ICD-9 code terms are listed in the practice patterns and Appendix D.

In summer of 2002, new rulings were established by CMS regarding coverage for individuals with 331.0, Alzheimer's and related disorders. It was recognized that individuals with these conditions have the potential to successfully complete and functionally benefit from a course of rehabilitation. However, the patient/client must be able to follow instructions: verbal, gestured, or a combination of the two, and demonstrate functional deficits that can benefit from physical therapy. As PTs do not "treat" Alzheimer's, it remains incumbent on the PT to justify the need for care based on functional deficits and prior level of function as in all patients/clients (i.e., 781.2 gait abnormality, 728.2 muscular wasting and disuse atrophy). The authors recommend that at least 2–3 PT diagnoses be included and that they are relevant to the deficits identified, the goals, and interventions.

III. MATCHING CODES

A. ICD-9 and CPT

Once the PT has established the appropriate treatment or PT diagnosis, it should be clear from the verbiage and the code number that they are related. The CMS 1500 form (see Appendix C) allows for services to be specified for each diagnosis.[3]

■ Example 3

Incorrect:

Medical diagnosis:	412 old myocardial infarction
PT diagnosis:	412 old myocardial infarction

Correct:

Medical diagnosis:	412 old myocardial infarction	
PT diagnosis:	781.2 gait abnormality, 780.79 overall body weakness and fatigue	
Treatment :	Gait training:	97116
	Therapeutic procedure:	97110

Correct:

Medical diagnosis:	457.0 Post-mastectomy lymphedema	
PT diagnosis:	457.0 Post-mastectomy lymphedema	
Treatment :	Manual therapy for drainage:	97140

Also correct:

Medical diagnosis:	344.0 quadriplegia	
PT diagnosis:	344.0 quadriplegia	
Treatment:	Therapeutic procedure:	97110
	Neuromuscular reeducation:	97112
	Therapeutic activities:	97530

IV. PROCEDURE SPECIFICITY

When selecting a code for a procedure, it is important to be as specific as possible. Select the code that best describes the intervention you are using, matching the code and documentation content (see Example 4).

■ Example 4

Incorrect:

Gait training: CPT 97116
Treatment: Balance and posture training

Correct:

Neuromuscular reeducation: CPT 97112
Treatment: Neuromuscular reeducation: Balance and posture training

A. Time

Most CPTs are defined in 15-minute increments, with each 15-minute segment described as a unit. Depending on the billing form used, the number of units may be required. The total session time should be recorded in the documentation entry itself.

Medicare Part B considers each AMA-defined CPT code as 8–22 minutes, not 15. The total time of the treatment session should be included in the documentation to accurately represent the time the patient/client actually received treatment. This practice is the same for non-Medicare billing purposes as well as liability.

Author's Note: As a general principle, If treatment exceeds 53 minutes or four codes, this must be justified in the documentation. For treatment that is provided between 38 and 52 minutes, three units would be billed. For timed services that exceed 23 minutes but are less than 38 minutes, two units should be billed. If a specific modality or procedure is less than 8 minutes, indicate this in the notes.

V. MODALITIES AND PROCEDURES

Although some physical agents/modalities, such as hot packs or cold packs, are generally not reimbursable alone because application of them is not necessarily considered skilled, they may be when rendered in conjunction with a procedure that is facilitated with their use. They must be included in the documentation even if not reimbursable.

VI. MODIFIERS

The use of modifiers allows the therapist to indicate when special consideration is needed to demonstrate the need for specific intervention. Modifiers may be used when treatment and evaluation are being performed on the same day or the patient/client has seen a physician and the PT. Some standard modifiers are listed below and can also be found in the AMA CPT manual and Medicare HCPCS manual. They would be used on the billing form, i.e., CMS 1500 when billing for physical therapy services.

- **GP:** indicates the physical therapist provided the services or care is being delivered under the PT's plan of care (POC).
- **GN:** indicates the speech language pathologist (SLP) provided the services or care is being delivered under the SLP POC.
- **GO:** indicates the occupational therapist (OT) provided the services or care is being delivered under the OT POC.
- **GA:** patient/client has been advised by an Advanced Beneficiary Notice (ABN) in advance that the service is not reasonable and necessary by Medicare standards and it is anticipated that Medicare will deny it.
- **GZ:** same as GA but the Medicare beneficiary has not been advised in advance. An ABN has not been provided to the beneficiary.
- **GY:** service or procedure is known to be noncovered by Medicare.
- **25:** evaluation and management performed on same day as treatment.
- **–59:** identifies a distinct service. If the physician has evaluated the patient/client the same day, this would indicate the PT evaluation was separate and distinct. It would also be used if two procedures were administered on the same day to the same area in distinctly unique unit times. For example, when billing manual therapy and therapeutic procedure the –59 modifier needs to be used for the second and subsequent codes. Otherwise the manual therapy code will be denied. This code is critical relative to the National Correct Coding Initiative (CCI edits). Although the CCI began with the CMS, it has been adopted by most payers…primary purpose is to indicate that two or more procedures are performed at different anatomical sites of different patient encounters.[5]
- **76:** treatment BID.
- **KX:** Requirements specified in the medical policy have been met. The KX code may be used when a therapy exception is appropriate or should be billed with any procedure code(s) that are gender specific for the affected beneficiaries. This modifier is used with the therapy cap exceptions. At the time of this revision, the exceptions were scheduled to be in place through 12/10. The cap limit in 2010 was $1860 and in 2011 was $1870, split between PT and speech language pathology services. A therapist can obtain information through the medicare administrative contractor to determine if a beneficiary has met their cap for a calendar year. All exceptions are automatic, but the documentation must support the skill need.

VII. BUNDLING

Although most procedures and modalities have separate and distinct codes, reimbursement may not be available individually. When a procedure or modality is not paid as distinct and separate, it is considered bundled. Medicare bundles hot packs and cold packs with all other services. CPT code 97602 for nonselective debridement may also be bundled. However, the provider should check with the specific carrier, payer, or Medicare Administrative Contractor (MAC) formerly (FI-fiscal intermediary) regarding bundled procedures and codes in the CCI edits.

VIII. COMMON PHYSICAL THERAPY/PHYSICAL MEDICINE: CPT/HCPCS THERAPEUTIC CODES/PROCEDURES

Because a billing code has been developed by the AMA, it does not mean that all codes or interventions are reimbursed by all payers. The provider has a responsibility to verify coverage. The codes included in this text while commonly used in physical therapy practice are not to be considered a complete list of applicable codes by any payer source. The patient's response to all procedures should always be included in daily entries.

97001: PT Evaluation. This code is used exclusively for PT evaluation including tests, measures, and analysis and synthesis, to establish a prognosis, POC, and appropriate goals based on the findings and anticipated recovery. It is not a timed code.

97002: PT Reevaluation. This code is used exclusively for PT reevaluation including tests, measures, and analysis and synthesis, to establish a prognosis, POC, and appropriate goals based on the findings and anticipated recovery, when a complete reevaluation is needed, and not in the course of ongoing treatment and or regular reassessment for daily recording. It is not a timed code.

> **Author's Note:** There is a distinction made between those modalities that require one-on-one administration by the therapist and those that do not. For example Ionotophoresis is a constant attended modality and requires one on one supervision of the therapist. Additionally, the specific body part(s) must be indicated in the documentation for all procedures and modalities. Deficits must be clearly identified, and goals objectively described, with an appropriate treatment plan or plan of care (POC).

97010: Hot Packs/Cold Packs. For Medicare purposes, this is a bundled code and will not be paid for separately. Justification must be clear in the documentation of the need for the hot pack or cold pack and the expected goal, even if used as an adjunct to another procedure. Specific parameters, including patient position and time, must also be included, as well as type and shape of pack. Condition of skin before and after treatment must be noted for liability purposes. Instructions should also be included for the patient of what to look for in skin changes after the session.

97012: Mechanical Traction. This code is used to describe mechanical traction that is set up for the patient and then requires general supervision and adjustment for a period of time. Justification must be clear in the documentation of the need for traction and the expected goal. All parameters including position and weight of pull must be included. For liability and safety purposes, the patient should be given a cutoff switch or means to call the therapist or assistant.

97014: Electrical Stimulation. This code is used for *unattended* electrical stimulation, once the patient/client has been set up. Justification must be clear in the documentation of the need for the stimulation and the expected goal. Specific parameters, including patient position and time must also be included, as well as the type of stimulation, electrode placement, and the machine type. Condition of skin before and after treatment must be noted.

CMS and HCPCS Codes for Unattended Electrical Stimulation:

- **G0281:** used for one or more areas for chronic stage III and IV ulcers of various etiologies that do not demonstrate measurable healing after 30 days of conventional management
- **G0282:** used for one or more areas for wound care other than G0281
- **G0283:** used for one or more areas for any indication other than wound care

97016: Vasopneumatic Device Therapy.
This code is used for the administration of Vasopneumatic Compression Device Therapy devices that require parameters to be set prior to use (i.e., mmHg based on blood pressure) and then general supervision over a period of time. Justification must be clear in the documentation of the need for vasopneumatic compression and the expected goal. Specific parameters, including patient position and time, must also be included, as well as appropriate measurements of edema using girth and/or volumetric measurement. It must be clearly stated when using girth where the measurements were taken. Treatment must indicate a linear progression of decreasing edema to enable function. Condition of skin before and after treatment must be noted.

97018: Paraffin Bath.
Justification must be clear in the documentation of the need for paraffin bath and the expected goal. Specific parameters, including patient position and time, must also be included. Precautions should be clearly indicated and the patient/client appropriately supervised. Condition of skin before and after treatment must be noted.

97020: Microwave Therapy.
This code has been deleted from the CPT coding as of 2006. If microwave therapy is administered, 97024 should be used. Justification must be clear in the documentation of the need for microwave therapy and the expected goal. Specific parameters, including patient position and time, must also be included. Precautions should be clearly indicated and the patient/client appropriately supervised. Condition of skin before and after treatment must be noted.

97022: Whirlpool Therapy (Non-Hubbard Tanks).
Justification must be clear in the documentation of the need for whirlpool therapy and the expected goal. Specific parameters, including patient position, type of whirlpool used, direction and intensity of jets, water temperature, additives, and time, must also be included. Precautions should be clearly indicated and the patient/client appropriately supervised at all times. Condition of skin before and after treatment must be noted. If the treatment is being used for wound care, specific conditions and measurements of the wound must be included, with clearly stated goals showing linear progression. If the treatment is being used to facilitate range of motion (ROM), or reduction in limb volume/edema, justification must be clear. For liability purposes, it should be made clear in the documentation that the patient was attended or safely monitored at minimum.

> **Author's Note:** As there are new wound care codes, use of them may be warranted. The use of whirlpool for wound care, in the advent of more effective and efficient procedures, is questionable in current practice for wounds.

97024: Diathermy Treatment.
Justification must be clear in the documentation of the need for diathermy treatment and the expected goal. Specific parameters, including patient position, settings, and time, must also be included, as well as appropriate padding to an area and removal of external metals, watches, and the like. Precautions should be clearly indicated and the patient/client appropriately supervised at all times. Short wave diathermy remains reimbursable by most payers. This code is appropriately used to bill for microwave treatment.

97026: Infrared Therapy. Justification must be clear in the documentation of the need for infrared therapy and the expected goal. Specific parameters, including patient position, settings, and time, must also be included. Precautions should be clearly indicated and the patient/client appropriately supervised.

97028: Ultraviolet Therapy. Justification must be clear in the documentation of the need for ultraviolet therapy and the expected goal. Specific parameters, including patient position, established dosage based on minimal erythemic dosage, and time, must also be included. Precautions should be clearly indicated, such as eye protection, and the patient/client appropriately supervised.

97032: Electrical Stimulation Manual. Justification must be clear in the documentation of the need for electrical stimulation and the expected goal. Specific parameters, including patient position, settings, type of probe or stimulator, and time, must also be included. Precautions should be clearly indicated and the patient/client appropriately supervised at all times. The skin should be inspected before and after treatment. This is an attended code and can be used for motor point stimulation.

97033: Electrical Current Therapy/Iontophoresis. Justification must be clear in the documentation of the need for electrical current therapy/iontophoresis and the expected goal. Specific parameters, including patient position and time, must also be included, as well as the medication used. Precautions should be clearly indicated and the patient/client appropriately supervised at all times. The skin should be inspected before and after treatment.

97034: Contrast Bath Therapy. Justification must be clear in the documentation of the need for contrast bath therapy and the expected goal. Specific parameters, including patient position, water temperatures, receptacle used, and time in each receptacle and total time, must also be included. Precautions should be clearly indicated and the patient/client appropriately supervised at all times. The skin should be inspected before and after treatment.

97035: Ultrasound (US) Therapy. Justification must be clear in the documentation of the need for ultrasound therapy and the expected goal. Specific parameters, including patient position, area treated, type of ultrasound (i.e., pulsed vs. continuous), transmission medium, intensity, and time, must also be included. Precautions should be clearly indicated and the patient/client appropriately supervised at all times. As US is usually administered by direct hands-on application, this should indicate constant supervision.

97036: Hydrotherapy/Hubbard Tank. Justification must be clear in the documentation of the need for Hubbard tank hydrotherapy and the expected goal. Specific parameters, including patient position, water temperature, intensity, and direction of jets, water additives, and time, must also be included. Precautions should be clearly indicated and the patient/client appropriately supervised at all times. (Refer to whirlpool.) Hubbard tanks or other full body whirlpools are no longer commonly used with the exception of some burn care.

97039: Physical Therapy Treatment. This is a nonspecific code and, therefore, should be avoided. It should be used only if a procedure is being used that does not fall into any other category. In addition to a detailed service description, information must specify the type of modality utilized and if the modality requires constant attendance.

97110: Therapeutic Procedure. All categories of skilled therapeutic exercise are covered by this code to one or more areas. It covers strengthening (not general in nature) and exercises to develop strength, endurance, ROM and flexibility. It is imperative that the documentation and POC include the term therapeutic exercise before listing the specific types employed with the patient/client. For justification of the need for skilled exercise, specific exercise parameters, applicable hand placement, technique name, tactile facilitation or other facilitation such as vibration or tapping, and verbal instructions (not cues) and patient/client response must be included. The exercises must be appropriate for the level of strength/muscle performance the patient/client demonstrates, and linked ultimately to function. Strength should be expressed in fractions, which are more universally understood by non-professionals than verbiage. One of the most common scales expresses strength in a range from 0/5 to 5/5, with 5/5 being the strongest and 0/5 representing no muscle contraction. Avoid using goals for strength that state "increase strength by 1/2 grade." Instead, link the strength to function and state the expectation.

■ Example 5

Strength:
Increase strength from 3/5 to 4/5 in L/R quadriceps and L/R hip extensors to enable stair climbing into home.

Range of Motion (ROM):
ROM should also be expressed in numbers. Goniometric measurements, using the appropriate goniometer, are the most reliable compared to visual estimates. ROM is best stated in fractions, with the available ROM, active (AROM) or passive (PROM), listed over the total "normal" ROM. If the full AROM should be 180° and the patient/client demonstrates 90°, it should be recorded as 90°/180°. Avoid using terms such as "increase by 10%." Instead, as in strength, list the numbers and link to function.

Increase ROM L shoulder from 90°/180° degrees to 160°/180° in order to reach for overhead objects.

97112: Neuromuscular Reeducation. Justification must be clear in the documentation of the need for neuromuscular reeducation. The code is used for reeducation of balance, coordination, kinesthetic sense, posture, and proprioception for activities performed in sitting and standing. It may also be used if a specific muscle is impaired, including motor control, and if muscle reeducation is necessary because of neuromuscular impairment. Some types of exercise, such as PNF or NDT, may fall under this category if being used specifically for neuromuscular reeducation. It is intended to use with neurological diagnoses. Since all payers do not reimburse for this code, the specific interventions would be coded as therapeutic exercise. CMS announced that physical therapists are able to bill for canalith positioning under this code 97112.

97113: Aquatic Therapy/Exercises. This code is intended for individual patient/client sessions that are in water. For justification of the need for skilled aquatics, specific exercise parameters and why the patient/client requires a water-based environment must be included.

97116: Gait Training. Justification must be clear in the documentation for the need for gait training (this includes stair climbing). Although many carriers and fiscal intermediaries allow the term ambulation to be used to describe "skilled walking assessment and intervention," the CPT code term is gait. For consistency, therefore, and indication that the activity is the same, the use of the term "gait" for assessment and training purposes is recommended. The term "walking" is never considered skilled and should be avoided unless the patient/client is being quoted. "Skilling" gait requires the assessment and training of all gait characteristics with appropriate goals including base of support (BOS) preferably described in inches; arm swing; swing phase; initial contact; stance; deviations; level of the pelvis; weight bearing and acceptance of weight on the limb; stride length; cadence; posture; assistive devices; balance; surfaces negotiated; safety; ability to change directions (forward, back, 180° turns R/L, 90° R/L) and negotiate or avoid obstacles; opening and closing doors; asymmetry; distance; sequencing; leg length discrepancies; extent of total effort patient/client is exerting if assistance is needed; and speed. Normal gait speed ≅ 82 m/min. Monitoring aerobic capacity/

endurance limitations by monitoring vital signs, the use of pulse oximetry, and instructing a patient/client in the Borg Rate of Perceived Exertion (RPE) scale, speed and demonstrating positive changes over time will strengthen the skill of the training and help support reimbursement.

■ Example 6

Gait Training: front wheeled rolling walker with rear skis, 2-point continuous pattern, minimal assist to prevent balance loss with directional changes and to control walker in forward direction, 2 repetitions; 100', 125', 3–4 minutes each repetition, even indoor surface, R/L 90° turns, verbal instruction for effective heel/toe pattern, erect posture, and to achieve consistent even step length and equal weight bearing.

Vital sign	Pre-gait	After 1st rep	After 2nd rep	After 3-minute rest
Blood pressure	126/82	130/84	130/84	130/80
Pulse	86 bpm	90 bpm	92 bpm	84 bpm
Respiratory rate	16	20	22	18

Author's Note: _____

Increasing distance alone for gait training will not justify skilled care.

_____

97124: Massage Therapy/Therapeutic Massage. Massage should be referred to as therapeutic massage in the documentation. The body part/area should be clearly stated as well as the relationship between the therapeutic and the expected outcome. It is usually used adjunctively to decrease spasm, increase joint range, mobilize scars or adherent tissue, decrease edema, and restore muscle function. Types of strokes and/or massage should also be included in the documentation, as well as body position and massage medium used: gel, lotion, etc. With appropriate justification, this code may be used for postural drainage techniques if it is necessary for it to be done by PT and can be used with both musculoskeletal and circulatory diagnoses such as swelling/edema of a limb. For myofascial release use 97140.

97140: Manual Therapy. This code includes manual therapy/mobilization/manipulation, manual lymphatic drainage, and manual traction to one or more regions. Justification must be clear in the documentation of the need for the specific procedure and the expected goal. Specific parameters, including patient position, methodology, and post-therapy procedures such as compression wrapping, must also be included. Precautions should be clearly indicated with the patient constantly attended as manual therapy is hands-on throughout. The coding is by 15-minute increments regardless of number of areas treated. Using this code with therapeutic will most likely require the use of the -59 modifier for billing purposes.

97150: Group Therapeutic Procedures. Used when patients/clients are receiving skilled services in a group (2 or more) with others requiring similar services (same POC). The PT must indicate in the documentation the specific treatment, how it will result in stated goals for the specific patient, and the size of the group. This is an untimed code. Only 1 unit of 97150 can be billed for each member in the group. See Appendix E on guidelines for group coding.

Author's Note: As of spring 2002, CMS/Medicare reviewed the group therapy code. They issued a transmittal indicating that even if all patients/clients are not receiving the same treatment, this code should be used if the PT is attending to multiple patients/clients in the same time period. The therapist must be in constant attendance, but not involved in one-on-one physical contact. However, according to the APTA, part of the session may be billed individually for direct one-on-one intervention, provided a component of the treatment was one-on-one (Transmittal: CMS 1753 CR 2126)

"CMS has established a correct coding initiative edit that prohibits billing for group therapy along with certain therapeutic procedure CPT codes (97110, 97112, 97116, 97140, 97530, 97532, 97533) in the same session unless a −59 modifier is used in certain settings. To be reimbursed for both services, the provider's documentation must support that the group therapy and the therapeutic procedure were performed during separate time intervals. In the fall of 2010, new group guidelines for provision of skilled rehabilitation in skilled nursing facilities (SNF) are going into effect. Although reimbursement is based on RUG level in SNFs, therapists should be aware of this change for documentation purposes."

97530: Therapeutic Activities, Direct. This category covers direct functional activities, such as lifting, carrying, reaching, catching, overhead activities, and bending, employed when a patient/client demonstrates limitations in strength, flexibility, range of motion, balance, and/or coordination. The documentation must show the relationship between the activities and the stated goals.

Transfer training or transitional movements may also be included in this category. Each type of transfer necessary for function should be included (i.e., sit to and from stand, stand and pivot, partial stand and pivot, sliding board use, standing disks, mechanical lifts, sit to and from supine, supine to and from long sit). The degree of patient/client ability must be stated clearly and reflected in the goals. Colloquially for physical therapy, patient/client ability has been stated in terms of assistance needed, which translates into patient/client ability. The terms are independent (I), supervised, minimally dependent or minimal assistance (up to 25% patient effort), moderately dependent or moderate assistance (up to 50% patient effort), maximally dependent or maximal assistance (up to 25% patient effort), and total dependence or total assistance (0 patient effort). For each of these, however, the documentation should include exactly what the percentage includes functionally. Medicare recommends the use of the terms limited and extensive, with limited corresponding to minimal, and extensive corresponding to all other more dependent terms. However, percentage of patient effort is required for all descriptions. Percentage should always be expressed in the evaluation to establish a baseline, with goals indicating decreasing percentage in a linear fashion. This covers dynamic activities and assumes one-on-one constant attendance. Essential functional activities—those activities that a patient/client needs to do rather than wants to do—are applicable in this category (see Example 7).

■ Example 7

Example of dependence/assistance:
Therapeutic Activities: Transfer training sit to/from stand from wheelchair; moderate assistance, verbal instructions and tactile facilitation to initiate stand and clear buttocks up to 6"; minimal assistance with walker stabilization to complete transition to stand; moderate assistance to facilitate eccentric control of extensors stand to sit and prevent "falling" into chair.

97532: Cognitive Skills Development. Justification must be clear in the documentation of the need for cognitive skills development, such as improved memory, reasoning, problem solving, and attention to tasks. This activity requires constant attendance with one-on-one care, billed in 15-minute increments.

97533: Sensory Integration. Justification must be clear in the documentation of the need for sensory integration. The code is used for enhancement of sensory processing, promoting appropriate responses between the patient/client and the environment. This activity requires constant attendance with one-on-one care, in 15-minute increments.

97542: Wheelchair Management Training/Propulsion. This code is used for skilled assessment, training fitting, and instruction and adaptation determination of either temporary or permanent confinement to a manual, power wheelchair or power-operated vehicle (scooter). When documenting for manual chairs, all appropriate aspects must be included, such as ability to transfer in and out of (including falls, bed, toilet, other chairs, other surfaces, ramps, cars/buses/trains), manipulation of any of the parts (brakes or power controls), terrain (even/uneven, indoor/outdoor), door opening and closing, all directions including turns, and folding/unfolding. The training of caretakers in all aspects of wheelchair use may also be applicable to this code. The same parameters are applied for power mobility appropriate for the types of controls and adaptations. Essential functional activities—those activities that a patient/client needs to do rather than wants to do—are also applicable to this category when "wheeled" mobility is indicated.

97601: Selective Debridement. This code includes removal of devitalized tissue from wound or selective debridement without anesthesia (i.e., high-pressure water jet, sharp debridement). Justification must be clear in the documentation of the need for selective debridement based on the description of the wound and devitalized tissue.

97602: Nonselective Debridement. This code includes general, nonspecific removal of tissue. For Medicare purposes, this is a bundled code.

97750: Physical Performance Test. Physical performance test covers performance tests, such as functional capacity assessments and other performance measures with written report (i.e., isokinetic testing).

97760 (Formerly 97504): Orthotic Management and Training. Justification must be clear in the documentation of the need for orthotic assessment training and fitting and the expected goal.

The type of orthotic and body area must be included (i.e., upper extremity [UE], lower extremity [LE], and trunk) and billed in 15-minute increments. Precautions should be clearly indicated and the patient/client appropriately supervised.

> **Author's Note:** A durable medical equipment (DME) number may be needed in order to bill for the actual orthosis. Treatment under this code may not be reimbursable for multiple sessions.

According to the First Coast Medicare Web site[4], orthotic training (CPT code 97504) for a lower extremity performed during the same visit as gait training (CPT code 97116) or self-care/home management training (CPT code 97535) should not be reported unless documentation in the medical record shows that distinct treatments were rendered. In addition, the casting and strapping codes should not be reported in addition to code 97504. If casting and strapping of a fracture, injury, or dislocation is performed, procedure codes 29000–29590 should be reported. Refer to the Local Medicare Review Policy (LMRP) policy (29580) for further guidelines regarding strapping.

97761 (Formerly 97520): Prosthetic Training. Justification must be clear in the documentation of the need for prosthetic training and the expected goal. The type of prosthetic and body area must be included (i.e., upper extremity [UE] or lower extremity [LE]) and billed in 15-minute increments. Precautions should be clearly indicated and the patient/client appropriately supervised. The pattern of use must be clearly indicated and any gait deviations, pressure concerns, and functional challenges for the LE listed. For the UE, pattern of use, pressure concerns, and functional challenges must be included.

97762 (Formerly 97703): Orthotic/Prosthetic Checkout Use.
This is for a patient that is already receiving care and have a new device or modification but does not need repeat intensive training.

97799: Unlisted Physical Medicine/Rehabilitation Service or Procedure.
This code would be used for an unlisted service.

HCPCS S8948: Laser low level.
Application of a modality (requiring constant provider attendance) to one or more areas; low level laser, each 15 minutes.

> **Author's Note:** There is no specific CPT code for low level laser therapy (LLLT). An alternative CPT code that can be used, but may result in non-payment is: 97799 which is unlisted service.

A. Other Billable Codes

94667 and 94668: CPT.
Respiratory procedures that require the hands on expertise of a therapist; 94667 is used for the initial examination and assessment and 94668 are used for subsequent intervention.

HCPCS:

- G0237: therapeutic procedures to increase the strength or endurance of respiratory muscles, which are conducted face-to-face and one-on-one, each of which is charged in 15-min units (includes monitoring); Interventions such as instruction in pursed-lip breathing, diaphragmatic breathing, and paced breathing would be included in this category.

- G0238: therapeutic procedures to improve respiratory function, other than those described by code G0237, which are conducted one-on-one and face-to-face, charged in 15-min periods (includes monitoring) and would include energy conservation techniques incorporating efficient breathing.

- G0239: therapeutic procedures to improve respiratory function, or to increase the strength or endurance of respiratory muscles, conducted with two or more individuals. This is considered a group code.

64550: Apply Neurostimulator.
Application of a neurostimulator may include a bone stimulator or functional electrical stimulation, but not TENS unit.

90901: Biofeedback Training/Any Method.
Biofeedback training/any method covers external methods. Justification and need must be clear in the documentation. Specific patient positioning, parameters, electrode or feedback device placement, time, and goals must be included.

90911: Biofeedback Training Peri/Uro/Rect.
Biofeedback training peri/uro/rect covers specific training for the perineals, urethral sphincter, or anorectal sphincter, with specialized equipment. Specific patient positioning, parameters, electrode or feedback device placement, time, and goals must be included. Medicare may cover this for incontinence with appropriate documentation and justification.

95831: Limb Muscle Testing, Manual; 95832: Hand Muscle Testing, Manual; 95833–95834: Body Muscle Testing, Manual.
Codes 95831–95834 are self-explanatory. It is the PT's responsibility to get clarification from the payer regarding

the use of these versus the PT evaluation code. In cases such as peripheral nerve injury in a limb, postoperative hand management, or spinal cord injury, these codes may be preferable to the evaluation code.

95851–95852: Range of Motion Measurements.
It is the PT's responsibility to get clarification from the payer regarding the use of these versus the PT evaluation code. In cases such as multiple trauma in which multiple ranges must be obtained, these codes may be preferable to the PT evaluation code. Range of motion (ROM) however, is usually included in a comprehensive initial examination and evaluation.

96000: Motion Analysis, Video 3d.
Justification must be clear in the documentation of the need for motion analysis, video 3d, and the outcomes from the assessment as well as goals.

96001: Motion Test with Foot Pressure Measurement.
Justification must be clear of the need for motion analysis of dynamic foot pressure measurement during gait. The goals and outcomes from the assessment should also be included.

96002: Dynamic Surface EMG.
Justification must be clear in the documentation of the need for dynamic surface EMG during walking and other functional activities. The goals and outcomes from the assessment should also be included. This is calculated in increments up to 12 minutes.

96003: Dynamic Fine Wire EMG.
Justification must be clear in the documentation of the need for dynamic fine wire EMG during walking and other functional activities for 1 muscle. The goals and outcomes from the assessment should also be included.

96110: Developmental Test, Limb; 96111: Developmental Test, Extremity; 96115: Neurobehavior Status Exam.
Generally, codes 96110, 96111, and 96115 are covered under the PT evaluation code. With appropriate certification, based on state licensing, PTs with special certification may perform and receive reimbursement for EMG/NCV under codes 95860–95937 from Medicare.

97535: Self-Care/Home Management Training.
Justification must be clear in the documentation of the need for self-care/home management training. This includes activities such as activities of daily living (ADL), meal preparation, use of assistive or adaptive devices and technologies, and safety. This code should be used for lymphedema management when the patient/caretaker is instructed in self-bandaging and skin care. Precautions should be clearly indicated and the patient/client appropriately supervised. Billing should be listed in 15-minute increments.

97537: Community/Work Reintegration.
Justification must be clear in the documentation of the need for community/work reintegration. Reintegration includes developing incremental activities of daily living (IADL) skills, such as shopping, negotiating transportation, managing monetary transactions, vocational and avocational activities, work environment and ergonomic considerations, and work task analysis. Precautions should be clearly indicated. This activity requires constant attendance with one-on-one care and should be billed in 15-minute increments. Medicare may not reimburse for all activities covered by this code based on the concept of essential function.

97545: Work Hardening.
Justification must be clear in the documentation of the need for work hardening and the expected goal. Specific parameters, activities, and time must also be included. Precautions should be clearly indicated and the patient/client appropriately supervised. This code is used for the initial 2 hours of work hardening. Medicare does not reimburse for work hardening.

97546: Work Hardening Add-on.
This code would be used for time beyond the initial 2 hours and is billed in 1-hour increments.

98960: Education and Training for Patient Self-Management. This is for training by a qualified nonphysician healthcare professional using a standard curriculum face to face:

> *As above, but 2–4 patients in a group: 98961*
> *As above but 5–8 patients in a group: 98962;* for example, a group of patients who are post total hip arthroplasty, posterolateral approach

> **Author's Note:** Before using any code to bill for procedures, check with the carrier/MAC to determine if the service is covered. Identification of a procedure by code does not automatically qualify it for payment.

B. Noncovered Conditions and Services as Listed on CMS Web Site

It is the responsibility of the therapist to be aware of medical conditions and services not covered by the third party payer. Regardless of the documentation, noncovered services will not be paid regardless of therapist efforts or goals. Examples of **noncovered** services and conditions in the **Medicare program** include:

1. Vertebral axial decompression (VAD) therapy is considered "investigational" and is a noncovered service under Florida Medicare.
2. General exercises to promote overall fitness and flexibility and activities to provide diversion or general motivation.
3. Work hardening/conditioning **(CPT codes 97545–97546)**.
4. Electrotherapy performed for the treatment of facial nerve paralysis in the application of electrical stimulation **(97014)**.
5. Electrotherapy for the treatment of facial nerve paralysis, commonly known as Bell's palsy **(ICD-9 code 351.0)**.
6. Diathermy **(97024)** or ultrasound **(97035)** heat treatments performed for respiratory conditions or diseases **(ICD-9 codes 460–519.9)** are investigational under the Medicare program.
7. General exercise programs to improve a patient's general cardiovascular fitness; pulmonary rehabilitation; cardiac rehabilitation; or a maintenance program of therapeutic activities.
8. Aquatic therapy with therapeutic exercise **(97113)** should not be billed when there is no one-on-one contact between therapist and patient.
9. Diapulse and Rolfing **(97799)** treatment is noncovered.
10. Noncovered ICD-9 codes, i.e., Bell's palsy.
11. Hot packs or cold packs unless bundled and an integral component of other intervention.

C. Evaluation and Management Clarification

Providers may report evaluation and management services on the same day as physical medicine treatments, provided the services are separately identifiable.

> **Author's Note:** *Some insurance companies initially approve the evaluation. The PT must submit documentation to receive approval for treatment visits.*

There is a clear relationship between CPT coding, ICD-9 (or appropriate ICD edition coding), and documentation. In order to receive reimbursement, the ICD code must be related to the treatment rendered. The treatment rendered must be described in verbiage that matches the CPT codes in order to appropriately code the billing. However, regardless of the accuracy of the CPT and ICD coding, the documentation must also support the medical necessity of the skilled PT intervention in an appropriate time frame. Unless there is devastating illness or injury, or the patient/client is in a preapproved program self prescribed time, most care should be planned for episodes of 30 days or less.

Understanding the basic concepts of coding and application of them will not guarantee reimbursement. It is up to the therapist to justify all care by entering into the record that skilled services were required, goals were reasonable and reached (preferably in a linear manner), care was reasonable and necessary, and the therapy was both effective and efficient.

IX. SUMMARY

The National Correct Coding Initiative (CCI) began in 1996 and in 1998 required the use of CPT codes for all Medicare billing of rehabilitation services, as do all payers.[5] CMS developed the HCPCS codes for those codes not included in the AMA CPT coding and to clarify other AMA CPT codes relative to the Medicare system. In order to ensure reimbursement, the correct procedural codes must be used for all physical therapy services, many of which are general physical medicine codes.

The correct combination of CPT codes, ICD-9 diagnostic codes, CPT matching verbiage describing the procedures rendered in the documentation, emphasis on function, ongoing justification of the medical necessity for skilled PT, and matched billing dates will assist the PT in ensuring reimbursement based on the documentation.

In those instances in which the PT is not performing the CPT coding or billing, it is critical that the individual(s) handling the billing understand correct coding. If the PT is familiar enough with the codes and appropriate terminology to use them appropriately, an "outsider" can more easily do the coding. Electronic or computerized systems can be designed to facilitate automatic coding, as inclusion of codes with correction description on preprinted forms.

REFERENCES

1. http://www.who.int/en/. Accessed April 15, 2011.
2. http://www.apta.org/Payment/Coding/CPTChanges/
3. http://www.cms.gov/MLNProducts/downloads/form_cms-1500_fact_sheet.pdf
4. http://www.medicine.fcso.com.
5. http://www.cms.gov/NationalCorrectCodInitEd/

CHAPTER 5 REVIEW QUESTIONS

1. What is a CPT code? Explain the application in physical therapy.

2. What is an ICD-9 code? Explain the application in physical therapy.

3. What is the relationship between the CPT codes and the ICD-9 codes?

4. What is the medical diagnosis?

5. What is the physical therapy diagnosis or physical therapy problem?

6. What is the relationship between the medical diagnosis and the physical therapy diagnosis (problem)? Provide at least one example.

7. What is a code modifier? Explain the role of modifiers in the billing process.

8. What are the time increments for CPT code procedures for Medicare billing versus non-Medicare billing?

9. Relative to CPT codes, explain the difference between attended and unattended procedures.

10. What are the risks of billing for noncovered procedures?

11. Describe the concept of HCPCS codes and their role in billing, reimbursement, and documentation.

12. When is code modifier -59 used? Provide an example relevant to physical therapy.

13. Does a CPT or HCPCS code need to be included in a daily medical record entry? Provide rationale.

6 Home Health Documentation

Providing physical therapy services in the home health setting involves creativity, flexibility, and solid documentation skills. Physical therapists (PTs) need to employ their full scope of assessment skills in order to manage a medically complex individual without the support of a medical facility or quick access to individual staff.[1]

The legal and professional responsibility associated with documentation is an essential component of home health physical therapy. PTs must stay current with continuously changing regulations and laws regardless of payer source. According to the Home Health Section of the American Physical Therapy Association (APTA), home health care is a medically oriented, skilled, and intermittent service provided in the home that may include nursing, physical therapy (PT), occupational therapy, speech therapy, social services, dietary/nutrition counseling, pharmacy services, and/or home health aides.[2] Home health services are typically provided for individuals who meet homebound criteria. Patients are most often senior citizens, disabled persons, or children with variety of diagnoses including orthopedic, neurological, cardiovascular, medical and other. Patients are typically restricted to an environment such as the patient's home, caregiver's home, assisted living facility, skilled nursing facility in extended care beds, group home, residential facility or the like. Home health offers more autonomy than other settings in which a PT is rendered and provides needed services for individuals who have difficulty leaving their homes.[3]

Reimbursement for outpatient services such as Medicare Part B, that are provided in homes as a result of patient preference or lack of transportation typically follow the guidelines set forth by the outpatient facilities and usually require a co-pay as patients are not homebound.[4] Reimbursement for home health services varies and can be based upon prognosis, the patient's living situation, or insurance. Although Medicare A covers home health, non-Medicare payers may limit or exclude physical therapy as a covered home health service, resulting in the patient paying privately for therapy in the home, or being forced to obtain outpatient services. In all cases, PTs and PTAs should continue to document using principles consistent with APTA Guidelines: Physical Therapy Documentation of Patient/Client Management [BOD G03-05-16-41].[5] Since documentation regarding pediatrics is covered in another chapter, this chapter will focus primarily on documentation for the geriatric client receiving services covered by Medicare A and provided by home health agencies (HHA), as most payers follow Medicare guidelines.

In 2008, Medicare reported a record number of home health participants: over 37.5 million aged 65+, and over 7.7 million disabled.[6] Over the past decade, home care documentation by therapists and assistants has undergone a massive transition that includes revisions to the primary tool used to assess patients, and a push toward 100% electronic records.[7,8] Clinicians must be familiar with specific regulatory requirements from national, regional, and state levels, and be aware of medication management, depression screening, case management, and diagnosis coding. Documentation for each treatment is highly scrutinized for skill level and medical necessity, and may be subject to review or audit by a growing number of government agencies and third party payers.

I. THE OASIS AND REGULATORY GUIDELINES

According to the Home Health Section of the APTA, the PT and PTA must be able to produce timely and appropriate documentation as it relates to home health, including Medicare Part A OASIS related documents.[2] The Outcome and Assessment Information Set (OASIS) was created in 1999 to better monitor the quality of home health using a standardized, reproducible assessment instrument.[7] It was designed to provide a thorough analysis of the patients' needs on admission to care and discharge, by either a nurse or therapist and to determine payment for home health providers. The OASIS tool has undergone numerous revisions based on input from multiple task forces, government agencies, and clinicians. The most recent revision, OASIS-C, became effective on January 1, 2010. Throughout this chapter, the OASIS-C will be referenced with the unique challenges it presents to physical therapy.

Information regarding the most recent Medicare updates on OASIS and Medicare documentation requirements for home health is available at the Centers for Medicare and Medicaid Services' (CMS) Web site at http://www.cms.gov/center/hha.asp. This site includes the latest user manual for the OASIS-C as well as any updates from the CMS. The CMS publishes a Medicare National Coverage Determinations (NCDs) manual, which describes the specific services and treatments that may be reimbursed by Medicare can be found at http://www.cms.gov/manuals/downloads/ncd103c1_Part1.pdf.[9] The CMS assigns regional intermediaries responsible for administering the Medicare program and processing claims, to serve as Government Benefit Administrators (GBA) such as Palmetto GBA, Cigna GBA, and Cahaba GBA. Based on CMS policies, these agencies establish guidelines referred to as Local Coverage Determinations (LCDs), that identify the GBA's interpretation of CMS directives and determine Medicare coverage and policies regarding payments. More information about these groups can be found at their respective Web sites.

II. ELECTRONIC DOCUMENTATION IN HOME HEALTH

Advances in technology are changing the method of physical therapy documentation, and home health providers are in the process of converting to paperless alternatives. One reason for this shift involves the CMS proposal of monetary incentives to organizations that convert to electronic health records as early as 2011.[10] Electronic documentation in home care provides clinicians with useful tools to increase accuracy, consistency, and efficiency. The improvement in communication among clinicians and disciplines provides opportunities to review patient records in order to gain a more thorough assessment. Many electronic systems have built-in mechanisms to insure that documentation is accurately completed.

Although electronic documentation includes the same components as any written record, using electronic resources reduces many challenges of handwritten communication, including legibility, patient scheduling, failure to appropriately articulate goals, inconsistent care plans for supportive personnel, as well as lost forms and records. Clinicians may be able to document and print home exercise programs, search the internet for information and locate patients' homes using built-in mapping programs.

Many different models of portable, handheld devices are available. The devices currently on the market can be programmed to meet the specific needs of the home health agency (HHA). One such advancement, telemonitoring, which provides live visual and auditory feedback, may soon be a reality for home physical therapy to record exercise programs and compliance, exertion levels, or respond to patient's concerns about their care. Cardiac home programs have already instituted telemonitoring of vital signs and other information from their patients with overwhelming success.[11] Systems should provide adequate means for physical therapy professionals to enter narratives that distinguish their unique services and skills without records appearing rote from patient to patient.

III. MEETING THE REQUIREMENT FOR HOME CARE

In order for patients to qualify for the Part A home health benefit and be eligible to receive services, a beneficiary must meet four requirements:[12]

- Be confined in the home (homebound)
- Under the care of a physician
- Receive services under a plan of care (POC) established and reviewed by a physician
- Be in need of skilled nursing care on an intermittent basis or physical therapy or speech–language pathology; or have a continuing need for occupational therapy

IV. DOCUMENTATION FOR HOMEBOUND STATUS

According to the CMS, homebound patients are those that require a "considerable and taxing effort" to leave their home.[12] At the onset of care, a physical therapist must determine or verify and document a patient's homebound status. These patients may leave for medical appointments and other infrequent but necessary outings, and documentation should demonstrate an inability for the patient to function normally outside of their home. Clear written justification of reasons that a patient is homebound is required at each therapy session. In most cases, the functional status of the patient should serve as validation and is critical in the documentation.[13]

Examples of documentation for homebound status include:

- confinement to a wheelchair or bed following any injury, or with pathology such as a stroke or spinal cord injury;
- ambulation with a walker or crutches with assistance or constant supervision;
- vision deficits requiring assistance;
- any medical condition limiting stress or activity, such as cardiac surgery;
- physical deficits, such as loss of lower extremity strength or muscle performance, that may limit function in public settings.

In addition to the above criteria, whenever possible, just as in outpatient, the PT should use standard tests and measures to document in the most objective manner the functional deficits that limit the patient and progress over time. An example is the Borg Rating of Perceived Exertion (RPE), a 15-point scale ranging from no exertion to maximal exertion.[14] A patient could be assessed and then instructed in the use of the scale. If the patient leaves their home for specific events, the events should be documented with the patient report of their RPE. Progress can be measured over time by the patient reports.

Although the CMS does not specify events that would lead to disqualification as homebound and therefore reimbursement, they do indicate that each occurrence should be infrequent and of short duration.[12] Examples of documented home absences include:

- physician appointment;
- dialysis, chemotherapy, radiation therapy;
- adult day care;
- religious event;

- hairdresser;
- reunion, funeral, graduation, or unique event.

In a question posed to the CMS in April 2010 concerning a patient's ability to drive a car while receiving home care services, the CMS responded

> Homebound status is determined on an individual basis, looking at the patient as a whole. If the net effect of driving indicates that the individual has the capacity to get their health care routinely outside of the home, then it could challenge their eligibility. The fact that a patient is fit enough to drive raises questions as to whether the basic statutory requirement is met. Because individual circumstances can vary greatly, necessitating determinations on a case-by-case basis, we are reluctant to issue a specific policy that relates to driving in every possible occurrence. Inherent in such a policy would be judgments about the particular circumstances under which it may be appropriate for an individual to operate a motor vehicle. We believe that such determinations must continue to be made on a case-by-case basis.[15]

A focus on documentation of homebound status has been undertaken by internal and external auditors for Medicare and will be discussed later. If patients meet the criteria for homebound status, PTs can proceed with an initial examination and evaluation.

V. EVALUATION IN HOME CARE: OASIS-C START OF CARE (SOC)

Since January 1, 2010, the OASIS-C document is required at the initial or start of care (SOC) evaluation for all Medicare and Medicaid patients.[16] The OASIS manual created by the CMS as well as updates can be found at the following Web site: http://www.cms.gov/HomeHealthQualityInits/14_HHQIOASISUserManual.asp

The reimbursement from the Medicare GBA for a 60-day period is determined by the information provided in the OASIS-C. Therefore, all of the care that will be provided to the patient by the HHA should be accurate and complete. According to the CMS, a registered nurse (RN), PT, or speech therapist (ST) may complete the OASIS-C for SOC.[16] The assessing therapist may need to consult with other clinicians treating an individual patient, or individuals more knowledgeable in certain components of the OASIS-C to ascertain the best responses to each question. The CMS also conducts regular webinars to address concerns with the OASIS-C and responds to questions posted to their Web site. Most HHAs also provide training and testing on accurate OASIS completion by all professionals who may be required to use it.

The OASIS-C is a combination of over 100 multiple choice and short answer questions, although not all questions are applicable to every patient. According to the CMS, the time required for completion ranges from 20 to 125 minutes with a mean of 49.61 minutes.[7] For this section, specific components of the SOC that pose unique challenges to the PT are addressed.

A. Documenting History and Demographics

The first series of questions involve the background of the patient and include the following:

- HHA provider number and state
- Physician NPI (National Provider Identification) number
- Start of care (SOC) date
- Patient name, state, zip code, insurance number (HICN—health insurance claim number), social security number
- Patient race/ethnicity
- Discipline of person completing assessment
- Date assessment completed and the date the assessment was ordered
- Location of patient prior to assessment (hospital, home, SNF) and discharge date

- Medical and social history
- Inpatient procedure and diagnoses for past 14 days, if applicable
- Current diagnoses using ICD coding

B. Documenting International Classification of Diseases (ICD) Codes

ICD codes represent the diagnosis, surgical, history, and procedure codes that are related to the patient being evaluated.[17] Therapists should be knowledgeable about the ICD-9 codes currently in use in the United States, in order to accurately plan the care of the patient and reflect the diagnoses being treated. The medical diagnoses may be the same or different from the PT treatment diagnoses, as presented in an earlier chapter. PTs should be familiar with the most commonly used functionally oriented and impairment oriented code verbiage. Although the PT may not be the one assigning the numeric ICD code, as long as the verbiage is consistent, a "coder" employed by the agency can accurately assign it. Many of the electronic documentation systems contain some form of assistance with ICD coding. The order of the documented codes should list the most severe condition being treated first then the lesser severe to the least severe. The home health PT must document all present diagnoses; medical and treatment, prior medical and surgical history; past and recent, all current dietary habits, social history, and medications and/or supplements, both prescription and over the counter. All of this information facilitates the selection of the most appropriate ICD codes.

C. Documenting Risk for Hospitalization

The CMS included a question in the OASIS to gain better understanding of the patient's potential for being admitted to a hospital while in home care.[16] Therapists can select none, one, or multiple choices for hospitalization risk. These options include the following:

- Recent decline in mental, emotional, and behavioral status
- Multiple hospitalizations
- History of falls
- Taking five or more medications (which increases the risk for falls)
- Frailty indicators such as weight loss or exhaustion

It is expected that patients discharged to home would be medically stable. However, with diagnostic related group (DRG)-based reimbursement to hospitals and prospective payment systems (PPS) in SNFs, this may not always be the case, hence the CMS OASIS question regarding short-term prognosis.

D. Clinical Depression

In 2010, questions were included in the OASIS that concerned clinical depression. The depression component was added to better understand the psychological needs of home health patients, as it was believed that depression was not properly identified and assessed in elderly clients.[6] This requires the HHA to select a standardized tool to screen for depression, but not medically diagnose. The CMS includes Pfizer's PHQ-2 scale which asks about frequency of decreased interest in activities, and frequency that the patient feels down, depressed, or hopeless.[15] Other commonly used depression screening tools include the Geriatric Depression Scale and the Cornell Scale for Depression in Dementia.[18,19] As depression may interfere with function and progress, early detection and appropriate medical management will benefit the patient. Therapists should include in their documentation descriptions of behaviors that may be indicative of depression as well, especially if a patient is not achieving appropriate functionally oriented goals in the expected duration of care.

E. Diabetic Foot Care and Heart Failure

The CMS added two new components to the OASIS requiring further assessment and documentation by physical therapy in 2010. If a patient has a diagnosis of diabetes, the CMS expects additional information to be included in the POC that is directed to diabetes related conditions. This includes two items: monitoring for the presence of skin lesions on the lower extremities and feet and providing education on proper foot care. The PT has three choices of response: "no," inferring the patient has diabetes and these interventions are not on the POC; "yes," the patient is a diabetic and these interventions are included; or "NA," the patient is not diabetic.[16]

The CMS also requests information at discharge concerning symptoms of heart failure. If the patient has a diagnosis of heart failure, the CMS asks whether he or she exhibits any symptoms of heart failure since the last OASIS assessment. As in diabetes, there is the option of three responses: "no," has the diagnosis without symptoms; "yes," has diagnosis and has symptoms; or not applicable, "NA," the patient has no diagnosis of heart failure.[16] These questions, although simply stated, can be easily misinterpreted and answered incorrectly by the PT. Someone may hastily select "no" to a question if the patient does not have the diagnosis of diabetes or heart failure when the appropriate response is NA. If an appropriate history is obtained or medical record review conducted, the PT should be able to respond correctly.

F. Pain Assessment and Management

Medicare regulation requires that clinicians use a standardized assessment tool for the assessment of pain.[16] The tool should be appropriate for the communication and cognitive level of the client in order to record an accurate response. The tool should also express the range of answers from *no pain to severe pain*. Examples of such tools include the following:

1. Numeric Pain Intensity Scale: patients use a 0/10 to 10/10 scale to assess degree of pain at rest and with acquity.

2. Simple Descriptive Pain Intensity Scale: patients choose words like "mild," "moderate," and "severe" to describe the pain intensity.

3. Visual Analog Scale (VAS): patients select a point on a 10-cm vertical or horizontal line that indicates pain intensity.

4. Wong-Baker Faces Pain Intensity Scale: patients can select a picture of a facial expression that best matches their pain level. This scale is used more in pediatrics or with adults who are unable or unwilling to use other types of scales.

The initial examination and evaluation should, as in all settings, include appropriate questions that qualify pain including the location, what makes it better and what makes it worse, a description of the quality of the pain, i.e., sharp, dull ache, throbbing, stabbing, when it is the worst and what the patient does, if anything, to manage the pain.

In addition to using a standardized tool, clinicians must document the frequency that the pain interferes with the patient's activity and the intensity.[16] A patient may report a decreased pain rating because they are *not* performing an activity. A patient may not perform an activity such a gardening if he or she experiences knee pain, so the clinician must ask and document what behaviors (including frequencies) would be performed if pain was reduced. However, leisure activities such as gardening and returning to gardening are not justification for skilled PT. Clinicians should also observe and document their clients' facial expressions during activities to further evaluate pain. Pharmacologic and/or nonpharmacologic interventions may control the pain so that it does not interfere with activity or movement. These interventions should be documented since they could be temporary and limit the patient's activity level. Patients' pain over time and the decrease of the pain should be included in continuum of care documentation and should reflect positive progress toward goals as function increases.

G. Documenting Wounds and Pressure Ulcers

The documentation requirements for wounds and ulcers may vary based on reimbursement, practice settings, and by how the skin area is classified. The CMS has specific guidelines for recording pressure ulcers to gain a better understanding of the risk and status of their clients.[16] In the OASIS document, the clinician must assess the risk of the patient for developing pressure ulcers. As with other sections in the OASIS, the utilization of a standardized tool, i.e., Norton, Braden, etc., is preferred to determine risk, or the therapist may base the evaluation of risk on clinical factors such as mobility, incontinence and/or nutrition. The CMS reports their intent is to capture the home health agency's best practice regarding the integumentary system.[16] If one or more pressure ulcers are present, the clinician must document how many, the stage of each unhealed ulcer, and the measurements (cm) of the largest ulcer. Standard guidelines for documentation of any open wound include size/measurements, drainage, odor, color, and description of tissue both in the wound and in the peri-wound area.

The clinician must also document in the OASIS any venous stasis ulcer. These areas are caused by poor venous circulation and are often associated with stasis dermatitis.[16] If a surgical procedure was performed, the clinician must also identify if a surgical wound is present. For each of theses concerns, the therapist is requested to describe the status of the most problematic observable pressure ulcer, stasis ulcer, and surgical wound with one of the following:

a. Newly epithelialized (epithelial tissue has completely covered the wound surface)

b. Fully granulating (granulating but epithelial tissue has completely covered the wound surface)

c. Early/partial granulation

d. Not healing (≥ 25% necrotic or avascular tissue)

And for pressure ulcers only:

e. No observable pressure ulcer (covered by dressing, cast, etc.)

The documentation of other types of skin lesions or open wounds that require intervention should be listed.[16] Examples of these lesions include skin tears, burns, PICC line sites, rashes, diabetic ulcers, trauma wounds, and ostomies (bowel ostomies excluded). PTs should address these lesions in a narrative format to describe both the location, intervention and goals if part of the PT POC.

H. Documenting Medications and Medication Management

In order to participate in the Medicare program, certain medication standards must be met by the HHA.[12] One of these requirements concerns evaluating current medications. According to the CMS, all current medications must be reviewed to identify any potential adverse effects and drug reactions, ineffective drug therapy, side effects, drug interactions, duplicate drug therapy, and noncompliance with drug therapy.[16] Therapists may utilize office-based nurses to assist with medication review or acquire appropriate education through continuing education on pharmacology or other means. There are pocket guides that can be used for easy access to drug information or download applications for cell phones or other portable electronic devices. The OASIS dictates that the information be obtained and included by a representative of the home health agency at the time of the initial OASIS, but not by the PT unless the PT is performing the initial OASIS. The degree to which a PT should be engaged in issues related to medication management, including high-risk drug education, and management of oral and injectable medications varies by state. However, there should always be documentation of collaboration with nursing and other health personnel including the physician. From a prevention of medical errors perspective, the PT should be attentive to behaviors exhibited during therapy sessions, which may be side effects of the medications, potential negative interactions, and if indeed a drug prescribed for a medical condition is for that condition.

I. Documenting Function

A major component of the patient evaluation and OASIS is documentation of function and ability to perform specific tasks.[16] Accurate reflection of the patient's ability to perform certain tasks assists in the determination of reimbursement and outcome reporting to government agencies. Each task may be limited by physical, cognitive, or sensory impairments, and/or environmental barriers. This is critical in physical therapy documentation for Medicare and all other third party payers.

The physical therapist must document the patient's ability to perform the following functional tasks: (Note: some of the ADL information may be gained by interview, as long as either the patient or caregiver is competent to answer appropriately)

a. Grooming (washing hands, face, hair, teeth, nails, etc)

b. Ability to dress upper body

c. Ability to dress lower body

d. Bathing (wash entire body)

e. Toilet transferring (ability to get to and from toilet or bedside commode)

f. Toilet hygiene (ability to maintain perineal area or ostomy site, and adjust clothing)

g. Feeding or eating (ability to eat, chew, and swallow)

h. Ability to plan and prepare light meals (also includes safely reheating delivered meals)

i. Ability to use the telephone (dial and communicate effectively)

j. Transitional movement/transferring (ability to move safely from bed to/from chair, sit to and from stand, transition from supine to and from sit, or position self in bed)

k. Gait: ambulation/locomotion (ability to walk or use wheelchair safely on a variety of surfaces including directional changes, negotiating doors, curbs, etc.— without using the word "walk" unless quoting a patient or caregiver.)

For each functional item, responses are ranked from the most independent to the most dependent. For example, the most dependent response for ambulation is *bedfast* and the most independent response involves walking on even and uneven surfaces and negotiating stairs (with or without railing), both with neither human assistance nor assistive device. The CMS explains that these questions identify the patient's ability and not necessarily actual performance.[16] If the ability fluctuates, the clinician should select the response that describes the ability for the client to safely perform the task over 50% of the time. The best method to determine the correct response, especially for mobility, is observation and assessment of the specific activity. The condition in which the task is performed is critical to evaluating safety. A patient may be able to quickly transfer in and out of a bathtub in dry, clothed conditions but may have difficulty with this task in bare feet with soap and water. Clinicians should refer to the CMS OASIS-C Guidance Manual for further delineation of each functional question.

VI. MEDICAL NECESSITY IN HOME CARE

The GBAs (Government Benefit Administrators) provide two guidelines that demonstrate physical therapy services are reasonable and medically necessary. These guidelines are designed to assure that the treatment provided requires the unique set of skills of the PT or PTA. For a treatment to be deemed medically necessary, the documentation must provide the "complexity of the treatment" and "why the treatment is medically appropriate, based on the beneficiary's condition."[20]

This is consistent with all venues that provide physical therapy to Medicare beneficiaries.

Included in the complexity of the treatment are five components:

1. *Tests, measures, assessment*

These can include such procedures as orthopedic special tests, goniometric measurements, manual muscle testing, balance tests, standardized testing, postural assessment, cranial nerve testing, developmental tests, or other tests that require the knowledge of a PT or PTA to complete. Note: only a PT can perform an evaluation.

2. *Planning, interventions, changes*

This stage demonstrates how the knowledge gained through testing and observation is used to create a treatment plan, select specific interventions, and adapt to changes in the patient's condition. For example, if the patient scored a 10 on a Tinetti gait and balance test, the therapist would conclude that the patient is at a higher risk for falls and decide to select interventions that address balance in the patient's treatment plan.

> **Author's Note:** When using a standardized test and measure such as the Tinetti, in addition to attaching the completed test to the initial examination and evaluation, the identified deficits should be summarized in the body of the evaluation. Goals should be established consistent with the specific functional problem and match the treatment. The standardized test can be re-administered throughout care to monitor progress and at minimum, should be repeated at discharge.

3. *Teaching and assessment of patient's ability to follow through*

The documentation following treatment needs to show an improved ability for the patient or patient's caregiver to continue the treatment plan.

4. *Continued need for assessment and teaching*

This component is usually the most difficult for PTs and PTAs to write. The goal is to understand the functional problem, and determine what skills are required to change the behavior. For example, instead of assessing a sit to stand transfer as "requires moderate assist," one could report "patient unable to shift upper body forward in order to stand. Instructed in foot placement and provided verbal instruction/cues and tactile input at shoulders for patient to stand. Patient able to perform sit to stand 5 times, with the 5th repetition requiring contact guard." Although this example is noticeably more lengthy, it provides the skills (verbal cues, tactile cues), the assessment (contact guard), and that more treatment is warranted for the patient to be safe and independent. A patient must be able to repeat a skill multiple times in order to be functional.

5. *Avoid documenting repetitive modalities and interventions*

This documentation practice exists in all settings, but since the home usually contains limited exercise equipment, the tendency to repeat exercises and interventions increases. The CMS and the intermediaries are more concerned with the patient's behavior than a PT documenting "ther ex" every treatment session. If the use of a modality improves function, document the new behavior of the patient, or if the gait pattern of a patient improves, select different surfaces for the patient to perform gait and gait related activities.

In order to better document why PT treatment is medically appropriate, the GBA further reports that three conditions should be met:

Patient's needs, functional changes, or changes in condition

Documentation should include the rationale for selecting treatment options. For example, if a patient wants to return to safely bending down to don clothing or pick up objects and safely negotiate in the bathroom for personal hygiene, therapy would include gait and balance training on unlevel or uneven surfaces, positional changes, and upper and lower extremity therapeutic exercises including stretching, strengthening, etc. The narrative should also include what functional tasks may be affected by the patient's diagnoses.

1. Prior level of function (as immediately prior to the current episode of care as possible). The determination of past performance is helpful to evaluate changes in behavior.

2. Document any other condition that may support need for therapy in situations that would not ordinarily need a therapist. For example, a patient with a pelvic fracture may be able to ambulate with family after being instructed by the

therapist. However, the patient requires the therapist to support the trunk and guard the patient because of the fracture and risk for falling.

VII. PLAN OF CARE

If the determination is made that physical therapy treatment is appropriate for a patient and medical necessity requirements are met, the PT can establish a plan of care (POC). The POC should convey the predicted functional outcome over a specified duration of time.[1] In home care, the time duration determined by the PT may span an entire 60-day episode for patients that have significant medical need. Some clients may only be homebound for 1–2 weeks and then discharged to outpatient PT or discontinued from care. The POC may be derived separate from the OASIS, but most electronic documentation systems create the documents simultaneously. One should note that although one clinician is responsible for completing the OASIS, the POC should contain the following information from all disciplines:

1. Patient-centered goals written in measurable, functional terms with a projected date of completion.
2. All interventions to be provided to the patient by the home health agency.
3. The duration and frequency of all disciplines. For example, skilled nursing 1wk1, 2wk2; physical therapy 1wk1, 3wk2, 2wk2, 1wk2; occupational therapy 2wk5; home health aide 3wk4.

> **Author's Note:** 1wk1 means that the frequency for week 1 was once. 3wk2 means 3 times a week for 2 weeks.

4. The anticipated discharge plan for the patient. For example, outpatient PT; home with caregiver with appropriate instructions.
5. For Medicare clients, all of the current diagnoses and medications are included in the POC.[12]
6. Physician orders that may differ from those listed on the referral to home care. These may include frequency and duration of services, modalities, supplies, and interventions.

The POC should be thoroughly reviewed prior to sending to the referring physician for signature. If the POC contains orders that are different from the referral as in #6 above, verbal communication/contact with the physician needs to be performed and documented describing these differences at the time of the evaluation. If there is no record of physician approval for the changes, an agency may not be entitled to payment for services until after a signed POC is returned. Agencies should check with their intermediary for specific guidelines regarding the POC.

A. Writing Goals for the POC

The home environment provides physical therapists the opportunity to write realistic and functional goals for their clients. Not only can the therapist observe what tasks the patient is able to perform or not perform, but is also able to note the many obstacles that prevent the task from being completed safely. Clinicians often have to simulate environments in the hospital or rehab setting that more often than not, provide a poor substitute for the patient's specific needs. One example of this difference involves narrow doorways. In the hospital or other inpatient settings, most rooms have wide doors to accommodate beds and wheelchairs. Physical therapists may encounter narrow doors in the home where the patient cannot maneuver their walker or wheelchair. Goals that address these practical conditions should be included.

In the home, therapists should discuss with the patient and their caregivers specific behaviors that are required for the patient to function safely. Goals should not only include necessary functions like bathing and dressing, but may include leisurely functions such as arts and crafts, or even home maintenance tasks such as gardening and house cleaning. However, home maintenance or leisure should not be the primary focus of the goals. Goals should focus on the patient's functional needs in the home and immediate surroundings. Insurance providers expect PT services to provide a significant change in function in a reasonable amount of time.[1] Therefore, a time frame for each goal and outcome should be determined. Goals may be classified as *short term*, which can be accomplished in a few days or a week, or *long term*, which implies weeks or even months. The CMS does not require the headings of short or long term, but rather the identification of time period. In either case, all goals should involve the collaboration of the patient and/or caregiver, and should be updated at regular intervals as the patient improves (or declines).

When writing goals for homebound patients, the physical therapist should consider the following:

1. What was the patient's previous level of functioning?
2. What types of equipment, devices, orthotics, etc. are needed?
3. Is there anyone else available to assist the patient to meet the goal?
4. How long is the patient expected to be homebound?
5. How is this goal going to be measured in order to demonstrate improvement?
6. How many visits are needed to reach the goal?
7. Based on the findings from the evaluation, how much progress/improvement can be expected in a reasonable time frame and still meet the legal requirements for reimbursement?

■ Example 1

Examples of measureable short-term goals:

Patient will ambulate 20 ft from the bed to the bathroom in dim lighting with full weight bearing on both lower extremities with supervision and without the use of an assistive device to reduce the risk of falls in 1 week.

Patient will perform sit to stand at the kitchen table with contact guard assist in 3 days to improve safety at mealtimes.

■ Example 2

Examples of measureable long-term goals:

Patient will negotiate 4 stair steps with supervision using a railing on one side only in 3 weeks in order to go from the kitchen to the garage.

Patient will be able to stand for 10 minutes at the bathroom sink without upper extremity support and without loss of balance in 4 weeks in order to perform personal hygiene.

B. Documenting Interventions in the POC

The PT should include the interventions needed to meet the goals or describe the plan for the duration of treatment.[1] If a PTA will be treating the client, interventions should be appropriate and clearly understood by the PTA. When selecting interventions for a patient, the PT should consider the patient's medical and social history, cognition and learning ability, and discharge plan. Outside agencies may review this POC, so if a particular treatment is known only by a select group of people, it needs to be described in detail that is easily comprehended.

Some poor examples of intervention documentation include transfer training, modalities prn, and Back in Action Program. Each of these interventions could be improved by providing more information describing the equipment required, progression of the treatment, or components of the program. The PT should remember that with Medicare Part B patients interventions should be preceded by the CPT code verbiage. Some improved examples of interventions are as follows:

1. Therapeutic activities: Training and education for car transfers using a midsize SUV—progressing to SBA with caregiver.

2. Electrical stimulation: attended: Functional electrical stimulation to right quadriceps for 1 week to facilitate knee extension in gait.

3. Therapeutic procedures: Therapeutic strengthening exercises for trunk and hips with gradual progression of trunk extension. Increase resistance by 1 lb when patient is able to perform 10 repetitions of each exercise with decreased assistance to stabilize pelvis.

VIII. TREATMENT/VISIT NOTES, PROGRESS REPORTS, AND REASSESSMENTS

In home care, each visit requires a written record to be completed on the same day as the visit. Whether hand written or electronic, each visit note should correlate to one or more goals and interventions from the POC. In addition, visit notes provide the opportunity to explain any training or education that was given and the patient's response to that teaching. Typically, PTs and PTAs also discuss any collaboration with other providers working with this patient and plans for the next visit.[1] The record should also include the communication between the PT and the PTA.

For each treatment, PTs and PTAs should document the progress toward goals.[16] This progress can be in percentages, amount of assistance needed, progression to least restrictive device, etc. Communication to other disciplines working with the client is imperative to prevent any duplication of services and assist in the progression of the patient. For example, if the client can now achieve gait to the bathroom safely, then the OT or COTA may be able to progress from bed/chair baths to tub/shower baths. This may also apply to the home health aide and their ability to mobilize the patient safely to the bathroom. Documenting progress at each treatment allows the clinician to evaluate over time if the treatment is effective.

Vital signs should be documented at a minimum pre and post interventions, as well as intermittently as needed. Stabilization of respiratory rate and pulse over time is a good indicator of progress relative to aerobic capacity/endurance.

If the patient was taught the rate of perceived exertion, dyspnea scale or another tool was used, they should also be administered and documented in ongoing entries.

In most therapy practices and for most payers, the format of the report may be SOAP, narrative, or template, based on provider policy, and PTs are required to complete progress reports. The progress report differs from a daily note in that it provides a summary of the treatment and the amount of improvement (or lack of improvement) since the last evaluation or progress note, as well as describes the current status of the patient. The report should justify the need for PT and be closely related to the current POC. Progress notes may be requested by third party payers at any time or by physicians prior to an office visit by the patient. Although PTAs may gather data to be included in the progress note, the note must be written by the physical therapist to comply with APTA policy, Medicare guidelines, and applicable state law.[5]

The PT should be seeing the patient every 10 days on the average both in order to document progress and to be able to document the discharge appropriately. On November 2, 2010, the CMS released a final ruling on the payment update and policies related to the Home Health Prospective Payment System for the 2011 calendar year. The new reassessment documentation requirement will begin on January 1, 2011 and enforced on April 1, 2011. It states that a physical therapist reassessment in rural and non-rural areas under extenuating circumstances must take place at defined points during the course of treatment prior to the 14th and 20th therapy visits and at least every 30 days. This reassessment must include objective measurements of function and successive comparison of measurements. More information can be obtained at http://www.cms.gov/HomeHealthPPS/Downloads/Therapy_Requirements_Fact_Sheet.pdf.

Unfortunately, all home health patients do not always improve. If a client does not progress either by reaching a plateau where there is no change, or by declining in function, the clinician should consider the following:

1. Has there been a change in the medical condition? Has the disease worsened?
2. Is there a medication complication?
3. Is the treatment provided ineffective?
4. Were the initial goals unrealistic?
5. Should someone else treat the patient?
6. Should the patient be referred to a physician or other health care provider?

The lack of progress does not automatically indicate that an insurance company will deny payment. Clinicians should document their decision-making abilities when they evaluate progress and provide comments on why they believe the patient's behavior has a change or plateau. This type of documentation helps to demonstrate the level of skill required to manage these clients. It may be necessary to revise the goals of the treatment.

A. Documentation of Skill

Home health, not unlike other settings, requires therapists and assistants to document the unique skills they provide the patient during each visit. Since it is highly unlikely that a clinician would report that they lack skill, the most plausible explanation for the lack of documentation is the knowledge of how to indicate skill in their treatment notes. According to the CMS, skilled rehabilitation services require the technical or professional knowledge of the clinician, or the supervision of the clinician to be safe and/or effective.[12] If the treatment could be provided by a family member, or caregiver of the patient, without supervision, the treatment is most likely nonskilled.

In order to prevent a denial for lack of skill, the PT and PTA should verify in each note that there exists documentation of what unique skill he or she provided during the treatment. A typical visit note may include many actions that the patient performed, such as gait, transfers, or exercises, but to meet this objective, there should be no question of what skill the PT or PTA performed. The best way to document would be to precede the patient performance with the interventions preceded by the CPT verbiage, as discussed previously.

Examples: Poor

1. Patient ambulated 100 ft with rolling walker without loss of balance.
2. Patient performed HEP as per written instructions.

Examples: Good

1. Patient able to ambulate to the mailbox 40′ with front wheeled rolling walker with PT facilitating weight shifting at the pelvis to lengthen LLE stride length and L hip flexion.
2. Patient required verbal instruction to complete 25% of exercise program correctly today and able to remember and perform 75% of the exercises with supervision.
3. Patient required moderate assistance and tactile facilitation techniques to perform right hip flexion exercises secondary to 2/5 muscle strength.
4. Patient able to perform sit to stand from the patient's 20-in.-high sofa with tactile cues on bilateral shoulder 3/5 times for adequate forward lean and verbal instructions for foot placement; heels posterior to knees.
5. Patient able to demonstrate gait with large based quad cane using R hand, on deep pile rug 15′ forward and negotiate R 180 degree turn with verbal instruction without loss of balance, required moderate assistance with trunk stabilization to prevent secondary loss of balance with 180 degree turn to L.

In addition to skill, the documentation should not be repetitive in nature for each visit, and not repeat itself for each following visit.[1] When utilizing electronic documentation or flow sheets this is more critical. If the same boxes are checked on the EMR at each visit, the notes will look the same visit after visit, even though the treatment may be different. Programs that allow you to read and edit the visit note prior to submitting may resolve some of these concerns, as do the systems that allow free style entry. As discussed earlier, if the treatment plan needs to be changed, document the justification and reasons for the change to demonstrate skill level. These suggestions may only take a few extra minutes to complete but can save hundreds or even thousands of dollars from third party denials.

IX. RECERTIFICATION, RESUMPTION OF CARE, AND DISCHARGE

Recertification and resumption of care are two concepts that are closely related to the OASIS document addressed previously, and critical to documentation.[12] A recertification occurs when the 60-day episode ends and the provider identifies that the patient will need continued home health services past the 60-day threshold. The provider would then conduct another OASIS assessment that is submitted to the CMS reporting the current status of the patient and need for additional services. A resumption of care occurs when a patient is within their 60-day episode and is admitted to and released from a hospital with a greater than 24-hour stay. The provider would complete another OASIS document that identifies the current status of the patient and any new diagnoses or procedures from the hospital stay.

Although both of these document tools are similar to the OASIS SOC document, the responses should clearly reflect the improvement or decline in function, the update of goals and interventions, the change in patient status, and the revision of diagnoses and procedures. For each of these documents, the assessing clinician is responsible for obtaining and documenting orders for all services to be recertified or resumed. Frequency orders for PT visits or additional discipline orders such as for home health aides, do not carry over the 60-day period or the 24-hour hospital stay.

In any setting, discharge planning begins at the time of the initial examination and evaluation. Since homebound status currently plays a critical role in reimbursement for Medicare patients, therapists must predict which goals can be reached and to which setting the patient will be discharged. For Medicare patients, a discharge OASIS is required at the time of discharge from the home health agency with a few exceptions such a hospital admission or death.[16] This document contains nearly identical questions to the SOC OASIS and a few additional questions concerning interventions provided. These additions such as diabetic foot care and depression interventions were described earlier. The responses at discharge are reviewed by the CMS and other agencies to determine whether or not the patient improved in any component of the evaluation. Individuals may review outcomes of any home health agency contracted with Medicare by visiting http://www.medicare.gov/HHCompare. The information is provided in aggregate; not by individual patient. Because the last clinician (SN, PT, OT, or ST) treating the patient completes the discharge OASIS, the other disciplines should each be encouraged to write a discharge summary containing progress achieved to be included in the final OASIS. Frequent communication among disciplines is vital to obtaining the most accurate responses at discharge. The discharge summary, or summation of care, should address all problems identified at SOC in the initial examination and evaluation; the interventions provided, the goals established, the status at discharge and whether the patient met their goals. If the patient did not meet the established goals or interim modified goals, the reason they did not must be addressed. There must also be a discharge plan. Example: Patient will continue physical therapy as an outpatient; Patient will continue with home exercises as instructed until modified by an outpatient therapist; Patient instructed to call agency if any questions.

X. COMMUNICATION AND SUPERVISION

The importance of communication cannot be stressed enough in home care, and although it occurs on many levels, every day, for every patient, communication often fails to be documented every time it occurs. Communication involves anyone associated with the care of the patient including doctors, pharmacists, transportation companies, medical equipment companies, etc., all subject to HIPAA regulations. The opening statement to this chapter described home health as being "without quick access" to others.[1] Therefore, a concerted effort must be made to conduct regular case conferences with every discipline involved with a particular client and document the discussion and outcome in the medical record. If a patient is being treated by a PT and PTA, routine communication is warranted to ensure that the POC is followed and the appropriate level of supervision is conducted. With the easy access to cell phone technology and computers, it is possible in any home care situation to communicate. It is imperative to remember not to be tempted to discuss patients via phone or email in public places where conversation can be overheard or computer screens viewed by others.

Presently, the CMS does not provide specific supervision requirements for the PTA by the PT. Home health agencies are directed to review the physical therapy practice act of the state in which they are located for guidance. State practice acts do vary in supervision requirements and failure to perform what is legally required could subject an agency to severe fines and penalties.

XI. HOME HEALTH AUDITS

Audits in home health are regularly performed by the state in which the agency is licensed. However, there are now a number of government agencies that are playing a role in the auditing of Medicare payments. The most prominent group is the Recovery Audit Contractors (RAC) launched in 2005 in California, Florida, and New York, and was nationwide by 2008, which is discussed in Chapter 1.[2,21] These companies are contracted by the Department of Health and Human Services to identify underpayments and overpayments to providers of Medicare Part A and Part B, and are paid through a contingency of recovered funds. More information concerning RAC can be obtained at www.cms.gov/RAC/. Although physical therapy has not been the primary target of these audits in the past, the profession should anticipate increased numbers of audits for utilization, as well as those discussed earlier in this chapter: legibility, lack of medical necessity, lack of skill, etc. As the audits are conducted using the documentation, this is additional justification for appropriate, objective, skilled documentation.

A. Documenting Medicare and Insurance Appeals in Home Care

Medicare intermediaries perform regular audits of its providers. The most common first step is issuing an additional documentation request (ADR) to the provider.[22] The provider must submit the requested documentation as requested by a specified date. The requesting agency may accept the documentation, request additional information, deny payment, or request a full or partial refund if a payment was made. If a denial is issued, the provider has two options; accept the denial and make remuneration, or appeal the decision. When appealing a denial, one must follow the directions of the agency issuing the denial policies and procedures of that agency. If the services were justified and supplemental documentation is available, then an appeal is the appropriate action. When preparing the appeal, any or all of the following documents to support the appeal should be provided:

1. Supportive documentation for other treatment dates not in question
2. Progress reports or summaries
3. Communication with physician or other health care professionals
4. Nursing notes, or notes from other disciplines
5. State Practice Act

6. APTA's Guide to Physical Therapist Practice

7. Communication with the insurance carrier

8. Additional explanation

For more information concerning Medicare appeals, go to *Appeals and Grievances* at http://www.cms.gov/home/medicare.asp.

B. Pay for Performance

One topic that is gaining momentum in home health is pay for performance (P4P). P4P involves increased revenue to providers who achieve or exceed predetermined benchmarks of quality and/or cost.[1,23,24] This incentive payment has led numerous home care providers to institute changes in their processes for patient care. The improvements include the following:

1. Transition to electronic documentation

2. Enhancements to technology

3. Higher standards of practice

4. Addition of standardized testing and outcome measures

5. Improved patient satisfaction

6. Ensuring their practitioners are appropriately equipped

At present, the CMS is conducting research on P4P and has implemented components of the program in physician offices and medical practices.[24] Over the next few years, therapy providers should anticipate further clarification on this topic. Clinical documentation will play a key role in the evaluation and determination of payment for this program.

XII. CONCLUSION

Home health documentation is constantly evolving based on federal and state regulations. This section is not intended to be a substitute for learning the specific requirements for Medicare or non-Medicare providers, nor is it comprehensive in addressing all of the documentation concerns in home health. PTs and PTAs must be vigilant in keeping up with these changes to be successful in this field of practice. Though the home health documentation responsibilities may seem overwhelming, it is not dissimilar in content to the requirements for other venues. The benefits and rewards of working with people one on one in the comfort of their homes ameliorate the documentation challenges.

REFERENCES

1. American Physical Therapy Association. Defensible Documentation Resource – An Introduction. http://www.apta.org/AM/Template.cfm?Section=Documentation4&Template=/MembersOnly.cfm&NavMenuID=3366&ContentID=64544&DirectListComboInd=D. Accessed July 20, 2010.

2. American Physical Therapy Association. Home Health Section. *Guidelines for the Provision of Physical Therapy in the Home*, 2nd ed. http://www.homehealthsection.org/displaycommon.cfm?an=1&subarticlenbr=21. Accessed August 14, 2010.

3. American Physical Therapy Association. Home Health Section. Information for Consumers and Other Visitors. http://www.homehealthsection.org/displaycommon.cfm?an=1&subarticlenbr=11. Accessed August 14, 2010.

4. Centers for Medicare and Medicaid Services. Medicare Claims Processing Manual. Chapter 5 – Part B Outpatient Rehabilitation and CORF/OPT Services. http://www.cms.gov/manuals/downloads/clm104c05.pdf. Accessed August 7, 2010.

5. American Physical Therapy Association. Guidelines: Physical Therapy Documentation of Patient/Client Management. (BOD G03-05-16-41). http://www.apta.org/AM/Template.cfm?Section=Home&TEMPLATE=/CM/ContentDisplay.cfm&CONTENTID=31688. Accessed July 20, 2010.

6. Centers for Medicare and Medicaid Services. Medicare enrollment: national trends 1966-2008. http://www.cms.gov/MedicareEnRpts/Downloads/HISMI08.pdf. Accessed July 10, 2010.

7. Centers for Medicare and Medicaid Services. OASIS – Background & History. http://www.dhss.mo.gov/

HomeCare/OASIS/OASIS-CBackgroundHistory. pdf. Accessed July 10, 2010.

8. U.S Department of Health and Human Services. Achieving a Transformed and Modernized Healthcare System for the 21st Century. CMS Strategic Action Plan 2006-2009. http://www. cms.gov/MissionVisionGoals/Downloads/ CMSStrategicActionPlan06-09_061023a.pdf. Accessed August 28, 2010.

9. Centers for Medicare and Medicaid Services. Medicare National Coverage Determinations Manual Chapter 1, Part 1 (Sections 10–80.12) Coverage Determinations. http://www.cms.gov/ manuals/downloads/ncd103c1_Part1.pdf. Accessed July 10, 2010.

10. U.S Department of Health and Human Services. Centers for Medicare and Medicaid Services. Fiscal Year 2011. Justification of Estimates for Appropriations Committees http://www.cms.gov/ PerformanceBudget/Downloads/CMSFY11CJ.pdf. Accessed August 20, 2010.

11. Cardiovascular monitoring devices. Oximeter. Federal Register 2006;21(8):55733–55734. Codified at 21 CFR §870.2700.

12. Centers for Medicare and Medicaid Services. 2010. Medicare Benefit Policy Manual Chapter 7 – Home Health Services. http://www.cms.gov/manuals/ Downloads/bp102c07.pdf. Accessed July 10, 2010.

13. Federal Bureau of Investigation Detroit. Press Release. *Home Health Agency Owner Pleads Guilty in Connection with Detroit Fraud Scheme*. February 17, 2010. http://detroit.fbi.gov/dojpressrel/pressrel10/ de021710.htm. Accessed September 4, 2010.

14. Borg G. *Borg's Perceived Exertion and Pain Scales*. Champaign, IL, Human Kinetics, 1998.

15. Centers for Medicare and Medicaid Services. *Could You Clarify CMS' Policy about the Homebound Status of Home Health Patients Who Can Drive?* April 4, 2008. https://questions.cms.hhs.gov/app/ answers/detail/a_id/9070/~/could-you-clarify- cms%E2%80%99-policy-about-the-homebound- status-of-home-health. Accessed August 7, 2010.

16. Centers for Medicare and Medicaid Services. OASIS-C Guidance Manual. http://www.cms.gov/ HomeHealthQualityInits/14_HHQIOASIS UserManual.asp. Accessed July 10, 2010.

17. Centers for Disease Control and Prevention. Classification of Diseases, Functioning, and Disability. http://www.cdc.gov/nchs/icd.htm. Accessed September 4, 2010.

18. Yesavage JA, et al. Development and Validation of a Geriatric Depression Screening Scale: A Preliminary Report. *J Psychiatric Res* 1982:17(1);37–49.

19. Cornell Scale for Depression in Dementia. www. ncbi.nlm.nih.gov/pubmed/3337862. Accessed August 28, 2010.

20. CAHABA Government Benefit Administrators, LLC. Documenting Medical Necessity of Physical Therapy. http://www.cahabagba.com/rhhi/coverage/ home_health/pt_doc.htm. Accessed August 21, 2010.

21. American Physical Therapy Association. Home Health Section. Regulatory and Legislative News. http://www.homehealthsection.org/displaycom- mon.cfm?an=1&subarticlenbr=34. Accessed August 21, 2010.

22. Centers for Medicare and Medicaid Services. MLN Matters. https://www.cms.gov/MLNMattersArticles/ downloads/MM4022.pdf. Accessed September 4, 2010.

23. Delaune MF, Bemis-Dougherty A. *Documentation in Physical Therapy Services*. PT Magazine, Feb 2007. http://www.apta.org/AM/Template.cfm?Section= Current_Issue1&Template=/CM/HTMLDisplay. cfm&CONTENTID=42468. Accessed August 16, 2010.

24. Centers for Medicare and Medicaid Services. U.S Department of Health and Human Services. Development of a Plan to Transition to a Medicare Value-Based Purchasing Program for Physician and Other Professional Services. Issues Paper. Public Listening Session. December 9, 2008. http://www.cms. gov/PhysicianFeeSched/downloads/PhysicianVBP- Plan-Issues-Paper.pdf. Accessed September 4, 2010.

CHAPTER 6 REVIEW QUESTIONS

1. What criteria are need for Medicare part A home care benefit?

2. List some examples of when a home bound patient can leave the home.

3. What is the OASIS used for and what categories are examined?

4. What does the ICD-9 code represent?

5. Under the OASIS how can the PT objectively document pain?

6. List 5 functional tasks that can be assessed under the OASIS.

7. Under Medicare how often should the PT be seeing the patient?

8. What are the things the PT should consider if the patient is not progressing?

9. Describe pay for performance in home health.

7 Legal Issues in the Medical Record

I. INTRODUCTION

"Effective patient care documentation is as important as the delivery of care itself."[1] The process of health information management by healthcare professionals presents challenges and legal responsibilities. In all documentation, physical therapy professionals must abide by professional standards, ethical codes, accreditation standards, and legal requirements in creating a permanent record of patient/client data.

Physical therapists are responsible for creating, maintaining, and disclosing patient care medical record information as authorized by the patient or as dictated by law. Legally, the records created serve as the best evidence of patient information obtained and shared, the care rendered, the role of the healthcare provider, and whether the professional and legal standards of care were met or breached. For these reasons, physical therapists who document and collect patient health information (PHI) need to understand medical record/health information laws to ensure that they act responsibly and in compliance with applicable laws, and identify when expert legal advice is indicated.

The significance of documenting patient care accurately, comprehensively, concisely, objectively, contemporaneously or within reasonable time, and legibly cannot be overemphasized. Content substantiates billing for reimbursement and need for present and future physical therapy/medical services. The consequences of altered, incomplete, or nonexistent records can be legally and personally catastrophic. Practical application of risk management (prevention of any type of loss—financial or otherwise) and quality care includes proper documentation. The medical record frequently is the most important document available in defending against or preventing legal actions, including but not limited to personal injury suits, criminal cases, workers' compensation actions, disability determinations, and claims of negligent or improper healthcare (medical malpractice), and is generally admissible at a trial.[2] It also serves to communicate with others as to the patient's status and progress in therapy.

II. CHANGING ENVIRONMENT

The changing healthcare environment, growth of managed care organizations (MCOs) and likelihood of increasing government involvement, the widespread use of technological advances, trend towards national PHI data banks, and direct access PT permitting primary care provision, therapists are assuming new duties and greater responsibilities in roles as healthcare providers and in healthcare organization delivery systems.

With the dominance of managed care, the decisions regarding care issues, such as visit authorization are constant. Working within stringent allowances for treatment periods will continue to be a challenge for clinicians. As a result, physical therapists need to be effective advocates for their patients to ensure appropriate approval of treatment and payment. The ability to document defensively is essential, as the contents of the medical records could negatively impact defensibility against claims or authorization for additional care.

Documentation may not solve the dilemma of extending treatment for those who have been terminated by third-party payers, but proper recording of patient care may validate the need for more treatment while protecting against risk of liability.

III. MEDICAL RECORD AS A BUSINESS AND LEGAL DOCUMENT

The medical record is a permanent record, whether manual or electronic, of substantive and objective evidence of patient information obtained and medical care rendered by providers when legal wrongdoing is alleged. The record forms a basis from which an expert witness can formulate an opinion as to whether acceptable standards of care were met. It may also provide substantive evidence of work or functional capacity in workers' compensation hearings and other administrative proceedings. The recording of informed consents may serve to protect healthcare providers and organizations by demonstrating evidence that a patient understood the risks and benefits of a procedure and made an informed decision to proceed with or terminate care. Inclusion of patient goals or those of a responsible party for therapy and their participation in the decision-making aspects of care will verify patient or caretaker autonomy. In cases where patients/clients have signed advanced directives, appropriate documentation protects providers who must carry out the directives.

Author's Note: Unless therapy services are being provided in a hospital, skilled nursing facility or through a Medicare-certified home health agency, it is not common practice to have a copy of the patient's "Do Not Resuscitate" (DNR) directives in the medical record. It is recommended that this be included with patient/client information on the initial patient visit.

Generally, laws, regulations, and standards contain requirements for medical recordation relevant to end-of-life decision making. The medical record should clearly detail pertinent information concerning the patient's decision and plan prior to the physician's order to withdraw or forego life-sustaining treatment.

The patient care record is a routinely generated business record that serves as the legal record of the nature, extent, and quality of care given to the patient, as well as who rendered the care. Therefore, the medical record has both business and legal significance and as such serves to protect the patient and the professional. Primary healthcare providers are required by legal, business, and ethical standards to record and safeguard clinically relevant patient history, examination and evaluative findings, and treatment-related information in PHI records. State and federal laws, organizational policies and procedures, and customary practices in the setting, should be consulted to determine who can legally enter PHI in the medical record. This information may be entered electronically or manually, and the record maintained electronically or in hard copy for time dictated by law.

IV. THE LAW

A. Statutes

Laws define and govern relationships among private individuals and organizations. Four primary sources of law are constitutions, statutes, administrative agencies, and court decisions. The U.S. Constitution is considered the supreme law of the land because it establishes and grants power to the three branches of federal government (legislative, executive, and judicial) and restricts actions of federal and state governments. Amendments one through ten of the Constitution are called the Bill of Rights. The 14th Amendment places due process requirements on state governments, as does the 5th Amendment on federal government, and as such, they assure equal protection under the law. The power related to the regulation of healthcare traditionally falls upon the states, as protected by "police powers" assured under the 10th Amendment, which reserves states' rights to regulate behaviors for the general welfare, morals, health, and safety within its boundaries. State powers have been declining with the growth of federal government involvement in healthcare regulation. With respect to regulation of hospitals and healthcare professionals, constitutionally protected rights of privacy and liberty are often at issue. Arguably with the recent passage of "Obama Care" we now have a protected right to access to health care for more of our population.

> **Author's Note:** The Obama health plan was passed by Congress in March 2010 and is expected to be phased into practice over the next 4 years. Many of the specifics of the plan are not known as of the publication of this book.

Laws enacted by legislatures (U.S. Congress, state, and local legislatures) are called statutes and codes. For situations in which federal and state law conflict, valid federal law supercedes. When state and local laws conflict, valid state law supercedes. Medical record laws are generally governed by state legislation and regulation, and as a result may vary from state to state. Applicable medical information provisions are found in laws for healthcare information confidentiality, healthcare provider licensure (practice), communicable diseases, child and elder abuse, peer review, fraud, and the dying process.

Courts interpret and determine whether statutes and regulations are constitutional and render decisions in matters not controlled by existing laws.

B. Administrative Rules and Regulations

The legislature (federal or state) delegates authority to healthcare agencies to regulate professionals, professional practices, and enforce laws because it lacks the time and expertise to address the complex issues involved. These regulations are enforced as laws, and violation of a regulation is often accompanied with violation of comparable law. Additionally, healthcare agencies may provide guidelines related to patient care documentation. The Joint Commission on Accreditation of Healthcare Organizations (JCAHO) and the Centers for Medicare and Medicaid Services (CMS)/Medicare expect that documentation in patient medical records be timely, accurate, complete, legible and be free from abbreviations.

V. MEDICAL MALPRACTICE

Since the 1970s, there has been a "malpractice crisis" characterized by excessive numbers of lawsuits and verdicts in favor of patient/clients primarily against physicians and large organizations. Physical therapists are increasingly vulnerable to lawsuits with the expansion of professional practice into primary care, direct consumer access, clinical specialization, and responsibilities delineated in the *Guide to Physical Therapist Practice*.[3] Effective, systematic communication with patients/clients and other health professionals involved in care, with appropriate documentation, helps to reduce risk.

The legal bases for imposing liability on physical therapists are professional negligence, breach of contract, strict product liability, strict liability, and intentional misconduct. Professional negligence or medical malpractice occurs when the delivery of patient care falls below the acceptable standard of care; minimal standards of ordinary, reasonable practitioners acting under similar circumstances. When a therapist performs or fails to perform something during examination, evaluation, treatment, or follow-up, that other similarly situated therapists would not find acceptable, and harm (adverse outcome) comes to the patient, professional negligence exists. In pursuing a successful action for medical malpractice, the injured party or plaintiff must prove it by a preponderance of the evidence or that it is more likely than not that:

1. the therapist (defendant) owed the patient a special duty of care;
2. the therapist breached or failed to exercise that duty of care;
3. the violation of the standard of care caused physical and/or mental injury to the patient;
4. the patient suffered legally recognizable damages for which money can be awarded as compensation to make the patient whole again.

The important message is that accurate, complete, timely, and concise documentation not only may save patient lives, but writing consistent with these criteria may save a professional career. In an action for malpractice, the written treatment record may be the sole objective evidence of whether care to the patient was in compliance with acceptable standards or was substandard.

A. Terminating Care/Patient Abandonment

In most situations, healthcare providers can decline to initiate care but the same choice does not apply to discontinuing care that was initiated. When a healthcare provider or organization unilaterally terminates a professional relationship with a patient inappropriately without the patient, his/her representative or healthcare surrogate's consent, when there remains need for continued service, legal abandonment occurs. Legally actionable abandonment based on professional negligence or intentional misconduct may result under a variety of situations ranging from temporarily leaving a patient unattended to terminating service when a patient has not achieved rehabilitative goals or progress towards goals has plateaued.

Patients are able to unilaterally terminate care without consequence (excluding responsibility for cost of care) because they are not bound by legal or ethical standards. However, the physical therapist must exercise certain steps to avoid potential liability for patient abandonment. Unilateral termination of the professional–patient relationship is legal when the patient voluntarily makes an informed election to end the relationship, or there is mutual agreement. Termination of care unilaterally is legal when the patient's medical condition has resolved or therapy goals are met. Discharging a patient at other times places the physical therapist at risk for inappropriate premature discharge. To prevent claims of unjustified, unilateral termination, physical therapists must carefully document all activities in the patient's care record.

Typical situations that result in abandonment include nonpayment of charges, failed reimbursement, and personality conflicts between practitioners and patients.[4] Under managed care, practitioners are becoming increasingly liable for patient abandonment due to patient inability to pay for continued intervention. To avoid legal issues of abandonment, good practice would be to advise the patient when a third-party payer has preauthorized a specific number of visits, and to record same in the medical record. If the therapist decides to seek reconsideration for additional visits, care must be taken not to promise the patient/client that it will be obtained. If more sessions are not granted but were promised, the therapist may be held responsible for "abandoning" the patient/client if the patient believed additional care was needed. Alternatively, the therapist can offer the option of private pay. If the patient/client declines, this can be documented to avoid the appearance or accusation of abandonment.

Author's Note: A recent Supreme Court ruling declared that a health maintenance organization's denial of payment for services rendered does not indicate that care may not be needed. Denial of payment does not equate with denial of care. Therefore, there arises an ethical dilemma if a professional believed care should be given or continued. CMS Medicare regulations indicate that if a professional believes care should be continued even if reimbursement is not, it is incumbent on the professional that care be continued.

When anticipating the need to unilaterally discontinue care, the practitioner should be honest with the patient in explaining the reasons for termination care and provide assistance with transferring the patient's care to another provider and providing the patient records.

Physical therapists are held to the same standards of professional performance and abandonment regardless of the form of reimbursement or whether services are provided pro bono (free of charge), and documentation principles should be consistent regardless of payment.

VI. CONFIDENTIALITY, PRIVACY AND SECURITY, AND ACCESS

State Medical Record Access Laws ensure the confidentiality of the patient–provider relationship and impose a duty to guard against unauthorized disclosure on licensed health providers and covered entities (organizations and health plans). Additionally, the Health Insurance Portability and Accountability Act (HIPAA), passed in 1996, imposes a higher level of privacy, security, and confidentiality on all providers of healthcare than ever before. HIPAA privacy standards establish an individual's right to access their health information, limit when access can be denied, and list legal requirements for compilation and storage of patient medical information. HIPAA also requires healthcare organizations to designate a privacy officer to oversee and implement all health information privacy policies and procedures because the standards in their entirety are complex.

Prior to the HIPAA privacy rule, there was no generally applicable federal legislation protecting confidentiality of medical or personal information. There was a lack of conformity of existing regulations governing access, use, and disclosure from state to state.

In addition to HIPAA, accrediting agencies such as the Joint Commission, have also developed standards to assure security and confidentiality of the patient health data collected.

Computerization of patient information has enabled the immediate data exchange among authorized providers, payers, employers, and consumers both regionally and nationally. The use of electronic format in disclosing patient information is cost effective and promotes quality (and safety) of patient care. However, computerized records create challenges in protecting patient privacy as a result of the continual erosion of release guidelines. It is also becoming increasingly difficult to determine who owns and is responsible for protecting against unauthorized access to the medical content.

In 2003, the healthcare provider, as generator of the documentation, became owner of the medical record which was released or accessed only in accordance with the law. The ownership of the medical record is less clearly that of only the individual provider in managed care settings where the individual providers are employees of larger healthcare organizations. Under Florida law, for example, the employer may be the record owner.[5]

Healthcare personnel must access patient medical records for care reasons, administrative purposes, and defense against lawsuits. However, all personnel are legally required to safeguard the confidentiality of the records and prevent unauthorized use of the information. Generally, facilities have established policies and procedures to ensure that confidentiality of health information is maintained.

Specific state laws allow reporting of PHI without patient authorization when reporting vital statistics or matters affecting the public health, safety, or welfare. Some examples include reporting child and elder abuse or neglect, presence of communicable diseases, and victims of violent crimes. Since these requirements vary among the states, knowledge and understanding of reporting requirements for the state in which the provider practices is a necessity.

To comply with HIPAA rules regarding disclosure, healthcare providers must obtain the patient's consent to access, use, or disclose personally identifiable health (PHI) information for purposes of treatment, payment, and healthcare operations (TPO). The HIPAA privacy rule, in general, requires that patients have a right to a notice of privacy practice explaining how private health information will be used and disclosed. The notice should explain the individual's rights and covered entity's legal duties with respect to the private information. In most applications, patient consent must be obtained at the time the healthcare services are provided. According to HIPAA, the consent must be in plain language.

Consent for disclosure of PHI should be obtained in writing and it ordinarily does not specify a date of termination or revocation of the consent. With patient consent, only that information minimally necessary to accomplish the intended purpose can be revealed. Patient authorization is required for use or disclosure of information beyond the minimum necessary for treatment, payment, or support of healthcare operations. At a minimum, the disclosure should specify what information is to be disclosed, to whom it is being disclosed, and why it is being disclosed.[6] See HIPPA Disclosure Authorization Form CS-1786 (Appendix B).

The HIPAA privacy rule requires that healthcare providers and other covered entities must limit use, access, and disclosure to maintain patient privacy. The same standard applies to use of information by individuals working for the facility. Any staff requiring access to the record should be identified in institutional policies.

Protected health information under the privacy rule is expansive and includes information transmitted or maintained by electronic media or other form or medium. The privacy extends to any health information in any form or medium, including paper, electronic or digital imaging, and oral forms. The privacy standard also refers to designated record sets: health records, billing records, and various claim records used to make decisions about individuals.

As with many rules, patients are free to waive their privilege to privacy and nondisclosure of health information. It is recommended that any such waiver be written. Healthcare providers and facilities may be subject to civil and criminal liability for disclosing PHI that has not be authorized by the patient or required by law. HIPAA privacy and security violations may result in civil and criminal penalties of fines ranging from $25,000 for multiple violations of the same standard in a calendar year to $250,000 and/or imprisonment up to 10 years for knowing misuse of PHI.

Because insurers and MCOs generally require patient information before making utilization review or reimbursement decisions, some states have laws or have adopted the National Association of Insurance Commissioners Insurance Information and Privacy Protection Model Act (NAIC Model Act), which requires that confidentiality of information be preserved and that disclosure is limited to particular circumstances.[7]

Regardless of general laws, access to certain patient records, for example patients with alcohol and drug abuse problems, is expressly controlled by state and federal laws. Many states have special laws addressing and limiting staff access to records of mental health and HIV? AIDs patients. Only those personnel with a need to know and directly involved in a patient's care are permitted access under law.

The Privacy Act of 1974 places restrictions on the type of information a federal agency may collect about citizens and legal aliens, requires that individuals be informed as to the purposes and uses of the information, and limits how the information can be used (5 USC sect. 552a).[8] The Act also ensures that individuals can access and make copies of their records.

Hospitals operated by the federal government and MCOs that provide health insurance to government employees are subject to the guidelines of the Privacy Act. Healthcare facilities that receive federal funding may be subject to the Act, as well. Requested changes may be made to the information or explanation provided for denial of the request. Under certain circumstances, the Act permits the disclosure of information without consent.

The Freedom of Information Act (FOIA) allows public access to information about the operations and decisions of federal administrative agencies.[9] Specific categories of information are available to the public, subject to nine specific exceptions. Of the noted exceptions, personnel and medical files are relevant to healthcare in that disclosure would violate rights to privacy. Requested records must be made available promptly and there are rules establishing when and where the records can be inspected and the fee for copying. Laws permit the patient or patient representative to examine and copy the medical record. This requires a written request and payment of reasonable clerical costs for copying the record. State laws provide that records only need to be made available at reasonable times and places.

HIPAA was amended by the American Recovery and Reinvestment Act of 2009 aka "the Stimulus Bill." A portion of this law, called the Health Information Technology for Economic and Clinical Health Act, or HITECH Act, was designed to further federal government interests in proliferating the use of electronic health records (EHR) by healthcare providers and organizations but maintain confidentiality of PHI. It also imposes a 60-day breach notification for unauthorized disclosures of patient medical information.[10] With the new health care reform bill signed into law on March 22, 2010, clinicians and organizations can expect further changes that will impact health information technology and transmissions, and documentation requirements.

A. Responding to a Patient Request for Release of Health Information

There are many reasons for a patient to request his or her medical records other than for a potential malpractice claim. It may be prudent and a good risk management procedure to meet with the patient to answer questions directly and in layperson's terms. This type of meeting may prevent the filing of a claim or avert litigation. It is well accepted knowledge that the chief complaint among litigants for bringing legal action against providers is the lack of communication. Prior to any patient meeting, it is wise to consult with appropriate risk management personnel.

Copies of healthcare records and other PHI should not be disclosed to third parties unless the patient authorizes the release in a signed document. Therapists should request a copy of this signed release from a third-party payer prior to releasing a copy of the patient's record.

Generally, disclosure of the medical record of a minor requires authorization from one parent or legal guardian. Parents typically are permitted access to a child's medical information. Under certain circumstances, the minor may be able to authorize release of medical information.

The Internet is increasingly being used for transmission of clinical information. Every healthcare provider and organization should exercise care to maintain patient confidentiality. Policies and procedures should enforce confidentiality standards and ensure appropriate secure technology. The primary risks in using the Internet are related to unauthorized access and unauthorized disclosure of healthcare information. The American Health Information Management Association (AHIMA) has developed guidelines for Internet use and security concerns. Healthcare providers using the Internet should comply with the AHIMA standards and applicable state or federal regulation.

VII. Legal Requirements for Medical Records

A. Record Security

It is important to safeguard medical records not only to protect patient confidentiality but also to prevent intentional alteration, removal, destruction, or falsification. HIPAA requires records be stored in a secure, restricted location, not to allow removal of the record from the premises unless court ordered, and to supervise patients and their representatives when examining the record. If a physical therapist (PT) or physical therapist assistant (PTA) is engaged in home health care, they must take care to also safeguard their records as they move patient to patient, home to patient, and home or patient to referring agency. This is applicable to hardcopy and electronic records.

B. Required Records

Healthcare providers must keep a medical record for each patient according to proper record-keeping procedures. Failure to abide by this requirement may result in liability. Institutional policies incorporating state laws, when applicable, should designate the types of patient care information to be included in each patient record, the length of time for record retention, and the proper methods for destruction of the record.

Patient medical records consist of personal, financial, social, and medical data. Personal information contains identification information such as full legal name, date of birth (DOB), sex, marital status, next of kin, person to contact in an emergency, occupation, and physician name(s). Information about the patient's employer, health insurance carrier, types of insurance coverage and policy numbers, and Medicare and Medicaid numbers are considered financial and are used for billing purposes. The patient's race and ethnicity, family relationships, community activities, and information about lifestyle or court orders are considered social data. The continuous recordations of the history of treatment form the clinical record. This may consist of patient complaint(s), medical and family histories, results of physical or other medically related examinations, course of treatment, diagnosis and therapeutic orders, informed consent, clinical observations, progress notes, consultation reports, nursing notes, reports of diagnostic tests and procedures, and operative reports.

The medical record may be hand written, typed, dictated, or computer-generated, but should be consistent in format and content data for each discipline within an organization. The record should be a complete, accurate, and current account of the history, condition, and treatment of the patient, including outcomes and all other appropriate information in chronological order.

C. Content Requirements and Maintenance

Required content in patient healthcare records vary and generally depend on relevant state and federal laws and regulations, accreditation standards, organizational and system requirements, patient clinical settings, and professional guidelines such as those contained in the *Guide to Physical Therapist Practice* (APTA, 2001) and the APTA *Defensible Documentation for Patient/Client Management* available at www.apta.org.

Therapists, assistants and other practice personnel responsible for documentation or any information which goes in the medical record, should know the rules and regulations for record content as required by the state in which they work. With the advent of technology, access to state and federal regulations is available through the Internet.

Healthcare providers who participate in federal reimbursement programs must comply with the federal regulations for record content and maintenance which may require a clinical record for each patient be maintained in accordance with professional standards, and to be promptly completed, filed, and retained [42 CFR sect. 482.24 (hospitals); 42 CFR sect. 418.74 (hospices); and 42 CFR sect. 484.48 (home health agencies)]. In facilities participating with CMS compliance, specific criteria for record content must be met. Conditions for CMS records are similar for all settings in which Medicare beneficiaries receive physical therapy.

Accrediting organizations also impose maintenance standards for records. The JCAHO requires the content of the health record in accredited organizations and hospitals to include member identification, diagnoses, plan of care, medical history, appropriate physical examinations, immunization and screening status, results of treatments, procedures and tests, referrals or transfers to other practitioners, and evidence of advance directives. For home health accreditation, records must contain patient's height and weight, dietary restrictions, documentation as to suitability of home for services provided, documentation of patient and family education, and list of individuals and organizations involved in the patient's care, as well as the information required by federal regulation such as those for the Medicare program in the OASIS (Outcome and Assessment Set).

Most facilities have adopted formal written policies concerning the content of medical records. For PTs, it is good practice to adopt and follow the content criteria established in the APTA *Guide to Documentation* (see Appendix E) in conjunction with the most current applicable state, federal, and accreditation requirements associated with medical records. As laws change, it is important to monitor for new pertinent laws and regulations, which is required of all PTs and PTAs.

D. Formats

Practitioners should ensure that the content and format used for documentation of patient/client information is understood by others involved in the care of the patient. It is up to the facility, department, or therapists to determine which format is selected. Additionally, from an organizational perspective, there should be consistency in content and format within a department and between therapists. Quality improvement (QI) or quality assurance (QA) initiatives should ensure that content is complete and appropriate to ensure the record will serve all identified purposes (See Chapter 12). Regardless of the format selected, the content should be objective in nature with all information matching and relevant. The necessity of the need for skilled intervention should be clear based on identified problems, planned interventions, and relevance of functional goals or outcomes.

Interestingly, written goals represent professional judgment and not necessarily a guarantee or warranty of a specific therapeutic result. Legally, patient intervention goals are generally not actionable. However, actual communication of therapeutic promises including documentation of said goals, may create contractual obligations to patients and legal liability, if not achieved, so care must be taken and realistic goals must be agreed upon by all appropriate parties.

VIII. PROBLEMS, ERRORS, AND PRACTICE

Problems with documentation can have serious legal ramifications. Therefore, it is important that therapists familiarize themselves with common errors and the recommendations for averting adverse consequences, and employ proper documentation skills. See Chapter 4 for more information.

A. Illegibility

Illegibility is a common documentation problem and may result in inability to translate patient care information. The solution is for therapists to write legibly, print, type, or utilize alternative documentation systems not based on handwritten notation. Additionally, the record must be complete. This is reinforced in the Medicare guidelines, which require that all entries be legible and complete [42 CFR sect. 482.24(c)].

B. Patient's Full Name

The patient's full legal name, last name first, and identifying information should be on every page of the medical record. Failure to correctly identify a patient receiving care is negligence and can lead to liability. When the record is copied, the lack of patient identification on any page can result in inappropriate filing or loss of information.

C. Date and Time of Patient Care

The date and usually the time of patient care should be included in all records. This will support time billed for that patient and can be used as evidence in any patient dispute regarding date and time of visit. If treatment time is not indicated, total treatment time or units should be at a minimum.

D. Standard Forms and Formats

Standard forms and formats that are universally understood by other providers in the same facility or network should be used. Standardization helps to ensure appropriate content and consistency. Although many physical therapy practices have adopted their own interpretation of a SOAP note, SOAP note format is not required by any federal or state regulation, and indeed may be inconsistent between practices or even within (which may be legally challenging). The "S" component may lead to denials if inappropriate information is included.

E. Indelible Black or Blue Ink

Indelible black or blue ink should be used for documenting patient care to prevent tampering with entries, especially in the advent of legal action. However, the facility must determine which color will be used by policy and to ensure uniformity.

In the event the pen runs out of ink while documenting, a therapist must complete the note. If another ink color is used, an explanation in parentheses should precede the second part of the patient note stating that the original pen ran out of ink. This parenthetical explanation should be initialed. This procedure is necessary to avoid implications of spoilage of records in a potential lawsuit.

Computerized entries should be saved automatically to prevent subsequent loss or alteration of patient content.

F. Blank Spaces

Blank spaces or lines are unacceptable in the record, as blanks may infer lack of completeness or create the potential to add information. Therapists should use each line to document care, leaving no spaces between lines or by putting diagonal lines through large empty spaces. In computerized or electronic records, the format is often preset and the professional documenting may have to simply comply with what an individual entry field allows.

G. Signatures

Signatures (or initialing patient care corrections or flowsheets) on entries are required for authentication purposes and to acknowledge legal and ethical responsibility for the information contained in the entry. Entries should bear legible legal signatures followed by professional title to demonstrate a skilled professional rendered care. When signatures are illegible, better practice is to print name below the signature. In most states, computer signatures constitute legal signatures, but the therapist should seek legal counsel for verification. Licensure number is recommended. If a PT or PTA student is documenting, their name must be followed by the designation SPT or SPTA, and a cosignature by the supervising therapist or assistant should follow. Students should also print their names to facilitate identification if needed.

■ Example 1

Rebecca Rosenthal, SPT Eric Shamus, PT, DPT # 2345
Rebecca Rosenthal, SPT

Author's Note: The professional designation for a physical therapist, according to the APTA is PT. State law may allow RPT or LPT. However, an educational degree such as MPT or DPT is not a professional designation. Therefore, an individual who wishes to use their professional title and educational level would sign:

Debra F. Stern, PT, DPT # *1234*

If a student signature is required and it is not clearly legible, the signature should be followed by the printed name. Although this is good practice for PTs and PTAs as well, the license number would be used for identification if the signature was illegible, provided the numbers were legible.

Rebecca Rosenthal, SPT
Rebecca Rosenthal, SPT

H. Error Correction

Error correction commonly consists of a single line drawn through the erroneous content, initialed, and dated, preferably with the time. The most important rule is not to hide the mistake by whiting it out, scratching it out, blacking it out, or writing over it. The addition of the words "error" or "mistake" are controversial and create an image of sloppy patient care which may impair a defense in a malpractice claim.

■ Example 2

Active ROM of ~~Left~~ Right *DFS*, 4/30/10 shoulder flexion: 100°/180°

I. Addendums

Addendums can be made or added to the patient record and should always contain the date of the addendum. If the treating professional is entering an addendum to an entry, it should be preceded by the date of entry, and state "Addendum to entry of…"

Amendments made at the patient's request should be included as an addendum with a notation explaining that the change was made at the patient's request. Patient amendments that are deemed inappropriate should be discussed with the patient. Generally, if the requested change is not made by the facility, it may be a good idea to permit the individual to insert a statement of disagreement in the record. Some states allow this procedure provided notice of change or statement is given to designated persons within certain time periods.

Intentional alteration of a medical record or writing an incorrect record may subject a provider to statutory sanctions, including license revocation. Altering or falsifying a chart to obtain Medicare or state health reimbursement is a crime under federal law, punishable by substantial fine or imprisonment [42 USC sect. 1320a-7b (a)].

J. Acceptable Abbreviations

Acceptable abbreviations save time and facilitate accurate communication. However, problems arise and can result in medical errors when abbreviations have more than one meaning, are open to multiple interpretations, are illegible and resemble other abbreviations or words, or are not widely known. (Providing a key within the record to a repeating abbreviation may alleviate potential errors). These are some of the reasons JCAHO has recommended that in JCAHO-accredited healthcare organizations, abbreviations are not to be used at all. Physical therapy professionals should only use abbreviations that have been approved or are universally disseminated within their practice or organization. Actionable medical malpractice liability may be attributed to the healthcare provider who authors and/or reads erroneous information conveyed by use of unintelligible abbreviations that result in patient injury (see Appendix A).

K. Improper Spelling and Grammar and Wordiness

Improper spelling and grammar, and wordiness create negative impressions of practitioner and are construed as practitioner carelessness that contributes to findings of liability. All entries should be as accurate and concise as possible to avoid confusion or discrepancy.

L. Orders or Referrals: Written, Verbal, Telephonic, E-mail, Fax Electronic

Illegible physical therapy referrals must be clarified before seeing the patient or carrying out the referral. Therapists should document any and all inquiries and physician responses regarding ambiguities in diagnostic and treatment referrals. State laws, policies of the facility, accreditation standards, and customary practices govern whether care is elicited under verbal orders. For most therapists, laws require written referrals in order to ensure reimbursement. In direct consumer access states, written referrals from other healthcare professionals may not be required; but reimbursement may be declined. In hospital, rehabilitation, and skilled nursing home settings, written referrals are required by Medicare and Medicaid by a physician.

The person taking a referral verbally, via telephone, e-mail, or fax, should transcribe the orders or referral into the medical record. It is not sufficient to make a copy, for example of the faxed referral and insert it into the medical record without transcribing the content directly into the record. State law may dictate who may take and transcribe the order, but in most cases, it is the licensed physical therapist, and may limit the taking or transcription of orders to physical therapy related orders or referral only. The entry should include what the order is for, the time it was taken (i.e., phone, verbal face-to-face, phone message as voice mail, email, fax, other), the prescribing/referring/ordering individual's name, and the name of the person who entered it into the medical record. Verbal, telephone, email, electronic, or faxed orders/referrals require authentication usually within 24–48 hours by the prescribing professional, based on organizational and/or accreditation guidelines or requirements. This practice will enhance communication and protect both the referring physician and the therapist. Policies related to verbal orders should require that only personnel qualified to understand physician orders be authorized to receive and transcribe them. In direct access states, therapists are responsible for knowing laws regarding the need, if any, to refer patients/clients to a physician. Written orders are preferable because they create fewer chances for error.

M. Timeliness

From the legal perspective, timeliness of medical record entries is important. Late entries mean that the records are incomplete for a period of time. Documentation should occur contemporaneously or as closely as possible to when the actual care is rendered. The longer the time lapse between the conclusion of care and the time that the note is written, the less accurate it will be. Untimely documentation that results in prolonged care or extension of patient discomfort is professional negligence and provides opposing attorneys opportunity to challenge the accuracy of the entire content of the note. In the event a late entry into the medical records must be made, for example, when the record is unavailable, it should be designated as an "addendum" or "follow-up entry." Transcribed or dictated entries (whether transcribed and dictated by external service or directly into a computerized voice-recognition system) should be received within 24 hours by the time of the next patient visit and should be reviewed for accuracy and corrected as necessary. It is unethical to document care before it is given.

N. Identification of Information Sources

Identification of patient information sources must be recorded. Failing to denote another practitioner's responsibility for clinical information provided may result in legal liability solely to the writer of the note and leads to misinterpretations as to who is responsible for patient care. If a primary care provider receives and documents clinical information regarding an adverse change in patient status, the provider is obligated to reexamine the patient expeditiously and should document accordingly to reduce risk for legal liability for inappropriate monitoring of the patient.

O. Blame or Disparaging Comments

Blame or disparaging comments should not appear in the medical record, unless the writer is willing to risk potential actions for defamation. However, statements made by patients relevant to the clinical services or that were provided must be entered into medical records in quotations. Before documenting a patient statement that appears contradictory to the patient's self-interest, the therapist should have the patient confirm the statement. In such a situation, it is advisable to have a witness, and ethically, the statement must be documented in the patient record when it contains clinically pertinent information.

P. Objective and Specific Findings

Objective and specific findings should be documented, whereas subjective findings or opinions should not. It is recommended that writing ambiguous statements starting with "it appears" or "apparently" be avoided.

■ Example 3

Incorrect: Patient was apparently in pain following therapeutic exercise of the RLE (right lower extremity).

Correct: Patient C/O (complained of) proximal RLE "stabbing pain," 8/10, following therapeutic exercise of the RLE.

Important details should not be presumed. For example, "ROM WNL" (range of motion within normal limits) does not tell the reader what joints were examined and is, therefore, not sufficient.

Q. Informed Consent

Informed consent for examination and treatment must be documented in the patient medical record, preferably as a separate form. It may be verbally obtained by the therapist and documented. The concept of informed consent originates from the legal and ethical rights that patients have to direct what happens to their own bodies. Medical informed consent generally requires that the patient be given sufficient information concerning the nature and risks of the recommended and alternative treatments to make an educated decision. The general rule is that if patient consent is not given, the patient is not serviced. However, the patient must be competent to make an appropriate decision based on the information received. In some circumstances, such as under emergencies and compulsory treatments when a patient may not be competent to give consent, the law implies consent and temporary care is given.

The Patient Self-Determination Act, effective December 1, 1991, codifies a patient's common law right to control their healthcare decisions and binds all facilities and providers participating in Medicare and Medicaid programs. The Act ensures that patients are educated to make "informed decisions" and have rights to make "advanced directives." The Act respects ethical rights of persons to make autonomous decisions about their bodies. In accordance with this law, facilities and organizations should require written informed consent from patients, including written policies and procedures protecting patient rights and documentation of whether a patient executed advanced directives.

A well-written, properly executed consent form is strong evidence that informed consent was given, although it is not legally conclusive. To be a legally effective consent form, the document should be signed voluntarily, indicate that the procedure performed is the same consented to, and demonstrate that the consenting person understood the nature of the procedure, the risks, and probable consequences. This can be done with a short or long form. The short form is generalized and does not contain specific risks and benefits. It is advisable to supplement the short form by writing detailed notes regarding risks and benefits discussed in the patient medical record. The long form includes a detailed description of the medical condition, proposed procedure, consequences, risks, and alternatives. The danger in using this form is that providers rely on it and may substitute the form rather than explain the information to the patient to assure understanding. In the absence of a long or short form, at minimum a therapist should document that the treatment was explained and consent was given.

Generally, a person's consent constitutes authorization for a particular practitioner to perform a particular procedure, so deviation from that authorization may invalidate the consent. Further, refusal of consent to treatment by a certain practitioner removes that practitioner from engaging in the treatment.

For situations in which adequacy of information given is disputed, courts will apply standards of the reasonable physician, the reasonably prudent patient, or a subjective standard (i.e., what would this patient need to know and understand). The trend is to apply the reasonable patient standard, wherein the physician's duty to provide information is determined by the information needs of the average patient, not the specific patient or professional practice.

Persons with difficulties understanding English must have the form translated into their native language to avoid any question that the patient understood the content and was able to give an educated consent. Healthcare providers servicing multiple cultural and ethnic populations should have consent forms in primary languages. It is usually sufficient to have a form translated orally. It is important to have a medically trained translator (not a family or community member) translate the form or certify that the form and discussion of the procedure have been translated for the patient. If a medically trained translator is not available, an individual accompanying the patient may be the only option for translation, but there is a risk that the information conveyed may not be accurate or complete and who the translator was should be documented.

For minors, parent or guardian consent must be obtained before treatment is given. If the minor needs emergency treatment, a statute gives the minor the right to consent when parents cannot be located, or a court order is needed. Legally, either parent can give effective consent for treatment, except when parents are legally separated or divorced, at which time, the consent of the custodial parent is typically required unless there is an agreement or court order permitting the non-custodial parent or requiring both to consent. A provider can rely on the parent(s) to tell them who has authority to consent to the minor's care.

Special consent requirements beyond informing as to risks and benefits are needed when patients undergo experimental treatments or participate in clinical research studies. Federal, state, and local laws, in addition to institutional polices and procedures, impose strict requirements for obtaining patient consent and should be consulted.

When a patient's condition changes significantly, the original consent may no longer be valid and new consent should be obtained. Patient refusal of consent and withdrawal of consent for treatment should be documented and the physician notified.

Theories of Consent. There are two theories of consent violations. One theory is based on the common law development of battery or violation of an individual's right to be free from harmful or offensive touching. Another theory is based on negligence whereby patients consent to procedures without having sufficient information to make an informed decision.

Refusal of Consent. Refusal of Consent is the legal right of competent adults to refuse medical treatment. Legally, courts have upheld these decisions despite the basis of the refusal. It is advisable to seek the advice of legal counsel and institutional legal advisors and ethics committees for situations in which the refusal is a serious threat to health and endangers the patient's life.

When a patient refuses to sign the consent form but is willing to give consent orally, the fact that verbal consent was given and the reason for refusal to sign the form should be documented on the consent form, along with the witnessed signature, and placed in the medical record.

IX. HOME INSTRUCTIONS/INDEPENDENT EXERCISE INSTRUCTIONS/OTHER INSTRUCTIONS

Home instructions, home exercise programs, independent exercise programs, other instructions, and the like must be documented, copies maintained, and preferably contain the patient/client or responsible party's signature and a statement indicating that they have been received and understood.

Standardized programs should be kept as part of clinical procedures manuals on site. If the standardized programs are identified by name or number, the name or number should be included in the documentation. As part of the documentation, the therapist should include that the patient, family, or other caregiver understands, safely carries out, and is responsibly complying with home programs of care. All precautions or limitations to activities and follow-up instructions must be documented. Lack of follow-up could be construed as actionable abandonment.

X. NONCOMPLIANCE/NONADHERENCE

Noncompliance, missed appointments, refusal of care, or nonadherence with given recommendations must be documented. The documentation should be objective, including specific times and dates of violations, and circumstances/descriptions of noncompliance. If a patient fails to comply and goals are not met or they suffer harm, and this is documented, contributory negligence may be construed making the patient partially responsible for an adverse outcome.

XI. INCIDENCE OR OCCURRENCE REPORTS

Incidence or occurrence reports are records of events that are unexpected and should not be included in the record or identified. It is important to objectively document the incident in the record and obtain quality care for any injuries. Risk management must be notified in order to protect the facility against unwarranted liability and educate to prevent similar future incidents. Incident or occurrence reports preserve memories of incidents. Since the reports are considered more administrative in nature and purpose, they are maintained separately from the patient medical record. In some organizations, formal reports may not be kept. It is up to the organization and risk carrier how an incidence or occurrence should be recorded.

XII. COUNTERSIGNATURE

Countersignature is expected for student documentation and recommended in the APTA *Guide to Physical Therapist Practice*. The reason the note must be cosigned is to authenticate the note and make it legally acceptable. The need for a countersignature legally is to assure that a professional has reviewed the note, and if appropriate, to indicate approval of action taken by another practitioner. The person who counter-signs has the authority to evaluate the entry and typically has more experience or has higher training than the person making the entry. Countersignatures permit delega-tion of responsibility. Providers who countersign another's notes should carefully proofread the note before cosigning. The countersignature imposes legal responsibil-ity for the information contained in the note. Incomplete or inaccurate notes should not be countersigned until corrected appropriately. Physical therapy students' entries must be countersigned by a physical therapist. Physical therapist assistant students' entries much be signed by a physical therapist or physical therapist assistant. Once countersigned, the physical therapy student's or physical therapist assistant student's note is legally adopted by the supervising therapist as his or her own note causing him or her to share the legal responsibility with the student for what is written in note. Without evidence of that supervision inferred by countersignature, a student might be held as violating and engaging in the unlicensed practice of physical therapy.

■ Example 4

12/15/10 While PT was swinging wheelchair leg rest to remove it, it swung back and into the patient's LLE above the lateral malleolus. No bruising noted.

XIII. AUTHENTICATION

Authentication and signature is made by the provider who delivers the care. Handwritten signatures were traditionally required. More recently, rubber stamps and computer key signatures are accepted and permitted by some states, and com-puter or electronic signatures are allowed by state and federal authorities.

The CMS requires authentication of each entry for Medicare participation. The CMS does allow authentication by computer, but not all entities allow this type of "auto-authentication." Failure to obtain a physician's signature to the record in its final form constitutes deficiency (BNA Health Law Reporter, October 21, 1993).

Author's Note: Rubber stamp signatures are not allowed on Medicare docu-mentation. If rubber stamp signatures are allowed in any cases, the therapist or assistant should control the use of the stamp and not leave it behind if they leave the practice.

XIV. RECORD RETENTION AND DESTRUCTION

Therapists should check for applicable statutory and regulatory requirements dic-tating retention in their particular state. The general period for retention of medi-cal records varies and should minimally cover the statute of limitations or period within which a party may bring a lawsuit. If participating under Medicare, retention of the original record or legally reproduced form must be for a period of at least 5 years. About half of the states require that original medical records be preserved for 10 years. Some facilities require record retention beyond statutes of limitations, including rules for deceased patients and deceased or relocating therapists. For electronic records, back up should be performed regularly and measures taken to preserve the information electronically.

The statute of limitations on contract and tort actions should also determine how long to keep records. Statutes of limitation based on various legal causes of actions are not uniform and may vary from state to state. Although most lawsuits brought by minors are filed soon after the incident causing the injury, therapists should retain the records until a minor reaches majority and for an additional time equal to the state statute of limitations for tort actions. Generally, the medical record of a minor should be kept until the patient reaches the age of majority (18 or 21 depending on the state) plus the statute of limitations. For example, for a state in which majority is 21 years and the statute of limitations for medical malpractice is 2 years, records should be preserved for 23 years.

For medical research purposes, it is advisable to establish a long retention period for records. When research involves experimental or innovative patient care procedures, records should be preserved for extended periods of time, typically 75 years. This means that space for storage must be designated and recordation be in a format that will withstand this time. Storage of medical records on computers may be governed by licensure or accreditation laws, federal programs, or rules of evidence associated with admissibility of copies of patient records at trial.

The American Health Information Management Association (AHIMA) has established record retention guidelines to aid organizations in determining how well they measure up to industry standards. These guidelines include ensuring availability of patient information for continued care; legal requirements; research, education, and other legitimate uses; developing a retention schedule for patients, physicians, researchers, and other user needs; legal, regulatory, and accreditation requirements; specifying what information is saved, for what time period, and how to store the information; establishing compliance programs addressing all types of documentation generated from employee training, hot lines, internal investigations, audits, modifications to compliance programs, and self-disclosures; retaining documentation for sufficient time to prove compliance with applicable federal and state laws and regulations; and developing policies with legal advice.

AHIMA's recommended minimum time periods for which patient health records should be kept are the following:

- Patient health records (adults): 10 years after most recent encounter
- Patient health records (minors): age of majority plus statute of limitations
- Diagnostic images: 5 years
- Disease index: 10 years
- Fetal heart monitor records: 10 years after infant reaches majority
- Master patient index: permanently
- Operative index: 10 years
- Register of births: permanently
- Register of deaths: permanently
- Register of surgical procedures: permanently

Courts have held facilities liable for an independent act of breaching their duty to make and maintain medical records, and one court permitted an action despite running of the applicable statute of limitations when the plaintiff had insufficient evidence to sustain a medical malpractice action because the patient health record could not be produced.

Patient health information (PHI) records may be destroyed in accordance with state statute when the retention period expires or the record has been copied onto microfilm or computer, or otherwise converted into readable form. Some states require that an abstract of pertinent information in the medical record be created before destruction. Large facilities generally contract with a commercial enterprise for destruction of records. It is important that such an agreement contain terms dealing with the method of destruction, safeguards protecting confidentiality of information, indemnification, and certification that the records have been properly destroyed. Failure to apply a uniform policy to all records may result in a jury's interpretation that if the records were available, they would reveal that a patient received substandard care. Electronic records should also be destroyed in a manner that permanently deletes them from a system or database.

XV. MEDICARE AND MEDICAID

The conditions relevant to participation in the Medicare and Medicaid programs require that medical records remain confidential. These conditions apply to various types of facilities including hospitals, long-term care facilities, home health agencies, substance abuse agencies, and hospices.

XVI. DISCLOSURE OF MEDICAL INFORMATION FOR RESEARCH PURPOSES

Many states as well as the federal government have laws providing for disclosure of patient information for research projects, especially regarding research using human subjects. Most facilities have established institutional review boards (IRB) that evaluate research protocol, protect the confidentiality of the information obtained, decide whether the research will benefit society, and determine whether adequate safeguards exist to protect the human study subjects placed at risk. With existing HIPAA privacy and security laws, it is required to obtain written patient authorization for any release of the medical record.

XVII. SPECIAL DOCUMENTATION CONCERNS

A. Celebrity Patients

Special care to protect the PHI records of celebrity patients may be challenging since the personalities are often subject to the close scrutiny of the news media. Some facilities have established policies and procedures to assess the need for anonymity, by omitting the patient name from the record or replacing it with an alias or code name and maintaining the record in a special secure file.

B. Hostile Patients

Hostile patients are more likely to take legal action in the event of rendered problematic or perceived problematic healthcare. It is recommended to create a detailed medical record that leaves little ambiguity regarding the medical care given the patient. Avoid inserting derogatory comments about the patient's behavior in the record, including only objective descriptions and quotes from the patient. Negative remarks may be used in litigation to prove bad faith and/or bias on behalf of the practitioner.

C. Recording Indicators of Child or Elder Abuse

Documentation in suspected situations of abuse should be detailed and objective containing a description of all relevant findings. This is important as the documentation may be used for determination of abuse. The results of any assessment and testing should be included as well as a detailed history and identities of interviewers or other caregivers or family of the patient.

D. Designation of Health Care Surrogate or Healthcare Proxy

Most states have adopted a process and form, commonly called the designation of health care surrogate or health care proxy that permits an agent of a disabled or incompetent person to make healthcare decisions on behalf of the patient. This document is more flexible than a living will, which is limited to when the patient is terminally ill or comatose and unable to communicate. The health care designation or proxy can be used whenever a patient is unable to communicate a choice regarding a health decision and is not limited to specific life-sustaining measures.

E. Do-Not-Resuscitate Orders

It is common practice to document in writing in inpatient/hospital and skilled nursing facilities, patient and family desires to DNR or "No CPR." The DNR and No CPR are not effective until documented in the orders for patient treatment. Additionally, an appropriate consent form or refusal of treatment form should be signed by the patient, patient representative, or family member. Orders related to DNRs and No CPRs should be prominently displayed in the record so that it is common knowledge. Failure to note same that results in action taken may lead to legal liability. Although, not legally mandated, best practices may require documentation of inquiry as to existing DNR or No CPR orders for patients seen in outpatient settings. Failure to respond in accordance with existing advanced directive although not necessarily known to the treating clinician could pose liability if determined that the standard of practice would be to obtain this information by patient interview. Although it is not common practice in outpatient practices to note "DNR," it is critical to incorporate it.

F. Disagreeing Opinions Among Personnel/Staff

All healthcare providers have the duty to take reasonable actions to safeguard the lives of their patients. Using professional judgment, a PT may encounter a situation in which it is necessary to clarify or object to physician orders or inform the physician of contraindications to treatment. Documentation of professional disagreements should be done in a manner that is objective, factual, nonjudgmental, and could not be used as evidence against the physician or institution in a negligence lawsuit. For example, is it not appropriate to write, "Dr. Joe is negligent again or the order is incorrect…" Most facilities will have policies and procedures for documenting professional differences of opinion.

XVIII. SPECIAL DISCLOSURES

A. Records Sought by Managed Care Organizations (MCO)

MCOs often need access to PHI to monitor discharge planning, case management, utilization review, and credentialing of physicians. Requests for access are often established by way of policies and procedures to reduce liability for negligent access. These policies typically adopt applicable laws relating to keeping confidentiality of patient information.

B. Records Sought by Law Enforcement

The general rule is that healthcare providers and organizations should not release medical records or other PHI to requesting law enforcement agencies without written authorization of the patient. Unless there is statutory authority, court order, or subpoena, the police have no authority to examine medical records.

XIX. LEGAL ISSUES RELATED TO IMPROPER DISCLOSURE

Healthcare providers and facilities may be subject to civil and criminal liability for disclosing PHI that has not been authorized by the patient, court-ordered, or required by law. State statutes and regulations provide for criminal and professional disciplinary sanctions. State laws and common law usually allow wronged individuals to file civil suits and seek recovery of damages.

A. Causes of Action for Releasing Information Without Authorization

In order to sue successfully, a patient must be able to prove the elements of the legal cause of action. The legal theories pertinent to medical information liability are defamation, invasion of privacy, and breach of confidentiality. A suit for defamation is typically based on common law and the injured plaintiff must prove by greater weight of the evidence that (1) a false and defamatory statement was made about the patient; (2) the statement was published to a third party; (3) the publishing party knew the statement was false or acted with reckless disregard of its truth or falsity; and (4) injury was caused by the statement or the statement by nature was harmful. If accusing invasion of privacy, the patient must show evidence of the improper disclosure of patient information. Another legal theory often governed by state statute and used by patients to sue healthcare providers who disclose medical record information is breach of confidentiality, or breach of physician–patient privilege. Generally, a violation of this confidentiality results in liability for damages caused by the disclosure that may have resulted in the deterioration of a marriage, loss of a job, and suffering from emotional distress.

B. Medicare Disclosure

Section 4311 of the Balanced Budget Act of 1997 requires that if a Medicare beneficiary submits a written request to a health services provider for an itemized statement for any item or service provided and billed Medicare, the provider must furnish this statement within 30 days of the request. The law also states that a health services provider not furnishing this itemized statement may be subject to a civil monetary penalty of up to $100 for each unfulfilled request unless it can demonstrate that to do so would pose an undue burden. Since most institutional health practices have established an itemized billing system for internal accounting procedures, as well as, for billing other payers, the furnishing of an itemized statement should not pose any significant additional burden.

30-Day Period to Furnish Statement. You will furnish to the individual described above, or duly authorized representative, no later than 30 days after receipt of the request, an itemized statement describing each item or service provided to the individual requesting the itemized statement.

XX. RISK MANAGEMENT

A. Computerized or Electronic Medical Records

The trend in medicine is to use and rely on technology. The method of maintaining patient medical records in paper files with eventual transfer to microfilm for safekeeping is antiquated. An increasing number of providers use computers, computer networks, facsimile machines, and optical scanning and storage equipment to create, transmit, store, and retrieve patient healthcare information. Although computerization enhances the quality of patient care, there are risks related to maintaining confidentiality of the information and complex legal issues regarding the duties and rights of providers. Electronic data exchange from the number of computer links and electronic fund transfers has opened up the doors to potential healthcare fraud. The legal precedence and laws are not keeping pace with the advances in technology, and do not provide much guidance for health care providers and organizations. Licensure laws and regulations and Medicare and accreditation standards require providers and facilities to safeguard records and protect against unauthorized access. The legal confidentiality obligations are the same for electronic and paper-based systems. Most legislative protections governing confidentiality of PHI only apply when the medical record data identifies the patient. Therefore, cleansed, meaning properly de-identified, data may be used with very few restrictions.

There are legal questions regarding which state's law would apply to medical record information transmitted across state lines. Similarly, computerization of patient data increases risk of unauthorized disclosure. A breach of a computer system's security could result in numerous unauthorized disclosures and potentially catastrophic liability since a system can access, copy, and transmit substantial numbers of records in short times. Therefore, reasonable safeguards employing password access and encryption may set legal standards of what should be built into the systems.

B. Electronic Claims

Standards for processing of health claims electronically have been established under the Health Insurance Portability and Accountability Act of 1996 (HIPAA) and mandate compliance. See prior discussion in this chapter.

C. Telemedical Records

The delivery of healthcare services from a distance using interactive telecommunications and computer technology is called telemedicine. Clinicians providing telehealth services across state lines are subject to applicable state laws and state licensing requirements for health practitioners; however, which states' requirement must be satisfied has been the question and have not been finally resolved. It is likely that at a minimum, they will need to comply with requirements of their home state and state where the patient is located or fall within an exception.

The practice of using electronic signals to communicate medical information generates potential legal issues regarding accuracy from distortion of data, confidentiality, and security of health information. Airwaves are not secure and the confidentiality of PHI cannot be guaranteed. Presently, there are very few legislative or accreditation requirements pertaining to the creation or maintenance of telemedical records. Because there are so few statutory or regulatory guidelines, all relevant standards should be followed.

D. Electronic Mail

Electronic mail (e-mail) and texting is increasingly used to transmit sensitive PHI. Although the modes of e-mail transmission have occurred at a rapid pace, the implementation of related technological safeguards have not developed at a similar pace and are less than adequate, creating more challenges for keeping confidentiality and security of medical records. Providers who send electronic messages must be aware to exercise caution when transmitting patient information to avoid compromising the integrity of the data and to prevent a breach of patient confidentiality. Title III of the Omnibus Crime Control and Safe Streets Act of 1968, commonly known as the federal wiretapping law, provides protection against improper interception of electronic communications, such as e-mail, and imposes civil and criminal liabilities on violators.

If a healthcare provider uses e-mail, it is important to develop policies and procedures addressing recording, retention, and destruction of the communications and implement reasonable safeguards to preserve PHI confidentiality. E-mail communications should be included in patient medical records and the guidelines of documentation should be followed.

XXI. MEDICAL RECORDS IN LEGAL PROCEEDINGS

As stated previously, patient treatment records provide clinical information about the patient to the various healthcare providers involved in that patient's care. As a business record, it justifies to third-party payers reimbursement billed for services provided, allows for monitoring of quality patient care, sets forth needs for risk management, and provides a basis for clinical research and educational training. Legally, the records protect the patients, healthcare providers and organizations, and support staff. In litigation proceedings, the records may be the only written record of what transpired. As such, it could be effective for a positive defense against a claim of professional negligence or be the reason for an unfavorable decision against a provider. Failure to create or maintain the records is a breach of the duty owed to the patient. If a breached duty results in a patient's injury, then actionable malpractice may ensue.

Intentional failure to maintain records, or spoliation, is typically a criminal matter of fraud and obstruction of justice. A charge of spoliation can result in suspension or revocation of licensure and imposition of a fine. Healthcare providers must resist the urge to correct records that appear obviously erroneous. Changes to a record should be implemented in a manner as previously described. It is not difficult to spot an altered patient care entry. Common signs indicating alteration include differences in handwriting, use of different writing instruments, erasures and/or obliteration or correction liquid, and nonuniform crowding of words particularly between lines or in margins. Similarly, signs of rewritten patient care entries may include differences in paper type, binder holes or other markings that do not match the rest of the record, date and/or time discrepancies, subsequent entries that seem out of context or confusing, findings not known at the time, and handwriting style or quality inconsistent with the writer. To avert dangers of spoliation, facility risk managers routinely segregate original patient records involving patients in litigated claims.

XXII. DEFENSE: USE OF HEALTH RECORDS IN JUDICIAL PROCEEDINGS

Patient health records containing relevant information are usually admissible into evidence in judicial proceedings when someone is involved in the legal action. Under these circumstances, a court order by way of a subpoena duces tecum is issued to require production of the medical information. State regulations governing court procedure indicate whether original or copies of the health records, as routine business records, will suffice. A records custodian will need to testify as to the authenticity of any records produced.

XXIII. THE U.S. LEGAL SYSTEM

Laws define specific relationships and are classified as public or private. Public laws involve relationships between individuals or businesses and the government and define, regulate, and enforce respective rights of the parties. For example, Medicare is public law and involves the government in its relationship providing health insurance for individuals. In comparison, private law involves rules and legal principles defining rights and duties between individuals and/or private businesses. Private laws apply in matters involving contracts or torts such as malpractice. There are four sources of public and private laws: constitutions, statutes, administrative law, and judicial decisions.

The U.S. Constitution defines and establishes the powers of the legislative, executive, and judicial branches of government. It also includes 26 amendments, the first ten comprising the Bill of Rights. Additionally, every state has a constitution, which is regarded as the highest law of the state but subordinate to the U.S. Constitution. Statutes are laws enacted by state legislatures and U.S. Congress. Accordingly, Medicare and HIPAA are statutes since they were enacted by the U.S. Congress.

Administrative rules and regulations are developed by administrative agencies to which Congress has given powers. For example, Congress has directed the Secretary of Health and Human Services to promulgate rules to carry out the intent of HIPAA. Judicial decisions interpreting the Constitution and statutes form a major source of law and serve as a primary source for private law.

A. Legal Proceedings

Lawsuits against healthcare providers are brought by plaintiffs who file complaints against an individual or organization called defendant(s). The next phase of the litigation is discovery, at which time medical records are often produced and utilized to determine the strength or weakness of each party. In depositions, subpoenaed individuals, including the records custodian and authors of the records, may be required to produce records and other patient information, testify that health records were compiled in the normal course of business and have not been altered in any manner. At trial, the medical records are often entered into evidence. Should a verdict or court decision be appealed, medical records that were admitted into evidence at trial may be reviewed by an appellate court. If a PT or PTA is deposed as part of a legal action, they will be asked a series of questions. It is always best to answer with only the content read from the record; which should be legible and easy to read. The PT or PTA should not "try to remember." As this process, from the filing of a lawsuit to the actual trial, could take place years after the injury to the patient, proper documentation may prove very helpful in refreshing memory of what transpired and very important for defending the claim.

B. Professional Liability

Medical malpractice refers to the professional liability of healthcare providers involved in the delivery of patient care. Professional liability may arise from breach of contract, intentional tort, and negligence theories.

The provider–patient relationship is established by either an express or an implied contract. Under either type of contract, a legal, contractual obligation arises from the relationship created and a promise to provide services at a certain standard of care, whereby the healthcare provider agrees to diagnose and/or treat the patient in accordance with standards of acceptable practice and to continue treating until the natural termination of the relationship, such as patient gets well or dies, mutual agreement to terminate, patient terminates, or healthcare provider withdraws from providing care. When the provider–patient relationship exists, failure to diagnose or treat using reasonable care and skill may give the patient cause to sue for breach of contract.

Healthcare providers can also be held liable when they intentionally harm a person under the legal theory of tort or strict liability. Intentional torts are wrongful acts that result in injury to another.

Negligence occurs when a healthcare provider commits a wrongful act by failing to do what another prudent reasonable healthcare provider would do under similar circumstances. Other causes of action against healthcare providers may include assault and battery, defamation, invasion of privacy, wrongful disclosure of confidential information, and abandonment.

XXIV. RISK MANAGEMENT

AHIMA has published guidelines on health information management, health record documentation, and content based on the practice setting. To reduce risk, all facilities providing patient care should have policies ensuring uniformity of content and format of healthcare records based on applicable accreditation standards, federal and state regulations, payer requirements, and professional practice standards. In order to meet legal requirements, many guidelines should be followed, including systematic organization of health records to facilitate retrieval and compilation of information and quantitative and qualitative analysis of health records to confirm that state law, regulation, or healthcare facility licensure standards are upheld as related to documentation.

A. Computerized, Photographic, and Videotaped Patient Care Records

Increasingly more facilities are using computers to record patient data. The electronic records, however, pose a challenge to preserving patient confidentiality and create temptations to alter or erase prior patient entries. Therefore, facilities must develop safeguards to protect access to and unauthorized alteration of records generated.

Photographic documentation is also used by PTs to memorialize before and after treatments. The photographic evidence; hard copy, video, digital, electronic or other, must be preserved in accordance with statutory retention requirements. Copying of photographs is more expensive and more time-consuming than paper, although computer scanning may reduce the cost.

Video documentation or digital recording memorializing patient status and treatment is also used by physical therapists. Provided the videotape meets certain legal standards, it may be admitted into evidence if needed. Videotapes must be retained in accordance with statutory requirements. Photography or videotaping typically requires explicit prior written informed consent.

XXV. SPECIAL CIRCUMSTANCES REQUIRING DOCUMENTATION/SEXUAL ASSAULT AND BATTERY

It is important to obtain and safeguard results of examinations and care given victims of sexual assault or battery. Most facilities have written policies addressing recordation, storage, and transfer of PHI to law enforcement authorities. Any statements made by a victim should be included in "quotes" in the documentation and may be admissible in a future court proceeding. Records of sexual assault patients should be maintained separate from the general patient care records. Facility policies and appropriate laws should be followed regarding reporting.

XXVI. DOCUMENTATION OF PATIENT RESTRAINT USE

Providers must document certain things before using physical or chemical/pharmacological restraints on patients. This requirement resulted from the danger of misuse and neglect related to the use of such restraints, especially in skilled nursing facilities. Practitioners must document clinical justification (patient behaviors) for using restraints by including documentation demonstrating that less restrictive alternatives were inadequate, other health providers have been consulted, and that the patient's physical and mental conditions have been considered. The potential for harm must be documented if the patient/client goes without restraints. Documentation and policy for the use of physical and chemical restraints must be consistent with federal and applicable state laws. If not properly documented, there may be cause for legal action based on false imprisonment.

XXVII. REIMBURSEMENT AND DOCUMENTATION

Documentation requirements for reimbursement are generally administratively controlled and constantly change. For this reason, it is important for therapists and assistants to familiarize themselves on an ongoing basis with applicable requirements. Legal issues involve whether the documentation constitutes larceny (theft) by fraudulent or deceptive practices. Healthcare fraud occurs when there is an untruthful representation of a material fact. Billing for services not rendered, waivers of patient copayments and deductibles under Medicare Part B, violations of anti-kickback and self-referral laws, over utilization or unbundling of services, upcoding, or miscategorizing coding to enhance payments by third-party payers, if done knowingly, can result in an allegation of fraud. Inadequate patient care documentation may support or create a claim for fraud leading to investigation, sanctions, and liability with the Department of Health and Human Services (HHS). The penalties for reimbursement fraud range from civil fines to criminal convictions, administrative penalties, exclusion as Medicare and Medicaid providers or other third-party payer systems, suspension or revocation of licensure, and professional association actions for ethical violations. Ignorance is not considered a reasonable explanation if a treating professional is unaware of changed regulations.

XXVIII. PROFESSIONAL GUIDELINES

The APTA *Guide for Professional Conduct* illustrates ethical principles for therapists relative to documentation practices.[11] Professional conduct standards require that the physical therapist–patient relationship is confidential and cannot be communicated to others without prior written consent from the patient, that peer-reviewed information cannot be released without written permission of the therapist, and that disclosure of medical information without patient consent may be done when necessary to protect the welfare of others in compliance with applicable laws. Physical therapists cannot delegate to less qualified persons activities requiring the skill, knowledge, and judgment of a therapist. Ideally, documentation interpreting health information, examinations, diagnosis, development of the plan of care and goals, identification of precautions and contraindications, reevaluations, discharges, readjustments to plans of care, and follow-up planning are best done when the physical therapist personally records. However, if support staff is used purely to transcribe and the physical therapist signs and/or counter-signs such notes, it may be legally sufficient. Ethically, the code specifies that the supervising therapist perform "identification and documentation of precautions, special problems, contraindications, goals, anticipated progress, and plans for reevaluation."[11]

XXIX. SUMMARY

Healthcare practitioners will be held accountable for knowing, comprehending, and applying relevant state and federal laws and regulations to their specific practice settings. As pertinent laws and regulations are constantly evolving and changing, a practitioner has a professional responsibility to continually update their knowledge. Documentation that is appropriate, complete, and accurate, not only contributes to quality patient care and prevents medical errors, but assists with defense against malpractice actions. Medical records containing inappropriate, incomplete, and inaccurate information may result in verdicts against the healthcare organization and provider.[12]

REFERENCES

1. Scott RW. *Legal Aspects of Documenting Patient Care for Rehabilitation Professionals*, 3rd ed.. Subury, MA, Jones and Bartlett Learning, 2006.

2. Pagano MP. *Authoring Patient records: An Interactive Guide*. Subury, MA, Jones and Bartlett Learning, 2001.

3. APTA. *Guide to Physical Therapist Practice*, 2nd ed. Alexandria, VA, American Physical Therapy Association, 2003.

4. Scott RW. *Health Care Malpractice: A Primer on Legal Issues for Professionals*, 2nd ed. New York, McGraw-Hill Companies, 1998.

5. Fla. Stat. Ch. 456.057. http://www.leg.state.fl.us/statutes/index.cfm?App_mode=Display_Statute&Search_String=&URL=Ch0456/SEC057.HTM&Title=->2008->Ch0456->Section%20057. Accessed July1, 2010.

6. HIPAA Disclosure Authorization Form, revised 5/2004.

7. National Association of Insurance Commissioners Insurance Information and Privacy Protection Model Act (NAIC Model Act). http://www.naic.org/ Accessed July 2, 2010.

8. Privacy Act of 1974. http://www.ftc.gov/foia/privacy_act.shtm Accessed July 2, 2010.

9. The Freedom of Information Act. http://www.justice.gov/oip/foia_updates/Vol_XVII_4/page2.htm. Accessed July 2, 2010.

10. HITECH, Title XIII in Division A, pages 112 through 165 and Title IV in Division B, pages 353 through 398.

11. http://www.apta.org/AM/Template.cfm?Section=Core_Documents1&Template=/CM/HTMLDisplay.cfm&ContentID=24781. Accessed July 10, 2010.

12. APTA Defensible Document. www.apta.org

CHAPTER 7 REVIEW QUESTIONS

1. What is informed consent? Explain the relevance to PT documentation.

2. What is HIPAA? What is the relevance to medical records keeping and PT documentation?

3. During what stage of litigation are medical records used? What are they used for?

4. While documentation cannot solve the dilemma of extending treatment for those who have been terminated by third-party payers, what role can it play in premature discharge?

5. What is authentication in documentation?

6. What is the "rule" for the use of abbreviations in documentation? What are the risks and benefits?

7. Explain how errors in documentation should be corrected.

8. What is the role of an addendum?

9. What is counter- or cosignature? In what circumstances is it applicable in PT documentation?

10. What are the benefits of dating and putting the time of treatment on an entry?

11. Are patients/clients entitled to copies of their records? Explain your answer.

12. What are the emerging challenges of protecting electronic or computerized documentation?

13. Explain the importance of legibility in the medical record.

14. A large hospital has PT services in multiple units; cardiac, orthopedic, general medical, trauma and pediatrics. Although the SOAP note format is used, the PTs and PTAs on each unit put different information in each category. Explain this is, or is not best practice.

15. Outpatient physical therapy facilities have historically not included whether a patient has a DNR. Should this be added to routinely obtained patient information? Provide rationale for your answer.

16. Jane Smith has just passed her national physical therapy board exam after completing a doctor of physical therapy degree and is licensed in Florida. How should Jane sign her medical record entries?

8 MDS Purpose and Components

The minimum data set (MDS) is a comprehensive assessment instrument designed to describe the medical condition, functional capacity, and treatment regimen of all persons residing/staying in skilled nursing facilities (SNFs)/nursing homes in the United States for more than 14 days.[1] The MDS and its companion documentation, the resident assessment instrument (RAI), are mandated by the Social Security Act for all persons receiving Medicare and Medicaid funding. Regulations were amended in the Omnibus Budget Reconciliation Act (OBRA) in 1987 to include all nursing home residents.[2] The form of the MDS in use since the fall of 2000 is version 2.0. In the fall of 2010, MDS version 3.0 was instituted along with a new set of resource utilization groups (RUGs) designed to guide the prospective payment for the care of Medicare A patients in SNFs.[3]

The MDS is used as a component of two separate processes. One process is the designation of prospective payment rates received by facilities for the care of each patient. The other is to provide assessment and reassessment data to be used in the RAI process that was also mandated by OBRA. MDS data are utilized by state and local agencies to monitor the quality and safety of SNFs. This section will outline the personnel involved, time frames for reporting, and the various applications of MDS/RAI data.

I. PERSONNEL REPORTING ON THE MDS

Federal law mandates that a registered nurse be designated for the coordination of MDS data collection and submission. By law, nurses may document all items of the MDS. Physicians, speech–language pathologists, occupational therapists, activities professionals, dietitians, and physical therapists may also complete MDS items. Information provided by all of the team members described above, including the patient, the family, direct care providers, such as nursing assistants, and ancillary service personnel may be used in the assessment process. Section Z contains a record of all of the persons completing a portion of the MDS and the specific sections they completed. Signing this section denotes legal responsibility for the accuracy of the information documented in the sections that are signed for.

II. MDS AND THE PROSPECTIVE PAYMENT SYSTEM

Prior to 1998, nursing homes were reimbursed on a cost basis. Reimbursement was based on the cost of the care provided with no consideration for the amount or type of services a resident actually received. This retrospective approach to reimbursement resulted in a more than 300% increase in healthcare expenditures by

TABLE 8-1 • Time and Frequency Requirements for RUGs

RUG Category	Therapy Minutes	Number of Therapies	Therapy Frequency	Actual Rehab Minutes	Estimated Rehab Minutes	Projected Rehab Days	Nursing Rehab
Ultra high	720	2 or more	At least 5 days	NA	NA	NA	NA
Very high	500	One or more	At least 5 days	NA	NA	NA	NA
High	325	One or more	At least 5 days	65	520	8	NA
Medium	150	One or more	At least 5 days	0	240	8	NA
Low	45	One or more	At least 3 days	0	75	5	At least two

Medicare in the early to mid-1990s. Since 1998, SNFs have been paid a prospective, per diem rate that is based on the care that a patient has received in the recent past and the care that the facility can predict they will need in the near future based on function. Actual cost of the services provided to a patient is not a factor in the reimbursement that a facility receives. Data collected using the MDS are used to place residents into one of 53 RUGs. Each RUG is associated with a corresponding per diem rate that is further adjusted for regional wage patterns.[4]

A. Resource Utilization Groups

The 53 RUG categories are divided into 7 broad categories, arranged hierarchically by cost. The rehabilitation plus extensive services category is the costliest, followed by the rehabilitation category. Extensive services categories are determined by nursing interventions that a patient receives. The balance of categories is determined by diagnoses that are associated with more extensive and costly care. Patients are placed into rehabilitation categories based on the number of days and minutes of therapy they receive during an assessment period. Time and frequency requirements for the various rehabilitation RUGs are summarized in Table 8-1. The process of determining a patient's eligibility for placement into the rehabilitation category, and their assignment to a specific rehabilitation RUG, is summarized in the next three sections. Two case studies applying the concepts discussed are presented at the end of the chapter.

The rehabilitation categories, extensive service categories, and the special care high categories qualify as skilled care under Medicare A guidelines. Rehabilitation clinicians should be familiar with the requirements for these categories because a patient must be receiving skilled care to receive Medicare A reimbursement. If a patient qualifies for skilled care based on rehabilitation needs only, the patient and/or their family must be informed immediately at, or prior to, discharge from care or when there is a reduction in therapy because Medicare A benefits will cease and alternate payment methods must be arranged.

B. ADL Index Score

Section G of the MDS is used to generate a composite score, called the ADL (activities of daily living) index, which describes a patient's ability to care for oneself and/or participate in one's care. Activities included in the ADL index are transfers, bed mobility, toileting, and eating. This score is used to assign patients to a subgroup within their RUG category. Patients with higher ADL index scores are more dependent; therefore, it is assumed that increasingly expensive care will be delivered to them.

It is important to consider that the MDS describes a patient's performance in their ADL across seven 24-hour periods and not a patient's best or potential for performance during an observation period. With this in mind, a rehabilitation professional's input should only be one component of the information used to determine the score for an ADL item. A patient's performance with all three shifts of nurses and nursing assistants must be considered and a representative score determined. Therapists should keep this in mind especially during a patient/client's initial examination and evaluation.

Assistance level descriptions differ from those used by most physical and occupational therapists. The ADL index is derived from a combination of two ratings for each activity. The first is a rating for patient performance, which is scored as follows:

0	Independent	Patient received help or oversight on no more than two occasions.
1	Supervision	Patient received help, oversight or cueing three or more times and physical assistance no more than two times.
2	Limited assistance	Patient highly involved in activity but requires limb maneuvering assistance three or more times and extensive assistance less than two times.
3	Extensive assistance	Patient performed part of the task but required weight bearing support or total assistance during the last 7 days.
4	Total dependence	Patient did not perform any part of the task.
7		Activity only occurred once or twice
8		Activity did not occur

Activity only occurred once or twice is to be used when an activity is becoming a new part of a resident's routine and not associated with a decline in function.

The "Activity Did Not Occur" rating should be used if an activity was not performed during the assessment period for reasons other than patient participation. An example of such a situation would be a patient that did not dress during an assessment period because of a sacral wound care regimen.

ADL support required describes the amount of staff assistance necessary for the patient to accomplish an activity. Items are scored as follows:

0	No setup or staff assistance
1	Set up only
2	One person assistance
3	Two or more person assistance
8	Activity did not occur

Assessment Reference Dates (ARD). Most of the observations on an MDS assessment describe a patient's condition over a 7-day period. Since various members of the interdisciplinary team may be completing the MDS at different times, the MDS coordinator must designate an assessment reference date. The assessment reference date is the final 24-hour period of the 7-day MDS observation interval. Because of this, all MDS documentation should be dated after the assessment reference date (ARD).

Grace Days. The MDS/PPS system allows for a certain degree of flexibility in the determination of assessment reference dates. Each of the MDS time frames described above has a range of possible ARD. All MDS may have an ARD before the assessment designated date (for example, the 30-day MDS may have an ARD as early as day 23).

The days beyond the designated day of an MDS assessment are called grace days. These dates are built into the system so that a facility can assess days that are truly representative of a patient's condition and treatment. Grace days can be used to accommodate decreased participation in care and therapy, associated with adjustment to a new facility and acuity of illness. Time away from the facility for tests, doctor visits, brief hospitalizations, and family visitation are accommodated for established patients as well. The grace day system also allows facilities to capture a representative number of therapy days and minutes for patients admitted late in the day or week.

III. SPECIAL TREATMENTS, PROCEDURES, AND PROGRAMS

MDS section O includes recording the number of days and minutes that the patient receives physical, occupational, speech, respiratory, and psychological therapy during the 7-day observation period. This record of the rehabilitation services that the patient received is used to determine the patient's eligibility for placement in a rehabilitation RUG for all MDS assessments except the 5-day MDS.

For physical therapy minutes to qualify for inclusion on the MDS, several criteria must be met:

1. Treatments must be based on an active treatment plan that was generated by a physical therapy evaluation performed on the patient as a resident of the SNF. A PT evaluation performed in the acute care hospital is not sufficient to initiate a course of treatment in a nursing home.

2. Treatments must be ordered by a physician.

3. All treatment minutes must be performed by a physical therapist but may include the assistance of a physical therapy student, aide, or volunteer.

or

Treatments must be performed by a physical therapy assistant under the supervision of a physical therapist.

4. Therapy provided to patients in groups of four or fewer persons by a PT or PTA may be included in section P if group therapy is less than 25% of the therapy received by a patient during the observation period.

It is critical that the time frame recorded in therapy documentation in the medical record agrees with the minutes and days of therapy entered in this item. In January 2000, the U.S. Office of the Inspector General (OIG) reported that Section O documentation along with ADL index scores are the two areas of the MDS that have the worst agreement with documentation in the rest of the medical record. The OIG made a point that the facilities inspected did not show a clear trend toward over-reporting therapy minutes, which suggests that facilities are not trying to defraud the Medicare system. As a result of this disagreement, the OIG recommended that these areas be scrutinized in further inspections and for revision of the items themselves.

A. Medicare 5-Day Therapy Supplement

Medicare 5-day assessments must include documentation on MDS section O if a physician has ordered PT, OT, or SLP services during the initial assessment period. This section provides an estimation of the amount of therapy a patient will receive during the first 15 days of an SNF stay. This section will be used to determine the patient's eligibility for rehabilitation RUGs for the first 15 days of a qualifying Medicare A reimbursed stay.

Predicted days and minutes of therapy are not used for placing patients in the rehabilitation very high and ultra high categories using the 5-day MDS. Actual performance of therapy, recorded in Section P of the 14-day MDS, is used to qualify for these RUG categories.

The procedure for determining estimated therapy days is as follows:

1. Count the days that a patient received at least one qualifying, 15-minute-long, therapy treatment through the ARD to determine actual therapy days.

2. Use therapy orders, treatment plans, and the policies of the facility to project the number of days the patient should receive at least one qualifying therapy treatment, starting the day after the ARD, through day 14 to determine the number of predicted therapy days.

3. Actual therapy days + predicted therapy days = estimated therapy days.

The procedure for determining estimated number of therapy minutes is as follows:

1. Count the number of qualifying therapy minutes that the patient received through the ARD to determine actual therapy minutes.

2. Use therapy orders, treatment plans, and the policies of the facility to project the number of minutes of therapy the patient should receive, starting the day after the ARD, through day 14 to determine the number of predicted therapy days.

3. Actual therapy minutes + predicted therapy minutes = estimated therapy minutes.

B. Resident Assessment Instrument Process

The MDS is used for an important set of processes beyond the MDS/PPS system. It is a data collection tool designed to cue facilities to develop care plans that will impact critical components of a resident's health and quality of life. MDS data are also used to assist state agencies in monitoring the quality and safety of SNFs.

Resident Assessment Protocols and Care Planning.

Scores on specific items in the MDS "trigger" a resident assessment protocol (RAP) for a given area. The trigger legend is a component of many printed versions of the MDS that indicate that an MDS item score identifies an area requiring further assessment by the interdisciplinary team. For example, a patient will trigger a RAP for pressure ulcers if they are scored as being incontinent of bowel, dependent in bed mobility, having diminished sensation, or being essentially bed-bound. There are 18 RAP areas, which are summarized in Table 8-2. RAP areas that will commonly involve evaluation and subsequent care planning by physical therapists include physical restraints, falls, decreased ADL, and pressure ulcers.

Discipline-specific documentation along with patient history and diagnostic testing information will be used to make decisions on the course of action necessary to address a given RAP area. If any of this documentation indicates the need for interdisciplinary intervention, a written care plan must be generated. All initial and annual MDS/RAI assessments must contain a RAP summary, which contains a summary of the information described above and the rationale involved in the decisions made. The MDS coordinator generates RAP summaries at the completion of the RAI process.

Quality Indicators.

The quality control component of the RAI is the care area assessment (CAA) system. This data is used by state agencies to track individual facilities performance against benchmarked quality standards for an area and to identify facilities that fall below critical standards. The CAA system also facilitates focused inspections by providing inspectors with lists of patients at risk for negative outcomes in the recent past. MDS data triggering a CAA results in the need for additional data to be collected and a care plan to address issues identified by this additional data collection. Physical therapy evaluations will typically be part of the data collection processes of the CAA for ADL falls, physical restraints, pain, and return to community (Table 8-3).

Time Frames for MDS and RAI Completion.

OBRA requires that a comprehensive admission assessment including the MDS and the entire RAI process be completed by day 14 of a patient's stay. This process is completed annually for all nursing home residents. Quarterly MDS reassessments are also completed for the duration of a patient's stay.

In addition, the Medicare/PPS system also requires that an MDS be completed on day 5 and day 14. With certain restrictions, either of these assessments can be used to fulfill the OBRA admission assessment requirement. MDS assessments are also required for day 30, 60, 90, and 100. The 90-day MDS may fulfill the requirements for the OBRA quarterly reassessment.

TABLE 8-2 · Resident Assessment Protocol (Rap)

1. Delirium	10. Activities
2. Cognitive Loss/Dementia	11. Falls
3. Communication	12. Nutritional Status
4. Communication	13. Feeding Tubes
5. ADL	14. Dehydration/Fluid Status
6. Urinary Incontinence/Indwelling Catheter	15. Dental Care
7. Psycho/Social Well-Being	16. Pressure Ulcers
8. Mood State	17. Psychotropic Drug Use
9. Behavioral Symptoms	18. Physical Restraints

TABLE 8-3 • Care Area Assessments (CAA)

1. Delirium
2. Cognitive loss/dementia
3. Visual function
4. Communication
5. ADL/functional rehabilitation potential
6. Urinary incontinence/indwelling catheter
7. Psycho/social well-being
8. Mood state
9. Behavioral symptoms
10. Activities
11. Falls
12. Nutritional status
13. Feeding tubes
14. Dehydration/fluid status
15. Dental care
16. Pressure ulcers
17. Psychotropic drug use
18. Physical restraints
19. Pain
20. Return to community referral

The 5-day MDS is used to determine the patient's RUG for the first 14 days of a patient's stay. Each of the subsequent Medicare PPS assessments is used to determine a patient's RUG for the period through the due date for the next assessment. Table 8-4 summarizes the PPS and OBRA reporting schedules.

Significant Change in Status Assessment. A new MDS with an RAI must be completed if the facility determines that the patient experiences a significant improvement or decline. A decline should resolve with time or standard medical treatment. The status change should also require the interdisciplinary review of the care plan, affect at least two aspects of the patient's care, and result in assignment to a new RUG category.

Other Medicare Required Assessment (OMRA). An Other Medicare Required Assessment (OMRA) must be completed within 8 days after all therapies have been completed for patients that satisfy requirements for another skilled care RUG. This assessment is designed to establish a new prospective payment for the balance of a patient's 100 days of Medicare skilled nursing.

TABLE 8-4 • Reporting Schedule

Type of MDS	Possible ARD	Determines Reimbursement for Days
5 Day MDS PPS and OBRA	Day 1–8 Includes 3 grace days	1–14
14 Day MDS PPS	Day 11–19 Includes 5 grace days	15–30
14 Day MDS PPS and OBRA	Day 11–14 No grace days if OBRA admission	15–30
30 Day MDS	Day 21–34 Includes 5 grace days	31–60
60 Day MDS	Day 50–64 Includes 5 grace days	60–90
90 day MDS PPS and OBRA quarterly	Day 80–92 Includes 3 grace days	90–100

IV. SUMMARY

Use of the MDS in SNF setting is challenging. However, it is necessary on an initial and ongoing basis for all SNF patients and residents in order to comply with federal regulations. Although this serves as an introduction to the instrument, clinicians should refer to the MDS 2.0 Users' Manual during their first attempts to negotiate the MDS and RAI system. Rehabilitation professionals should appreciate the importance of their contribution to the MDS process and its emphasis on function.

> **Author's Note:** The CMS has established new guidelines for rehabilitation services and the documentation of recorded minutes for each therapy service. The new "Group Rule" requires that each service provide 25% of a patient's minutes in groups on a weekly basis and that other care be rendered 1:1.

V. CHAPTER 8 REVIEW CASES AND EXERCISES

A. Case One

Mr. G. was admitted on Monday, January 14 at 9 a.m. after an acute hospitalization for CHF. He presents with decreased endurance, decreased high-level balance, and mild to moderate dementia. PT and OT evaluations were ordered on admission. After the evaluations, orders were received for PT and OT 5 times per week for 4 weeks. The MDS coordinator designated Friday, January 18 as the ARD for the 5-day MDS.

To determine the estimated number of therapy days for MDS Section T, item 1c:

1. Mr. G. received at least 15 minutes of therapy on 5 days through the ARD.
2. Mr. G. is scheduled for at least 15 minutes of therapy on 5 additional days through day 14.
3. 5 + 5 = 10 (actual days + projected days = estimated days).

To determine the estimated number of therapy minutes for MDS Section T, Item 1d:

4. Mr. G. received 75 minutes of PT treatment and 90 minutes of PT treatment through the ARD.
5. Mr. G. is scheduled to receive 90 additional minutes of PT treatment and 90 additional minutes of OT through day 14.
6. 165 + 180 = 345 (actual minutes + projected minutes = estimated minutes).

Based on the therapy performance and schedule described above, Mr. G qualifies for the rehabilitation high category.

ADL Index Score. Mr. G. requires set up for transferring, bed mobility, eating and requires physical assistance of one person for toileting 4 or 5 times per week.

These levels of assistance qualify Mr. G for an ADL Score of 6, which would place him in the rehab high A RUG. If Mr. G. received the same amount of therapy but was dependent for all tasks, he would qualify for the Rehab High C RUG.

B. Case Two

Mrs. S. was admitted for open reduction and internal fixation of a hip fracture on Wednesday, October 7. An OT and PT evaluation was ordered on the day of admission. OT completed its evaluation on Thursday, October 8. Mrs. S. began vomiting in the afternoon and did not receive her PT evaluation. Mrs. S. refused all therapies on October 9 secondary to nausea. The PT evaluation was completed on Monday, October 12.

The MDS coordinator designated Wednesday, October 14 as the ARD using all 3 grace days to accommodate Mrs. S.'s nausea and vomiting.

To determine the estimated number of therapy days for MDS Section T, item 1c:

7. Mrs. S. received at least 15 minutes of therapy on 3 days through the ARD.

8. Mrs. S is scheduled for at least 15 minutes of therapy on 7 additional days through day 14.

9. 3 = 7 = 10 (actual days + projected Days = estimated days).

To determine the estimated number of therapy minutes for MDS Section T, item 1d:

10. Mrs. S. received 90 minutes of PT treatment and 90 minutes of PT treatment through the ARD.

11. Mrs. S. is scheduled to receive 210 additional minutes of PT treatment and 210 additional minutes of OT through day 14.

12. 180 + 420 = 600 (actual minutes + projected minutes = estimated minutes).

Based on the therapy performance and schedule described above, Mrs. S. qualifies at least for the rehabilitation high category. Medicare guidelines require patients to actually perform the required minutes and days of therapy for the rehabilitation high and very high categories. If Mrs. S. performs all of her scheduled therapy days she will qualify for the rehabilitation very high category.

REFERENCES

1. http://www.cms.gov/MinimumDataSets20/. Accessed July 10, 2010.

2. http://www.ssa.gov/OP_Home/comp2/F100-203.html. Accessed July 10, 2010.

3. http://www.aahsa.org/article.aspx?id=462. Accessed July 10, 2010.

4. http://oig.hhs.gov/oei/reports/oei-02-02-00830.pdf. Accessed July 10, 2010.

CHAPTER 8 REVIEW QUESTIONS

1. Who is responsible for completing the MDS?

2. What is the role of the MDS in patient care in a SNF?

3. An individual is admitted to a SNF as a skilled patient. He remains in the skilled unit 100 days and then becomes a long-term resident for 2 months before being discharge to an assisted living facility. How many MDS reports will be completed in the 160 days? Provide rationale for your response.

4. How are the minutes of therapy services determined? Is there a difference between the first 5 days and ensuing days? Explain.

5. What are the RUGs and their relationship to physical therapy, occupational therapy and speech language pathology?

6. A patient is admitted to a SNF but following day 1, the patient is unable to participate in any of the therapy services and essentially remains bed-bound, secondary to low grade fever and emesis. Explain how this is dealt with in the MDS process.

7. Explain how each of the 20 CAA areas is related to physical therapy.

8. According to MDS and CMS guidelines, who can provide physical therapy services versus assistance with physical therapy services?

9. Explain the RAI and RAP processes and the relationship to the MDS.

10. Explain the relationship between the RUG level and reimbursement? Why is this PPS system more cost-effective that the previous cost-based system?

9 Medicare and Non–Medicare Content Principles

I. DOCUMENTATION CONTENT PRINCIPLES: FOCUS ON INITIAL EXAMINATION AND EVALUATION

According to the APTA *Guide to Physical Therapist Practice*,[1] there are 25 categories of tests and measures in physical therapy (PT): aerobic capacity, anthropometric characteristics, arousal/attention and cognition, assistive and adaptive devices, circulation (arterial, venous, lymphatic), cranial and peripheral nerve integrity, environmental/home and work (job, school, play) barriers, ergonomics and body mechanics, gait/locomotion and balance, integument integrity, joint integrity and mobility, motor function (motor control and learning), muscle performance (strength, power, endurance), neuromotor development and sensory integration, orthotic/protective and supportive devices, pain, posture, prosthetic requirements, range of motion (including muscle length), reflex integrity, self-care and home management (activities of daily living [ADL] and instrumental activities of daily living [IADL]), sensory integrity, ventilation and respiration/gas exchange, and work (job/school/play), and community and leisure integration or reintegration.

The physical therapist selects those tests and measures within each category most appropriate to the patient/client's signs, symptoms, and concerns using the clinical decision-making model. Ultimately focusing on movement and function.

For Medicare purposes, standardized tests and measures should be focused on activities related to necessary function versus leisure, and those problems or impairments directly impacting necessary or essential function. In the outpatient setting, objective standardized tests and measures are required on initial examination. Essential function includes: adequate aerobic endurance to perform activities such as transitional movements and transfers, bed mobility, gait on a variety of surfaces or if non-ambulatory or limited in gait, other locomotion (i.e., wheelchair, power-operated vehicle, or power wheelchair), negotiating doorways and different surfaces, avoidance of objects, safety, balance in standing and movements related to effective ADL performance. In some instances, tests and measures include IADL and negotiating public transportation if a beneficiary is still working, or receiving treatment on an outpatient basis. Pain, in the absence of dysfunction, is not a qualifier for skilled physical therapy. However, if the patient/client is reporting pain and it affects functions not necessarily apparent or measurable in the clinic, close attention must be paid to patient/client monitoring of improvement external to the clinic as a measure of success. Examples of this are sleeping through the night or if driving is necessary (even if it is to and from medical appointments), the ability to safely turn the head, sit for a prescribed length of time, and operate a vehicle safely. Lack of sleep secondary to pain, can result in impairment in judgment and fatigue, endurance limitations, depression, and weakness. Specific cardiac rehabilitation is not considered a skilled reimbursable Medicare-approved PT procedure, although respiratory programs may be in certain circumstances. Individuals with cardiac problems qualify for skilled PT secondary to weakness, functional decline, gait abnormalities, aerobic capacity limiting function, etc.

In the non-Medicare adult context, the concept of function may be more generic in scope, encompassing leisure and lifestyle. However, as in Medicare, pain as a sole diagnosis, in the absence of functional limitation may likely not be reimbursable unless the patient/client has been specifically referred for pain management or a pain program, and it has been preapproved by the payer. There may be limited reimbursement to instruct an individual in techniques that may help manage the pain and facilitate function, depending on the payer source.

Wellness programs are not usually reimbursed as skilled physical therapy in Medicare or non-Medicare venues. Specific cardiac and respiratory intervention may be covered in non-Medicare venues depending on the payer.

Standardized tests and measures performed at initial examination, depending on the specifics and how long a patient/client will be treated, should be repeated at intervals and at discharge. In some instances, the test itself can be used as component of therapeutic intervention. By repeating a test at the time of discharge, significant improvements made as evidenced by improvements in scores, facilitate reimbursement and justification of skilled services. This is true for quality of life instruments that may be questionnaires including confidence scales as well as more movement-related or functional tests and measures. Refer to example 1 for examples of standardized tests and measures.

■ Example 1

Questionnaire/survey instrument: OPTIMAL by Cedaron for APTA (confidence and functional report), SF 36 (quality of life, QOL), Oswestry Pain Scale (used frequently for pain assessment related to back pain), disease specific instruments i.e., Parkinson's, Multiple Sclerosis

Standardized functional tests: Timed Up and Go (TUG—for balance), Dynamic Gait Index (for gait ability under varied conditions), Romberg and Sharpened Romberg (static balance eyes open and closed; two legs, single leg), BERG Balance (functionally oriented balance test)

Author's Note: Standardized instruments should be "attached" to the documentation. Specific deficits should be summarized in the evaluation, record entries and surrender of case. Score totals may not be understood by the reader.

II. MEDICARE AND NON-MEDICARE

A. Skilled Content Recommendations; Initial Examination/Evaluation and Periodic Reports

Regardless of payor source, if billing with a CMS 1500 form the same content is required in the patient/client documentation. The data entered on the CMS 1500 does not include status or problems, but rather diagnoses and diagnostic codes, corresponding CPT codes (See Appendix C), and modifiers for clarification.

Author's Note: Content categories are relevant for all initial examinations and content as appropriate to non-Medicare evaluations (the shorter the form, the easier to find information). The CMS 700 series forms contain content for justifying care. The forms are not the actual bill.

The CMS 1500 billing form is a single page (see Appendix C) with boxes for patient identifiers, provider identifiers, onset date, start of care date (SOC), primary medical diagnosis, treatment diagnosis, (see Appendix B) visits from SOC, type of service modifiers, physician, and PT information. The CMS 700/701 also contains blocks of blank space for plan of treatment, functional goals (short and long term in weeks), plan frequency and duration, certification dates prior hospitalization (as applicable), initial assessment (history, medical complications, level of function at start of care, and reason for referral), and functional level (at the end of billing period). There are also progress report boxes to indicate whether to continue service or discharge (DC). In order to ensure appropriate completion, PTs should add written categories to the form. If entered in small enough font, adequate space is available if PTs enter only what is necessary.

Author's Note: In 2007, the UB-04 (CMS 1450 [See Appendix C]) replaced the UB 92. Organizations that qualify for a waiver according to the Administrative Simplification Compliance Act (ASCA) for electronic claims, can file claims manually using this form. CMS does not issue the form itself, but does provide guidelines for what the form must include.

Refer to Example 2 for sample content for CMS 700 series or initial examination.

■ Example 2

Initial examination/evaluation including plan of care

Patient demographics including SOC as indicated in introduction would precede the information below.

Initial Assessment (Fill in Blanks)

History of Current Illness

Past medical history:_____

Prior level of function (prior to current episode): _____

Reason for referral (should be functionally oriented and may match treatment diagnosis if functional): _____

Cognition (alert, oriented to person, place, time): _____

Follows _____ step directions:

    Verbal/gesture/combination: _____

Safety awareness: _____

Precautions:_____

Respiratory/cardiac status/aerobic capacity: _____

Balance:	Sitting: With/without back supported	Static:_____	Dynamic:_____
If used a device, Type:	Standing: With/without device	Static:_____	Dynamic:_____

Other categories: Systems

Strength: 0/5 to 5/5 scale: Extremities/trunk/cervical: _____

Other muscle performance: _____

ROM (expressed as fraction out of "normal ranges"): Extremities/trunk/cervical: _____

Tone: low, high, rigidity, spasticity (using Modified Ashworth Scale verbiage). Extremities/trunk/other: _____

Pain: location/grade 0/10 to 10/10, activity affected: _____

    Level at worst: _____ Least: _____

    What relieves or decreases it? _____

Willingness to move: _____

Skin integrity: _____

Sensation: light touch, pain, proprioception, other: _____

Coordination: _____

Motor control/quality of movement: _____

Bed mobility: _____

    Rolling: L/R: _____

    Supine <> sit: long sit and short sit: _____

    Scooting: side to side, up and down in supine: _____ in Sit: _____

Transfers: Sit <> stand: _____

Stand pivot: _____

W/C, chair <> bed/mat: _____

Gait: device, pattern, dependence: _____

WC management: manual, electric wheelchair, or power operated vehicle (i.e., scooter): _____

    Posture sit: _____ Stand: _____

    Standardized tests and measures: Summary of results: _____

    Other: _____

Rehabilitation potential (relative to PT): _____

Goals: Time defined: _____

Sample Plan of Care: Checklist on a CMS 700 form or other initial examination/evaluation form: Verbiage should match CPT/HCPCS categories as much as possible

_____ Therapeutic procedures: for specified body part, i.e., UE/LE/Trunk/low back: progressive strengthening/ROM/endurance

_____ Neuromuscular reeducation: balance training, proprioceptive training, coordination training (This category may be challenged by Medicare)

_____ Therapeutic activities: transfer training, functional training, bed mobility training

_____ Gait training

_____ Wheelchair training/management

_____ Patient/caregiver education/training (according to the APTA this should be CPT coded based on the content; i.e., instructions in home exercise under therapeutic exercise. It can also be billed or categorized as self-care)

_____ Self care management/Safety training

_____ Other (Fill in others as indicated based on CPT codes)

As all or most of this information using this basic format may be on one or two single pages with standardized tests and measures attached, it is not necessary to write a separate problem summary. However, in some settings, it may be a facility requirement. Reason for referral should include this information. However, each category with a deficit noted should have a corresponding short-term and long-term goal as indicated. Impairment-based goals should be included but linked to the functional end. Goals should also include the instructions the patient/client and caretakers need to know. Refer to Example 3 for integrating information on the initial examination and evaluation, regardless of payer.

■ Example 3

EXAMPLES FOR CATEGORIES ON INITIAL EXAM AND EVALUATION

Medical diagnosis: Contusion left hip (hematoma), low back pain

PT diagnosis: Gait abnormality, contusion, low back pain, muscle weakness, abnormal posture

Reason for referral: Dependent for gait, transfers, weakness BLEs, back pain impairing function, dependence for ADL, IADL since patient fell

Prior level of function: Lived alone in first floor apartment, I in all ADL & IADL, drove own car, I gait without assistive device

Muscle performance (Strength/quality of movement): BLE: 3+/5 proximal, 3/5 distal, with inability to perform repetitive movement against resistance, movements slow, hesitating

AROM: shoulders: 0° to 160/180° of flex/abd, fingers maintained in minimal flexion with arthritic changes noted, posture in standing forward flexed ~25° and R shifted; unable to extend or flex trunk secondary to CO severe pain 9/10 with any movement.

The categories indicated above may be adjusted depending on the type of clientele a facility sees. Remember that the treatment diagnosis must be consistent with the planned interventions, the deficits identified, and the short- and long-term goals. All categories indicated correspond to the categories in the APTA *Guide to Physical Therapist Practice*.[1]

III. PATIENT/CLIENT GOALS

According to the *Guide to Physical Therapist Practice*,[1] goals and expected outcomes are categorized together. Following are the categories of goals (based on increases or improvement) with summaries of the skills that should be considered when writing patient/client goals. Please note that although categories may be stated in broad, general terms, they must be stated specifically in the actual plan for an individual patient/client. These are applicable across all settings and are applicable to patients/clients throughout their lifespan. Refer to Example 4.

■ Example 4

GOALS:
STGs (2 weeks):
Patient will have a reduced Oswestry disability score of 30/100 and a reduced FABQ-W score of 8 in order to return to work and leisure activities.
Patient will have reduced pain as indicated by a NPRS score of 2/10 order to return to work and leisure activities.

Patient will increase muscle strength of abdominal and multifidi muscles to 3+/5 and 4+/5 to improve active spinal stabilization in order to tolerate standing for personal hygiene and work related activities.

LTGs (6 weeks):
Patient will have an Oswestry disability score of 10/100 and a reduced FABQ-W score of less than 5 in order to return to work and leisure activities.
Patient's pain complaints will be resolved as indicated by a NPRS score of 0/10 in order to return to work and leisure activities.
Patient will increase muscle strength of abdominal and multifidi muscles to 4+/5 and 5/5 to improve active spinal stabilization for reaching the plates in the upper cabinets at home.
Patient will accurately demonstrate home exercises & I perform to reinforce upright posture to spinal posture and stabilization to prevent reoccurrence of injury.

Patient will regain normal spinal mobility through the use of spinal manipulation in order to return to work and leisure activities.

Author's Note: For a single patient, "patient will" should be stated once, followed by a colon(:). It is understood that unless otherwise stated, all goals are patient related.

A. Impact of Pathology/ Pathophysiology/ Presenting Problems/ Impairments—Body Function and Structures (ICF Model)

The impact of the pathology or pathophysiology on movement is the reason the patient/client needs PT. This constitutes the PT or treatment diagnosis, PT problems, and the relationship between the medical problem and the resulting functional deficits. Patient pathology may lead to the need for reduction of edema or lymphedema, reduction of joint inflammation and swelling, reduction in soft tissue swelling or tone, enhanced wound healing, or tissue restriction reduction, all in order to facilitate movement and function. Refer to Example 5.

■ Example 5

UE Lymphedema: limited AROM, limited use of extremity, pain, limited ADL ability, unable to write, loss of fine motor control in hand

Palpable spasm paraspinals thoracic and lumbar regions limiting trunk movement and ability to stand or sit

Grade IV wound on R heel necessitating NWB gait and inability to drive car

The impact of PT on a patient/client's impairments—body function and structures, should be significant focused on facilitating function. Examples of changes as a result of PT include: increased muscle performance endurance and aerobic capacity; decreased energy expenditure or increased energy efficiency; increased ROM/decreased contracture, improved muscle performance (strength, power, endurance) for performance of specific activities for safety, gait, fall prevention; decreased breathing effort or increase in effective breathing effort with ability to sustain longer continuous activity; changes in motor control (synergy, patterns, coordination); stable or improved balance; increased postural control with decreased fall risk; improved integument and joint integrity; increased sensory awareness; improved gait and locomotion; increased weight bearing; optimal joint alignment and use (i.e., prosthesis, orthosis); optimal loading on a body part; increased ability to sit or stand for extended periods, ability to sleep through the night and enhanced tissue perfusion and oxygenation.

B. Impact on Functional Limitations and Disabilities/Functioning and Disability (ICF Model)

PT's impact on the patient's functional limitations includes decreased levels of dependence or need for assistance, improved ability to perform tasks, increased tolerance to positional changes, and increased performance of and independence in ADL and IADL with or without devices, return to work, leisure, school, and other responsibilities, i.e., that of homemaker or caretaker. (In the second edition of the *Guide to Physical Therapist Practice*[1] gait-related activities are listed under impairments.)

As the patient continues PT, his or her disabilities will be impacted in several ways. The patient's ability to resume performance of life roles, such as returning to work or school, returning home (if PT was inpatient), and resuming those leisure activities once challenging or impossible due to the impairment.

C. Risk Reduction/Prevention

As a result of PT, the patient should experience a reduction in risk factors associated with a lack of knowledge or understanding, as examples, to surgical precautions and weight bearing limitations. Another area of risk reduction would be enhanced awareness of surroundings for safety, compensation for sensory or vision loss, awareness of potential for skin breakdown, appropriate awareness of abilities versus inabilities.

Prevention or decreased risk of developing secondary problems may be critical in justifying skilled physical therapy. The necessity of protection of body parts in the absence of sensation or presence of vision impairment, reduction of pressure on tissues to prevent breakdown and infection, and increased understanding of assistive devices to prevent falls or other accidents, prevention of postural syndromes from pain and abnormal protective posturing, loss of function secondary to tissue restrictions, all benefit movement and patient/client function over time. When prevention of secondary problems/dysfunction is a component of PT, they should be clearly identified in the initial examination/evaluation.

D. Impact on Health, Wellness, and Fitness

A patient/client should gradually experience improved health status and increased overall wellness as an outcome of PT. Physical function and capacity are improved, allowing the patient to improve overall fitness and movement related activity, even in the presence of short-term, long-term, or permanent disability.

> **Author's Note:** The exception to this would be if the patient's declining and goals were being revised accordingly.

IV. PATIENT/CLIENT SATISFACTION RELATES TO GOALS

Although there are multiple factors to consider regarding patient satisfaction, the most relevant to goals of physical therapy, are improved sense of well-being, decreased stressors, overall improvement in movement/function and achievement of patient/client goals. The patient's satisfaction is based on the level and timeliness of goal achievement (see Tables 9-1, 9-2, and 9-3 for sample patient goals),

TABLE 9-1 · **Sample Patient Problems and Goals (Refer to the Endurance Scale at the End of this Chapter.)**

Deficit/finding/problem	Short-term goal, 2 weeks (include date)
Aerobic capacity limited to <1 minute continuous activity before becoming shortness of breath (SOB), RR 28	Increase to 3–5 minutes continuous activity and without SOB stabilize RR in 20–24 range and fatigue at rest
Impaired static sitting; unable to sustain upright without external support	Increased postural control and muscle performance of trunk stabilizers to reduce fall risk in sitting associated with COG changes, and sustain upright unsupported sitting
Dynamic sitting impaired; when challenged or leans in any direction beyond upright, is unable to resume upright (based on numeric scale)	Increase dynamic sitting balance with ability to I return to upright when leans out of COG to prevent falls associated with reaching and bending in sitting *(continued)*

TABLE 9-1 • Sample Patient Problems and Goals (Refer to the Endurance Scale at the End of this Chapter.) (*Continued*)

Deficit/finding/problem	Short-term goal, 2 weeks (include date)
Moderate dependence for standing with walker	Decrease dependence to minimal assist with pelvic stabilization to minimize fall risk in standing activities and facilitate activities in standing
Dynamic standing 1+ with rolling walker (See Kansas University Standing Balance Scale at the end of this chapter.)	Increase to 1 to begin decreasing fall risk on indoor surfaces
Rolling L/R modified with bedrails, limited assist 10% for lower trunk unable to sleep through night	Progress to limited assist 5% (tactile facilitation at pelvis) without rails to facilitate change of position for skin protection and to facilitate sleep through the night
Supine <> sit limited assist 25% to initiate unweighting of trunk and provide tactile facilitation	Supine <> sit with verbal instruction only
Scooting limited assist 25%	Scooting limited assist 10%
Transfers: sit <> stand limited assist 25% to initiate forward trunk flexion and unweighting of buttocks	Transfers: sit <> stand limited assist 10% to initiate unweighting of buttocks
WC <> bed/mat limited assist 25% to execute pivot	WC <> bed/mat with supervision/verbal instruction
ROM: bilateral dorsiflexion: 0° active	With verbal instruction, will perform exercises to be performed in room and at home to increase ankle ROM in order to facilitate performance of functional activities, i.e., sit to stand 10° of active assistive bilateral dorsiflexion
Strength 3+/5 to 4–/5 throughout extremities with impaired muscle performance; limited ability to perform repetitive activity against gravity or functionally	Strength consistent in 4–/5 range with increased muscle performance and ability to sustain movement and activity against gravity during functional gait, standing
Gait front wheeled rolling walker, rear end caps, step to, ↓ knee flexion L with swing, ↓ initial contact L/R, ↓ uneven cadence, forward flexed trunk, limited assist 25% for posture correction, stabilization of walker, tactile facilitation	Gait front wheeled rolling walker, rear end caps, step through pattern, initial contact with heels L/R, erect posture, limited assist 10%—supervision for stabilization of walker to prevent veering in forward direction
Gait with front wheeled rolling walker, rear skis level surfaces moderate (50%) assist to remain upright and propel walker, 10′, forward only	Gait with front wheeled rolling walker, rear skis, level surfaces to 80′ with safe/stable directional changes L/R 90° and 180° turns, to enable gait to bathroom and dining
WC management; moderate dependence, initiates rim movement only; unable to propel effectively **Note: ↓ = decreased**	I WC management on level and carpeted surfaces to allow safe locomotion and promote I mobility in the short term until safe with gait

TABLE 9-2 • Sample Patient Goals

2 Weeks: (can include actual date, or specify the number of weeks)

1. Contact guard: Gait with standard walker on even (or level) surfaces, WBAT, 50′, with ability to make 180° turn and step backward without toe drag, with single rest of 1 minute, at half normal speed: ~40 m/minute

2. Ability to open and close doors with round handles with limited assistance: 25% for standing balance while using walker

3. Supervision with minimal verbal instructions for safe transfers sit <> stand

4. Supervision with minimal verbal instruction for safe stand pivot transfer bed <> chair

5. Increased R dorsiflexion strength from 3–/5 to 3+/5 with elimination of toe drag to enable safe gait and decrease fall risk

6. Improve standing balance from _____ to _____ without walker to prevent falls when standing for activities that require both UEs (preclude holding walker); i.e., dressing, hygiene, kitchen related

7. Increase aerobic capacity with consistent O2 saturation of >95, for functional activity from _____ to _____

(continued)

TABLE 9-2 • Sample Patient Goals (*Continued*)

2 Weeks: (can include actual date, or specify the number of weeks)

8. I wheelchair mobility on even surface with ability to lock and unlock brakes, flip foot rests and leg rests, negotiate doorways and execute directional changes

9. Patient will demonstrate ability to perform exercises independently

3 Weeks: (can include actual date, or specify the number of weeks)

1. Stable, I gait with standard walker on even and uneven (rugs, concrete, grass) surfaces, with ability to execute turns spontaneously in all directions with heel/toe pattern 100′ without rest at normal speed of 82 m/minute

2. I ability to negotiate doors (open and close) without loss of balance

3. I transfers sit <> stand

4. Improve stand pivot transfers bed <> chair, toilet, shower from moderate (50%) assistance to minimal (25%) assistance with pivot component

5. Increase R dorsiflexion strength from 3–/5 to 4–/5 to eliminate toe drag/drop foot for sustained safe gait up to 100′ on even and uneven surfaces

6. Increase/improve standing balance from _____ to _____ for safe, stable standing for self-care activities, bathroom and kitchen tasks

7. I wheelchair mobility on even and uneven surfaces (rugs, concrete, grass) without need for interrupted propulsion

8. Patient will demonstrate home exercise independently

9. Stabilization of _____ spinal segment to enable full cervical rotation R/L to safely scan environment

10. Eliminate radiating low back pain with centralization to facilitate functional standing

TABLE 9.3 • Sample Patient Problems and Goals Note: **Limited = minimal**

68 y.o. male hospitalized for 5 days
Medical diagnosis: resolving left lower lobe atelectasis, HTN, pneumonia
PT diagnosis: gait disturbance, weakness, impaired aerobic capacity
Prior level of function: multiple falls over 6 months, lives with daughter in single-story house, ambulatory with standard walker
Precautions: cardiac, falls, universal
Alert, oriented to person, place, time;
Cognition: Able to follow single-step instructions
Vision: R cataract > reading glasses
Hard of hearing (B)
Safety awareness: poor
Skin intact, no edema noted
At rest: vital signs: BP: 135/85; RR 24: shallow pulse 90 BPM

Deficit/finding/problem	Short-term goal 2 weeks (include date)
Endurance poor (based on scale); Comfortable of rest; light, brief activity → fatigue and dyspnea standing tolerance 1-minutes	Increase to poor + to eliminate constant respiratory symptoms and fatigue at rest
Static sitting 3+/5	Increase to 4–/5 to reduce fall risk in sitting associated with COG changes
Dynamic sitting 3+/5	Increase to 4/5 to prevent falls associated with COG changes, reaching, and bending in sit
Static standing 2/5 on KUSBS scale (see Table 9.5)	Increase to 4/5 to minimize fall risk in standing activities; moving 1–2 inches in one plane
Dynamic standing with 2+/5 rolling walker	Increase to 3/5 to begin decreasing fall risk on indoor surfaces
Rolling L/R modified with bedrails, limited assist 10% for lower trunk	Progress to limited assist 5% without rails to facilitate change of position for skin protection and to facilitate sleep through the night
Supine <> sit limited assist 25% to position	Supine <> sit limited assist 10%
Scooting side to side limited assist 25% position trunk pelvis	Scooting limited assist 10%

(continued)

TABLE 9.3 • Sample Patient Problems and Goals Note: **Limited = minimal** (Continued)

Deficit/finding/problem	Short-term goal 2 weeks (include date)
Transfers: sit<> stand limited assist 25%	Transfers: sit<> stand limited assist 10%
WC <> bed/mat limited assist 25%	WC <> bed/mat with supervision
ROM: B LE within functional limits with exception of B ankles: 0 from neutral dorsiflexion	With verbal cues, will perform exercises to be performed in room and at home to increase ankle ROM and facilitate performance of functional activities
	ROM:10 degrees active assisted dorsiflexion
Strength: LE within 3+/5 proximal to 4–/5 distal, with limited endurance to sustain activities	Strength: consistent in 4–/5 range in order to sustain movement during functional activities; gait, standing
Gait: front wheeled rolling walker step to, ↓ knee flexion L with swing, ↓ initial contact L/R, ↓ cadence, forward flexed posture, limited assist 25%	Gait: with rolling walker level surfaces 50 to 80' to allow gait to bathroom and dining
WC management dependent	I WC management on level and carpeted surfaces to allow safe locomotion and promote I mobility in the short term

effectiveness of PT communication and caring and respect for the patient/client and significant others. Phone calls should be returned promptly and every attempt should be made to stay on schedule and communicate regularly.

Patient/client goals should be established at initial examination/evaluation, and assuming they are realistic in the LOS established, the PT should incorporate them into the overall plan. If the patient/clients goals are not realistic in the time frame available or established, the PT should redirect. If unable to redirect, the PT may have to consider not accepting the patient/client for care. If there is change in status of the LOS in physical therapy, goals should be modified.

V. PLAN OF TREATMENT WITH FUNCTIONAL GOALS

Since all patient goal information is on a single page on a CMS 700 series form (See Appendix B) or similar self-designed form, it is not necessary to write a separate problem summary. The reason for referral should include this information. However, each category with a deficit noted should have a corresponding short- and long-term goal as indicated. Impairment-based goals should be included but linked to the functional end. Example 6 lists several functionally oriented goals in PT.

■ Example 6

Functionally Oriented Goals

- Pain reduction from 8/10 to 1/10 during prolonged sitting for up to one hour correct desk chair, to allow resumption of work at computer station, with 10-minute break at the end of each hour and ability to repeat throughout 6 hours a day
- Resolution of disk protrusion with resultant resolution of right shifted standing posture to allow unguarded, pain free gait in order to resume ADL and IADL activities, leisure, work, family responsibilities
- Restore full, stable cervical rotation to allow safe independent driving: checking mirrors, backing up, in order to return to drive to work, etc.
- Increase UE elevation to 160° bilaterally to allow independent dressing including overhead garments, self-care activities, overhead reaching activities in kitchen, adjust auto mirrors

A. Intervention—Plan

The categories used in the intervention plan or plan of care should match the categories in the CPT and HCPCS codes. After stating the category, if it includes a variety of activities such as that for therapeutic procedures, the specific type of exercise would then be listed. This is not necessary in the general plan of care, but would be in the medical record entries especially for communication between therapists and between therapists and other individuals who require the information for continuity of care, continuation of services on subsequent days, and progression over time. Most facilities use the same categories repeatedly. The treatment diagnosis must be consistent with the planned interventions, the deficits identified and the short- and long-term goals. All categories indicated correspond to the categories in the *Guide to Physical Therapist Practice*[1] (see Table 9-4 for a sample intervention—plan).

TABLE 9.4 • Sample Intervention—Plan

Therapeutic procedures for UE/LE/trunk: progressive strengthening resistance; ROM active, active assistive and passive stretching

Neuromuscular reeducation: balance training, proprioceptive training, coordination training

Soft tissues mobilization: state body area

Therapeutic activities: transfer training, functional training, bed mobility training

Gait training:

    Wheelchair training/management

      Self-management: patient/caregiver education/training, safety training

      Other _____

VI. CONTENT: INITIAL AND ONGOING

A. Elements Guidelines for Essential Skilled Content

Documentation includes baseline or initial examination data, anticipated goals based on the identified patient/client problems, the interim status and progress described relative to the baseline and goals. All deficits must ultimately be linked to the function they impact.

Anthropometric. Anthropometric measurement is used in PT to describe overall height, weight, body mass index, hip to waist ratio, overall body type, extremity or extremity segment size, and how size relates to function. The therapist should describe fat distribution as applicable, presence of obesity, and weight control problems. Measurements must be objective. If a scale is not available, record observations and ask the patient/client's height and weight. From a wellness perspective, improvements should be noted over time, and decreases to facilitate movement may be goals, especially in bariatric care or wellness and prevention programs (note: wellness and prevention are not usually reimbursable by third-party payers).

Joint Integrity and Mobility. Joint integrity and mobility in PT is expressed in terms of joint play, end feel and range of motion (ROM). The ROM should be listed as a fraction of the measured and full range. These measurements should be taken at baseline, throughout care, and at discharge using the appropriate device: inclinometer, tape measure, or goniometer. If the measurements are visually estimated, be sure to indicate this in the record. Joint play is usually described with appropriate adjectives such as laxity, and end feel may be described as: bone to bone, soft tissue approximation, spasm, empty end feel, capsular end feel, and springy block. The position in which ROM was measured, if not the standard position, should be documented. Refer to Examples 7 to 10.

■ Example 7

R Shoulder flexion: AROM: 80°/180°, PROM 120°/180°

Deviations: from joint and body planes, with excursions in distances

Example 8

15° L genu valgum

5 inches of spinal excursion in forward flexion

Joint Motion: quality of motion, i.e., end feel, painful arc, bony block, capsular patterns, glide, laxity, or restriction

Example 9

Provocation responses/tests: + anterior drawer sign L knee

Patient description/reports of pain (objectively measure) or other during activities and movement

Patient CO pain anterior R knee at 5/10 at rest and 9/10 with weight bearing activities and active knee flexion.

Example 10

Patient CO (complains of) grinding in shoulders with elevation and functional use

Patient CO clicking in L knee during walking and cycling, with occasional "locking".

Muscle Performance. Strength should always be expressed as a fraction to indicate the finding relative to the "normal" which is 5/5 on the most commonly used scale. These measurements should be taken at baseline, progressively throughout care and at termination of care, based on a predetermined scale of 0/5 to 5/5 or scale of preference.

Manual Muscle Test (MMT) scale

MMT scale

0 = no strength;	2 = poor;	4 = good;
1 = trace;	3 = fair;	5 = normal.

Avoid verbiage only when indicating muscle performance because it is often misunderstood and considered better than it is.

At times, especially with impaired muscle performance strength expressed in numbers, since based frequently on a one time maximal isometric contraction against resistance, may be misleading. A patient/client may test at 4/5 on one rep, but be unable to repeat the resistance or use the strength functionally. In this case, clarification is needed in the documentation to ensure that it is clear therapy is needed. For example, patient tolerated moderate resistance x 1 rep for elbow extension, but was unable to repeat it in use with functional elbow extension. Refer to Examples 11 to 16.

Example 11

R quads 3/5 at initial examination

Goal: Increase R quad to 4/5 to enable safe standing without device as required for job

Interim statement of progress: Patient's R quad strength has increased from 3/5 to 3+/5 decreasing frequency of buckling with weight transfer on and off limb in standing

■ Example 12

R quads/knee extension in sitting: demonstrates moderate resistance at 4/5 one rep only, unable to functionally extend knee in upright or tolerate repeated resistance

■ Example 13

Active R SLR: 70°

In long sit: fingertip to toes with knees straight = 3 inches with CO pulling in low back musculature and hamstrings resulting in inability to don socks

■ Example 14

In standing, left trunk side bending limited secondary to R quadratus lumborum spasm

R quadratus lumborum tender to palpation

Trigger point or tender point location and radiation patterns as applicable, using finger pressure or a pressure meter designed for assessment

■ Example 15

Trigger point L upper trapezius with radiation into shoulder with moderate pressure, limiting ability to position head to read or turn during driving

Muscle contraction quality: smooth versus interrupted, tremulous or rigid or otherwise

■ Example 16

Unable to sustain smooth muscle contraction to oppose R thumb to R forefinger, assists with L hand

Unable to sustain smooth muscle contraction to control hand during attempts to write or use keyboard without error

Sustained muscle endurance to perform movement with multiple repetitions or sustained contraction

When abnormal tone is present, with or without synergy, using the 5/5 scale may also be misleading. Verbiage can include the Modified Ashworth Scale and a description of the patient/client's ability/inability to tolerate resistance within the range present or with description of the changes in tone.

Modified Ashworth Scale:

5/5: Normal tone: no increase or decrease
4/5: Slight tone increase, catch and release, or minimal resistance at end of range
3/5: Slight increase in tone manifested by catch, followed by minimal resistance
2/5: More marked tone through most of the range of motion but affected part(s) easily moved
1/5: Considerable increase in muscle tone, passive movement is difficult
0/5: Affected part(s) rigid in flexion or extension

Developmental and deep tendon reflexes should be identified in documents. See Example 17.

Example 17

R biceps reflex = 2+ (normal)

L patella reflex = 1 (hyporeflexive)

Electrical assessment over time: EMG, nerve conduction, etc.
   Synergic dominance and tone, abnormal reflexes and ability to initiate and isolate movement in relation to gravity and body position

Example 18

Unable to isolate elbow flexion and extension on table top for support, interfering with eating, writing, self-care; considerable increase in muscle tone of biceps, passive movement difficult and active movement absent (1/5 on MAS)

Modified Ashworth Scale: (MAS)
   5/5: Normal tone: no increase or decrease
   4/5: Slight tone increase, catch and release, or minimal resistance at end of range
   3/5: Slight increase in tone manifested by catch, followed by minimal resistance
   2/5: More marked tone through most of the range of motion but affected part(s) easily moved
   1/5: Considerable increase in muscle tone, passive movement is difficult
   0/5: Affected part(s) rigid in flexion or extension

Author's Note: Although the Modified Ashworth includes descriptions and numbers from 0/5 to 5/5, the numbers alone should be avoided since they may be confused for strength.

Sensory Impairment: Sensory impairments should be described by location and distribution. The implications of the impairments and potential for secondary problems are necessary to indicate need for skilled PT. See Example 19.

Example 19

Sensation absent in RLE in L5 dermatome, resulting in potential for injury, skin breakdown

Sensory integration with environment: state of system

Sensory Integration: Sensory integration is the process by which an individual integrates function within the environment. Impairments in this process are functionally debilitating and may require long term therapeutic intervention. See Example 20.

Example 20

Demonstrates tactile defensiveness to all external stimuli including clothing and touch.

Demonstrates increase in observable synergies in response to noise in room, interfering with ability to isolate movement and preventing functional use of extremities.

Developmental reflexes can impact movement patterns and posturing. See Example 21.

Example 21

R ATNR dominance preventing neutral supine positioning, unable to roll right or left.

Developmental level: described in terms of milestones usually indicated on standardized forms for standardized assessment.

Motor Function, Motor Control, and Learning. When evaluating motor function, motor control, and learning, the PT should observe movement patterns, postural control, and unprovoked movement. Objective tests and measures are encouraged for consistency of assessment and documentation.

Example 22

Demonstrates severe kyphosis in sitting, limiting UE elevation and diaphragm excursion associated with increased respiratory rate and accessory muscle use. Is able to correct trunk posture approximately 5° with passive positioning.

Coordination Skills. When evaluating coordination skills, include the quality of the movement, smoothness of movement, ability to perform a motor task with accuracy and speed in a functional context. Objective tests and measures are encouraged for consistency of assessment and documentation.

Example 23

Time to complete tasks: slowness when it interferes with function is justification of care, especially in tasks that need immediate response such as toileting.

Example 24

Patient transferred wheelchair to bed with minimal assist or limited assist of 25% in 5 minutes, stand/pivot to R, requiring assist with pivot moving forward in WC & erect sitting posture.

It is important to include sequencing and cuing instruction for task accomplishment or tactile facilitation/cueing.

■ Example 25

Requires 1 step instructions with tactile cues to execute sit to partial stand Recall/repeat ability to perform a task in a different context or at a different time.

■ Example 26

Able to perform stand pivot transfer from WC to Mat table with supervision; occasional verbal instructions.

Requires moderate or extensive assist at 50% from WC to bed at same height to unweight buttocks and execute pivot.

■ Example 27

Able to maintain erect trunk posture in response tactile facilitation and maintain for 2 minutes with verbal instructions.

Coma level description using standardized scales such as the Glasgow or Rancho Los Amigos.

Balance. The therapist should describe balance and/or record balance ratings on standardized scales or from computerized equipment. Always use functional terms rather than good, fair, or poor, which are not objective measurable terms. There are standard instruments such as the Berg balance, Timed Get Up and Go, Romberg, and Functional Reach, which assist in qualifying and quantifying balance. One can also use a 0/5 to 5/5 scale for describing balance in sit and stand, static and dynamic, but the scale should be included. See Table 9-5 for the Kansas University Standing Balance Scale (KUSBS).

TABLE 9-5 · Kansas University Standing Balance Scale (KUSBS)

KUSBS score ordinal

Description of patient performance for KUSBS scores

0	Performs 25% or less of standing activity (maximum assist).
1	Supports self with upper extremities but requires therapist assistance. Patient performs 25 to 50% of effort (moderate assist).
1+	Supports self with upper extremities but requires therapist assistance. Patient performs >50% of effort (minimal assist).
2	Independently supports self with both upper extremities.
2+	Independently supports self with one upper extremity.
3	Independently stands without upper extremity support for up to 30 seconds.
3+	Independently stands without upper extremity support for 30 seconds or greater.
4	Independently moves and returns center of gravity 1–2 inches in one plane.
4+	Independently moves and returns center of gravity 1–2 inches in multiple planes.
5	Independently moves and returns center of gravity in all planes greater than 2 inches.

Example 28

Maintains vertical position in standing for 60 seconds without cues or support. Self-corrects to vertical 50% of time with verbal cues.

Requires bilateral UE support to maintain balance during gait. Resting posture is 15° to right of vertical. Falls to left three out of five times when perturbed from right.

Consistently able to reach beyond base of support without falling.

Falls to left when changing direction of gait 80% of time and relies on constant cues to sequence.

Requires constant physical cues to weight shift during gait or loses balance.

Balance must be specific and described in sitting or standing, with or without support, type of support; or during a particular movement task or activity such as gait, rising from a chair, or reaching. Also describe the patient's ability to incorporate spatial relationships during movement.

Example 29

Patient is able to perform bilateral activities to both the right and left of midline in sitting.

Able to read 2" beyond neutral without loss of balance.

Describe behavior or painful reactions during specific movement tasks and the movements that aggravate or relieve pain.

Example 30

Patient experiences sharp, severe pain in L knee with initial attempt at single leg stance; a necessary gait component (midstance).

Pain. When documenting a patient's pain, use numbers from standardized scales for rating pain, a faces scale (smile versus frown), or any of the other measurement scales such as the Oswetry. The 0/10 to 10/10 scale is most commonly used to indicate no pain to the most severe. It is important to note areas of pain, and levels at rest and during activity, what relieves the pain, what increases it, and the type of pain described, i.e., dull ache, throbbing, sharp, stabbing. The Oswestry scale is a good indicator of how pain impacts function.

Pain reduction as a goal must be supported in terms of how the reduction in pain is related to change in functional performance and increased ability to perform specific movement tasks. When documenting pain reduction, it is important to relate interventions to specific goals.

The continued use of physical therapy interventions without documentation of meaningful, practical, and sustained benefits related to function is not acceptable and will not, in most cases, especially Medicare, be reimbursed. Use the suggested terminology examples in your continuing care documentation as well as any progress report to support your ongoing interventions and progress toward goals. It is not the format of the entry that matters, but the content.

Author's Note: No matter how well you qualify and describe a patient's pain, if pain does not impact function, physical therapy will not, beyond a very brief period, be considered medically necessary unless a patient is specifically in a preapproved pain program.

Describe patient's expression of sensory and temporal qualities of pain in response to tests of provocation or during rest or movement tasks.

Example 31

Patient reported stabbing pain with deep friction massage that lingered for 20 minutes after completion of treatment of the R biceps tendon.

Give location of tender or trigger points and determine sensitivity with a pressure point gauge or verbiage such as the following criteria for tenderness to touch of tender or trigger points: A good way to identify the points is with a body diagram.

    0 = none
    1 = mild, expressed, but no withdrawal
    2 = moderate, expressed plus withdrawal
    3 = severe, immediate exaggerated withdrawal
    4 = patient untouchable, withdraws without palpation

Somatosensory. To measure and document a patient's somatosensory functions, describe the patient's expression of sensation during sensory testing. This includes light touch, pain (sharp/dull), deep pressure, hot and cold sensitivity, and proprioception or kinesthetic sensation Barognosis, Stereognosis, 2-point discrimination, description of reported paresthesias or neuropathic symptoms such as numbness, tingling, burning or inability to "feel."

Example 32

Response to light touch is absent in L side, UE, LE, putting patient at risk for injury.

Document the patient's ability to describe position of body part with eyes closed (proprioception), to identify objects by touch only (stereognosis), to identify use of objects (praxis), neglect of body part, and expression of sensation in absent body part or phantom pain sensation.

Example 33

Impaired proprioception of L foot; great toe and ankle, impairing balance/postural stability safety in stand and during gait.

Unable to identify coin, comb, or pin placed in left hand.

Patient unable to determine use for cane;

Experiences severe phantom pain in L residual limb that limits all mobility.

Cranial Nerve Integrity. To evaluate and record the patient's cranial nerve integrity, describe provoked and unprovoked eye, tongue, and swallowing movements. It is also helpful to list the patient's visual field and hemianopsia and describe ability to form facial expressions, and evaluation of the strength of applicable cervical muscles. To complete the cranial nerve integrity evaluation, describe the patient's vestibular problems, such as nystagmus, vertigo, and past-pointing as will as postural stability/instability.

Posture. The patient's posture should be recorded and evaluated throughout the course of therapy if impaired, for the following positions: sitting, lying, standing, and during functional activity. In some cases, posture alone, or "postural syndrome," may be the root cause of the patient's problems, and correction may be the solution. There are ICD-9 codes related to abnormal posture.

■ Example 34

Patient demonstrates flexed trunk posture in unsupported sitting, with inability to correct secondary to trunk weakness, perceptual deficits, including (L) neglect.

In describing a patient's posture, include limb position, joint limitation, tone, and positions of comfort.

■ Example 35

Patient's relaxed standing posture demonstrates forward head, UEs forward of trunk, knee hyperextension, and bilateral pronated feet.

The posture evaluation should also include descriptions of muscle imbalances in relation to the vertebral curves (the cervical lordotic curve, the thoracic kyphotic curve, the lumbar lordotic curve, scoliosis).

■ Example 36

Thoracic curve decreased/flattened, cervical lordosis increased, resulting in back pain limiting ability to flex forward which is required for job performance. Include the functional implications.

Mobility. When evaluating a patient/client's mobility, it is important to consider all applicable aspects and types of mobility, including bed mobility, transfers, transitional movements, gait, wheelchair mobility (manual, electric, or power-operated vehicles/scooters). For babies or toddlers, the ability to creep, crawl, and cruise should be documented.

Describe assistance required by the patient in terms of the effort the patient is exerting, rather than the exertion by the physical therapist. The terms minimal assist (or limited), moderate assist (extensive), maximal assist (extensive), and total assist are commonly used. To better define these subjective terms, a percentage of effort scale serves as the basis of the FIM (Functional Independence Measures, taken from the Uniform Data System, which is available from Data Management Service, Buffalo General Hospital, SUNY at Buffalo, 100 High

Street, Buffalo, New York 14203). These percentages are related to the terms as follows:

Total assist (extensive assist) = patient exerts 0% of total effort

Maximal assist (extensive assist) = patient exerts some and up to 25% of total effort

Moderate assist (extensive assist) = patient exerts at least 50% of total effort

Minimal assist (limited assist) = patient exerts at least 75% of total effort

Contact guard = patient requires hands on guarding in the event assist is needed

Supervision or standby assist = patient has safety issues and requires someone close by for safety and occasional verbal instructions

Independence = patient is able to perform activity without assistance. If a device is used, it must be identified and may be considered modified independence as in the FIM grading.

Components of mobility. Bed mobility documentation should include descriptions of rolling left or right with or without bedrails, positioning self cephally or caudally, shifting body/body segments left and right, and whether the testing is performed on a bed or mat, as the treatment mats are firmer and easier than a bed.

Transfers. There are many types of transfers with multiple components. Break down the components of these functions to be specific. There are many small goals to be identified and achieved before an end result is evident. Include those components that are applicable to your patient. The following words and phrases should be used to describe transfers:

- Ability to self position toward edge of surface
- Sit to stand, with or without pushing or using UEs
- Stand to sit/sit to stand
- Stand and pivot
- Partial stand to pivot with or without a device
- Full stand to pivot
- Sliding board or standing disk utilization
- Use of mechanical lift or assistive device
- Supine to/from sit with roll to side-lying versus directly to long sit

The direction of the transfer must also be described, such as transfers to the left or the right or both directions as indicated for the needs of patient.

Although there is normal variation in motor planning for transfer and mobility activities, any posturing or reflexes, weakness or other impairments that interfere with the patient's activity must be addressed in the documentation and intervention.

Gait.
Gait assessment and training are unique to physical therapy. They are highly skilled services making it imperative that documentation refer to the normal phases of gait and description of deviations. Any use of a device, including assistive gait devices, prosthetics, or orthotics must also be included.

The following terms should be used to describe the gait pattern:

Traditional	Rancho Los Amigos
• Arm swing	Arm swing
• Heel strike	Initial contact
• Foot flat	Midstance

- Toe off   Terminal stance
- Swing   Preswing/swing
  - Width of base; base of support (BOS) normal = 2 to 4″
  - Cadence
  - Stride length
  - Posture
  - Weight bearing/weight acceptance/weight shift
  - Level of pelvis/pelvic movement
  - Stability of hips and knees
  - Trunk movement
  - Leg-length discrepancy
  - Varum or valgus in the LEs/hips, knees, ankles
  - Assistive devices, prostheses, or orthoses required
  - Distance, directionality
  - Ability to sequence
  - Surfaces and elevations negotiated
  - Quality of movement/motor control

> **Author's Note:** Never use the word walk, walking, walked in documentation unless quoting the patient. It is also preferable to use gait training versus ambulation, as other healthcare professional wheelchair management such as nurses document using ambulation.

Determining the type and adaptations for using a temporary or permanent (manual or electric) wheelchair, along with instructions for use and determining the ability to maneuver are all considered skilled services.

- The patient's ability to propel the chair in multiple directions for distances over varied surfaces and elevations, indoors, and outdoors
- Patient's ability to manipulate the parts (i.e., brakes and armrests, etc. or controls and type if power operated.)
- Chair model selected (including power, power-operated vehicles/scooters) and its fit
- Ability of caretaker to manage the chair, including pushing, folding, braking, and car transfers with patient/client in the chair and securing versus patient/client transfer out of chair into vehicle and then placing and securing chair on lift or into vehicle (Note: If caretaker is impaired, a lightweight chair may be justified)
- Ability of patient/client to manage the chair, including pushing, folding, braking, and car transfers
- Adaptations made/needed/recommended, including cushions, backs, headrests, leg rests, seat belts, or other stabilizing adaptations
- Ability to negotiate doors and other entrances and bathrooms/toilets
- Integumentary (skin) condition and ability to change position for protection from breakdown

Integument. The initial examination and evaluation should also include a description of any wounds, burns, scars, open areas, rashes, lesions, discoloration, hair patterns, dryness, cracking, or other conditions that impact function and present risk. Open areas must be measured and described. Wound measurements may be obtained with grids, pictures, picture grids, traces of the wounds, readings from a volumeter, water injection, syringe volume, or cotton-tipped applicator inserted to determine depth. Describe drainage, odor, temperature, color, bruising, scabs, skin tears, trophic changes, turgor, pigment, and skin and scar pliability.

Throughout treatment, repeated wound assessment is required to indicate response to treatment. Nail and nail bed integrity are included as is hair presence, absence and pattern.

Peripheral Vascular. When evaluating peripheral vascular conditions, describe color, skin temperature, skin condition, and pain resulting from ischemia or claudication, edema; pitting or nonpitting, capillary refill in fingers and toes, peripheral pulse integrity and any other pertinent findings.

Lymphatic or Edema. Record measurements at selected points throughout the limb. The points for measurement must be recorded as well as the circumferential measurements at the points. When possible, compare measurements to the uninvolved limb. Avoid terms such as minimal, moderate, severe, and less than or more than. Measurements should be recorded every inch along the involved extremity. If the breast is involved, measurements should be taken around the base of the breast and around the trunk at the nipple line. Lymphatic evaluations should also include descriptions of peripheral pulses (check for their presence and describe their strength), such as LE, femoral, popliteal, posterior tibial, and dorsal pedal. Describe the color, temperature, pain, and skin condition of the patient. Skin temperature and full integument assessment should also be included. Record the degree of pitting edema if present, using the following scale:

1+ barely perceptible depression (pit)

2+ easily identified depression (EID) skin rebounds to its original contour within 15 seconds

3+ EID skin rebounds to its original contour within 15–30 seconds

4+ EID rebound >30 seconds

Describe the rationale for and use of external elastic supports or intermittent compression, as well as lymphatic drainage and massage techniques and necessity. Describe the overall size of the body, extremity, or extremity segment and how problems with size relate to function. Describe uneven fat distribution and poor weight control, as well as abnormal size. Measurements must be objective by measuring, weighing, or volumetric displacement.

Progress and treatment documentation should include repeats measurements at each visiting addition to interaction provided.

Cardiopulmonary Status/Aerobic Capacity/Endurance. To record cardiopulmonary status and aerobic capacity/endurance, be as objective as possible, avoiding terms such as poor, fair, and good. Instead, describe the behaviors that led you to the subjective word. Pulse oximeter readings and vital signs, blood pressure while sitting, standing, and laying down if indicated as well as at intervals during the session, radial pulse (if a pulse other than radial is used, state which) should be included as well as respiratory rate, pattern, shortness of breath (SOB), and quality of respiration. Depending on the venue and reason for referral, auscultation of the heart and lungs may be necessary to include as well. The therapist should be able to determine normal heart and lung sounds, and deviations from norms or abnormalities and record them.

Document progress by repeating measurements at intervals during each session and include to stabilization/improvements in vital signs in goals. See Examples 37 & 38.

■ Example 37

Avoid describing aerobic capacity/endurance as poor, fair or good.

Document that: patient requires 5 minute rest after 3 minutes of therapeutic exercise to return from RR of 30 shallow, mouth open, to RR of 22, mouth closed; able to participate for 30 total minutes with appropriate rest.

Author's Note: By describing the time intervals, progression is easier to document as periods of activity tolerance increase and RR stabilizes in the normal range (12–20), or what is the baseline for a patient or SOB decreases. It is helpful to include teaching the rate of perceived exertion as an additional measure of activity tolerance and one the patient/client can self-monitor or Dyspnea Scale.

Establish an objective baseline from which to compare improvement in function. The following should be included in descriptions of aerobic capacity/endurance:

- Autonomic responses to activity
- Breathing patterns/quality
- Need for supplemental O_2 and volume needed
- Patient complaints in quotes
- Ability to increase treatment time or repetitions or tolerance for all interventions over time
- Rate of perceived exertion scales
- Respiratory rates
- O_2 saturation as measured by a pulse oximeter

■ Example 38

Patient is able to accomplish only 10 feet, minimal assist with 4-wheeled rolling walker before becoming diaphoretic and SOB. Pulse increases from 80 at rest to 120 after stand pivot transfer. After 10 reps of knee extension with a 5-pound weight, patient's breathing became shallow with RR of 32. Patient requires 5 minutes of rest for breathing to return to normal after every 5 minutes of exercise. Patient tolerates only 1 hour sitting in semi-reclined wheelchair. Requires 2 hours bed rest after every hour out of bed.

Author's Note: Vital signs that are monitored throughout a session can be documented in a table.

Describe cardiac status by comparing to baseline measurements at rest to measurements during activity. Examples of words and phrases include heart rate pulse, blood pressure, respiratory rate, breathing pattern, and O_2 saturation. Any abnormalities or complaints such as chest pain, SOB, and pounding in the chest, dizziness, and nausea should be recorded. The preexisting need for medications and history of medical problems, such as asthma and MI should also be included in the description. Unusual fatigue and other abnormalities must be described. Patient activity should be modified as necessary by recommending paced activity, energy conservation techniques, and rest periods. Pulse oximetry, EKG readings, and similar tests should be performed during treatment if patient/client is specifically referred for cardiac reconditioning. All information must be documented.

Describe baseline pulmonary function data to compare with data during activity as necessary. Pulmonary function data includes respiratory rate, breath sounds, congestion/cough, sputum color and consistency (if present), breathing patterns, chest deformity, unusual fatigue, difficulty breathing, abnormal breathing patterns, or chest pain. The pulmonary function data should also include paced activity and energy conservation techniques and pulse oximetry measurements (see Table 9-6 for an endurance scale noting that the description is what should be included in the documentation).

TABLE 9-6 • Endurance Scale (source unknown), Document using the Descriptions.

Good: Tolerates normal activity, using moderate to maximal resistance. Activity and position changes with no signs of fatigue, palpitation, dyspnea, or pain. Standing tolerance is 30 minutes.

Good−: Tolerates normal activity, using moderate resistance activity, and positional changes with only occasional or minimal fatigue, no palpitations, dyspnea, or pain increase. Standing tolerance is 15 minutes.

Fair+: Tolerates high to moderate resistive activity and position change with infrequent rest periods (20–30 minutes work period) and minimal fatigue noted; longer time or more resistance causes fatigue, palpitations, dyspnea, or pain. Standing tolerance is 15 minutes.

Fair: Tolerates light resistive activity for short to moderate length of times (10 to 15 minutes); needs occasional rest periods; longer time or more resistance causes fatigue, dyspnea, palpitations, or pain. Standing tolerance is 10 minutes.

Fair−: Comfortable at rest; tolerates nonresistive activity for short duration (5–10 minutes), needs frequent rest periods; longer time, or more addition of resistance increases fatigue, dyspnea, or pain. Standing tolerance is 5 minutes.

Poor+: Comfortable at rest; tolerates nonresistive activity for short duration (2–4 minutes); needs very frequent rest periods of longer time or addition of resistance to exercise causes fatigue, palpitations, dyspnea, or pain. Standing tolerance is 2–4 minutes.

Poor: Comfortable at rest; light nonresistive activity of brief duration causes fatigue, palpitation, dyspnea, or pain. Standing tolerance 1–3 minutes.

Poor−: Symptoms may be present at rest; if any physical activity undertaken distress is increased. Standing tolerance less than 1 minute.

Body Mechanics. To evaluate body mechanics, describe posture and movement patterns during all activities performed during the session which may be ADL, any transitional movements from position to position, work-related tasks such as sitting or lifting. Abnormal body mechanics may result in pain and dysfunction. Phrases and words used to describe body mechanics include abnormal body alignment, abnormal movement patterns, and inability to perform specific movement tasks. There are instances in which adaptation of a specific movement task is indicated, but a change in body mechanics is not feasible. This may be the case for specific pathology related to fused spine, limb contracture, or fused or limited joint movements kyphosis, scoliosis or movement contraindications such as with post posterolateral total hip arthroplasty.

Orthotics and Prosthetics. Describe orthotics and prosthetics in terms of the need for a device based on impairment in order to facilitate function. At times, a device may be used for cosmetic purposes only, but would not require rehabilitation unless instructions in skin care and application and removal are required for same, such as a static prosthetic arm. Once prescribed and obtained, describe how the devices are to be monitored for fit and function, and the patient must be appropriately trained to use the device. Documentation should include the type of device if the patient/client already has a device and condition of it, gait, posture, and/or body part description with and without device; alignment of the device itself relative to the body and its impact on function; ability to perform functional tasks with and without orthosis/prosthesis and need for assistive or adaptive devices; comfort; ability to apply and remove; skin integrity as a result of wearing the device; proper fit and prescription; and ability for self-care with device. Documentation should include prosthetic or orthotic training or check out consistent with CPT verbiage.

Adaptive and Assistive Devices and Equipment. General categories of prostheses and orthoses include AFO (ankle foot orthosis), rigid or dynamic; KAFO (knee, ankle foot orthosis); RGO (reciprocating gait orthosis); above-the-knee (AK) prosthesis; below-the-knee (BK) prosthesis; above-the-elbow (AE) prosthesis; below-the-elbow (BE) prosthesis; myoelectric prosthesis; lumbar supports; trunk orthoses; cervical collars; slings; and bivalve casts. There is a large variety of both custom and off-the-shelf splints and braces/orthoses for the elbow, wrist/hand, fingers, knee, and ankle/foot.

When evaluating the assistive devices, describe the devices and equipment in terms of the need for a device based on impairment and their role in facilitating function. Once obtained, documentation must address how devices must be monitored for fitness and function, and the patient must be trained to use the device. Phrases and words for this documentation include mobility, posture, ability or inability to use the device functionally, comfort, and self-care. Instructions to the patient/client regarding initial and ongoing skin inspection for under pressure should be documented.

Types of adaptive and assistive devices and equipment include walking aids such as walkers, canes, and crutches; wheelchairs; cushions; lift chairs; transfer disks; hospital beds; reachers; elastic shoelaces; and lap trays.

Activities of Daily Living (ADL).

Due to the multitude of ADL, it is necessary to describe which ADLs are addressed or identified as impaired in documentation. ADL specifically relate to self-care and function in the daily environment, but exclude work-related activities most activities outside of the home. Describe ADL in objective, functional terms that can be addressed and measured for evidence of improvement. ADL include household chores, personal hygiene, dressing, toileting, and retrieval of articles/items.

Information about ADL may be dependent on information provided by the patient during the initial interview or through observation. ADL scales, such as the Katz and Barthel's, are helpful and standardized for ADL skills. Depending on the facility and venue, the PT may or may not perform actual ADL examination and intervention.

> **Author's Note:** When the patient's main complaint is pain, it may be difficult to justify treatment unless it is related to the inability to perform ADLs. The patient's subjective description of improvement and pain relief may have to be relied on for determination of progress. Whenever possible, try to duplicate the ADL in the clinic to observe actual rather than reported performance.

Incremental Activities of Daily Living (IADL).

IADL activities range from averaging a checkbook, to shopping and riding public transportation. Although there may be medicare limitations, it is commonly performed in rehabilitation for neuromuscularly involved individuals. The Lawton scale and IADL interventions if performed by PT must be documented.

Functional Capacity.

Descriptions of results of functional capacity testing and work hardening and conditioning programs are typically completed on standardized forms or programs for accurate, consistent recording of the performance, and behavior of patients. When preparing functional activity data, avoid personal opinion (as in the initial evaluation). In this area—perhaps more than any other—the PT must rely on professional opinion rather than personal conclusions because patients involved in these programs are commonly patients injured on the job who are involved with the workers' compensation system.

VII. DOCUMENTING INTERVENTION/TREATMENT

An entry into the record should be made for each PT visit on the day the treatment was rendered, as close to treatment time as possible to insure accuracy, regardless of the payer source. The CMS currently refers to daily notes as "encounter notes," which must include the following according to CMS transmittal R52BP:[2]

"Date, total time spent in services represented by timed codes, total treatment time, signature and professional identification of individual performing the treatment, name of treatment/intervention, significant changes and/or unexpected occurrences, equipment issues." Optional inclusions, but are strongly recommended by the authors of this text, are meaningful self-report, any communication about the patient/client, and adverse reactions or response to treatment. The patient/client's full name should also be included on every new page as well as PT/PTA signature.

The APTA has a position that there should be documentation establishing the "physical therapist of record" who assumes the primary responsibility for the patient/client management. It also states that facilities should develop and implement a process to identify the physical therapist of record and "hand off" communication procedures. See the APTA position below:

PHYSICAL THERAPIST OF RECORD AND "HAND OFF" COMMUNICATION HOD P06-08-16-16 [Position][3]

Whereas, Recognizing that the physical therapist or physical therapist assistant providing care may change within a setting or institution, establishing a physical therapist of record and ensuring effective "hand off" communication help to ensure that the plan of care is continued and advanced in a manner that best benefits the patient/client; Resolved, The physical therapist of record is the therapist who assumes primary responsibility for patient/client management and as such is held accountable for the coordination, continuation, and progression of the plan of care; Resolved, That the American Physical Therapy Association (APTA) encourages practices and facilities to develop and implement a process to identify the physical therapist of record and "hand off" communication procedures; and Resolved, That APTA shall incorporate the concepts of physical therapist of record and "hand off" communication into appropriate Association documents.

The decision to use progress note format, commonly in the SOAP format, is an individual or organizational one. The significant difference between an encounter or treatment note and a progress note, are statements about progress relative to previous entries or established goals. Progress reports are episodic summaries that include progress toward goals in addition to a summary of interventions rendered over a prescribed period time. For Medicare purposes, progress reports are required once every 10 treatment days or at minimum once monthly. The PT of record must see the patient/client within the treatment period and write the report. In skilled nursing facilities, a progress note is required weekly.

Author's Note: Although progress notes/reports by the PT may be episodic, there must be a writer record/note for each patient/client encounter by the PT/PTA.

When documenting intervention and treatment, always be specific, using CPT codeable terms (see Chapter 5) to precede all interventions, unless the interventions themselves are codes, such as ultrasound or electrical stimulation (qualifying constant attendance versus unattended). This is applicable regardless of the format used: narrative, SOAP, flow charts, manual or electronic as templates. Include the location where the treatment was rendered, i.e., patient room, PT department, patient home, if anyone accompanied the patient/client or was present, and who that person was, and make sure the patient/client if not a minor gave consent, how long, and specific parameters and position for reproducibility. All verbiage used in the content section that preceded this section should be applied in context. In any entry for intervention, it is critical for reimbursement, audits, consistency, and coordination of billing with documentation of patient/client treatment sessions or visits, that the CPT code verbiage be included and precede the actual descriptions of what was performed.

Improvements in impairments should be stated in relation to the functional goals dependent on that improvement. For situations in which PT was administered in the OP gym, bedside, or home, clearly identify all intervention(s). Identify the specific equipment as indicated, with specific parameters (settings), time, and patient/client position. Describe the number of repetitions, dosage, distance, quality of movement/performance, deviations from norms, and degree of assistance needed to indicate skill needed. Increasing distance alone or increasing repetitions does not indicate skill. These should show progressions/improvements over time to indicate skill needed. Increasing distance alone or increasing repetitions does not indicate skill. If the same exercises, repetitions and resistance are administered for several days and the entries lack content that describes the PT skills required, reimbursement is at risk. Also list the specific area of the body treated and target tissues, problems, and purpose as well as patient/client position. Include in your entries the start and end time and the duration of the session, noting if rests were needed and if so include the length of the rest. The patient/client's response to treatment should always be included. In some settings, the number of minutes or units for individual interventions is required, or the actual treatment time i.e. 9:00AM–9:30AM. The concept of documenting in a skilled manner, always emphasizing the medical necessity should always be evident. Refer to Example 39 for time.

■ Example 39

Minutes for individual interventions:
15 minutes (1 unit)	Therapeutic exercise trunk
15 minutes (1 unit)	Soft tissue mobilization posterior trunk

Include vital signs in the intervention/treatment documentation as required based on history, condition treated, and precautions. It is also important to include any occurrence out of the "ordinary" or unique to that patient. Patient condition before and after treatment including response and effect on integument should also be documented.

In the record, the PT should also describe:

- contraindications and precautions and barriers, if any;
- symptom relief and improved function resulting from interventions;
- specific mode of treatment and parameters for application; with skilled role of PT/PTA
- immediate effects of intervention in terms of change in endurance, pain, sensation, reflexes, strength, and range and quality of joint movement; patient/client response.

Terminology should be skilled, but not so technical that it cannot be understood by other health professionals and most individuals needing access to the record.

VIII. SUMMARY

Regardless of the audience for PT documentation, the content and overall progress toward goals inclusive of the skilled role of the PT/PTA justifies the care given and establishes medical necessity. The physical therapist or assistant must convey what is known to be true, relative to the need for care. Historically, although PTs can verbally describe treatment being rendered, including the parameters and the medical necessity, the lack of ability to communicate this in writing has proven to be challenging and can result in denial of reimbursement.

In the initial examination and evaluation and ongoing, the PT must remember to include all areas of patient/client deficits that would justify the need for skilled care to ensure the patient benefits fully from the therapy. For example, a patient/client with a recent amputation requires gait and transfer training with and without the prosthesis, wheelchair training (at least early on), training on multiple surfaces in varied environments, adaptive driving, skin care training, prosthetic care training, therapeutic exercise, extensive transfer training including car transfers, ADLs, and IADLs. If patient/client is working, ergonomic assessment may be indicated as well. It they plan to return to work or continue working while receiving PT services, the ability to do so should be included as a goal at the onset of treatment.

A listing of all of the patient's deficits should be included in inpatient, home health, and outpatient documentation, with emphasis on what will addressed in the context of a specific venue and length of stay (LOS). For example, in a 3- to 4-day acute care LOS, treatment may focus on getting in and out of bed and gait for short distances, with instruction in activity the patient can do at home. In home health, in which homebound status is a concern, returning the individual to a higher level of function including aerobic capacity and muscle performance, in addition to safe transfers in the home, progression of gait to a variety of surfaces, and self-care may be emphasized, and so forth, as the patient progresses to outpatient. Additionally, emphasis should be placed on all comorbidities because they can potentially impact the need for skilled care and prolong the justification for care.

Regardless of venue, all components of the record should match. Critical to audits, is matching by the PT of patient/client goals to the goals of therapy, identifying all relevant deficits and establishing matching goals and interventions. The goals achieved at the end of the therapeutic LOS should match those established either at the initial examination and evaluation or as the patient/client progressed. If a peer or auditor can compare the initial examination/evaluation with the summation of care/discharge summary and quickly assess the progress, with emphasis on function, the record will more likely be viewed positively as representing skilled care. An auditor will also verify that all services billed have dates that are consistent with actual treatment days and documentation.

The key to successful documentation is not in what the therapist *knows*, but what the therapist or other designated personnel *documents*. If it is not written, it was not done. Furthermore, if it is not written correctly, it might as well not have been rendered nor recorded. From a reimbursement and liability perspective. Only the therapist can justify the need for care and support the need through appropriate, objective, and functionally oriented documentation. In situations in which the PT and the PTA work together, the communication between the PT and the PTA, must also be documented. All PT documentation must answer the question, but for physical therapy would the patient/client recover? As well as where the patient is functionally at every point in treatment.

■ Example 40

Smith, Pooja
1/2/11 10:00 AM: Spoke to Joe Morita, PT re:patient progress. Instructed to progress gait training with quad cane and emphasis multiple turn 90° and 180° B/L next week.

Allen Stem, PT # 0621

On the following pages are some documentation note examples from different settings.

1. Determine what context is missing & what is good
2. Identify why some notes would be denied for reimbursement

Initial Evaluation

Name: John Smith

DOB: 04-01-1965

Medical Diagnosis: 847.2 Lumbar Sprain

Date: 10/07/10

MR#: 60759

Physician: Frank Green, M.D.

Physical Therapy Diagnosis: Pattern 4F: Impaired Joint Mobility, Motor Function, Muscle Performance, Range of Motion, and Reflex Integrity Associated With Spinal Disorders

Patient/Client History: 45 y.o. male who injured his low back lifting boxes at work 1 week ago. Patient reports that he experienced sharp pain on the R side of the lumbar spine immediately following lifting and twisting a 45 lbs. box. He was brought to the ED by his supervisor, where he underwent radiographic evaluation that was negative, and was subsequently discharged. He followed up at the occupational health clinic the next day, received a prescription for Motrin 800 mg/tid, and was referred to physical therapy. He has no prior history of LBP.

Social Status/History: Married with 2 children, 8 and 11 y.o. Lives in one story house. Leisure activities include boating, fishing, and coaching soccer.

Employment: has been employed as a parcel delivery driver for 5 years.

General Health status: HBP, otherwise good.

Social/Health habits: smokes ½ pack of cigarettes per day, drinks 1 alcoholic beverage per day.

Family History: Mother had CVA 5 years ago, recovered fully

Medical/surgical history: unremarkable other than HBP

Current condition/chief complaints: Current pain rated as 5/10 on NPRS, aggravated by bending, standing, and prolonged sitting to 7/10, relieved by lying down to 1/10. Located in R lumbar paravertebral area, sometimes spreading into R buttock. Stiffness is noted when waking up.

Functional Status: Currently unable to work or perform leisure activities. Modified Oswestry score of 60/100. FABQ-Work score: 17.

Medications: Diovan 80 mg/qd, Motrin 800 mg/tid.

Systems Review:

Height 5'11", weight 202 lb, BP 140/85, HR 76. Systems review otherwise unremarkable (see health questionnaire attached).

Cognition: A&O ×3, normal communication skills, prefers written handouts for educational materials.

TESTS and MEASURES:

Observation: Increased lumbar lordosis, slight forward head. Decreased trunk rotation during gait.

Neurological testing: SLR negative, dermatome/myotome testing normal, DTRs normal.

Range of Motion:

UEs/LEs: normal

AROM Trunk: Flexion 45 deg (limited by pain)
        Extension 20 deg
        Sidebending: L 20 deg (limited by pain), R 30 deg
        Rotation: L 40 deg, R 30 degrees (limited by pain)
        Repeated motion did not reveal directional preference

(*continued*)

PIVM: PA Spring Testing limited 1/6 at L4-5, 2/6 at L5-S1

Strength:

UEs/LEs: Gross strength normal

Trunk: Lumbar Multifidi 4/5 bilat.

Transverse/oblique abdominals 3/5

Palpation:

Increased muscle tone of R paravertebral mm.

PROBLEM SUMMARY:

Patient presents with localized R paravertebral pain/muscle tone, ROM deficits of the lumbar spine, increased lumbar lordosis, and weakness of spinal stabilizing musculature. Patient also has a high level of disability, as indicated by the Oswestry and fear-avoidance behavior scores and inability to work or participate in leisure activities.

PROGNOSIS: Since patient meets 4 out of 5 inclusion criteria of the Spinal Manipulation Clinical Prediction rule, there is a high likelihood of good treatment outcomes.

GOALS:

STGs (2 weeks):

Patient will regain normal spinal mobility through the use of spinal manipulation in order to return to work and leisure activities.

Patient will have a reduced Oswestry disability score of 30/100 and a reduced FABQ-W score of 8 in order to return to work and leisure activities.

Patient will have reduced pain as indicated by a NPRS score of 2/10 in order to return to work and leisure activities.

Patient will increase muscle strength of abdominal and multifidi muscles to 3+/5 and 4+/5 to improve active spinal stabilization.

LTGs (6 weeks):

Patient will have an Oswestry disability score of 10/100 and a reduced FABQ-W score of less than 5 in order to return to work and leisure activities.

Patient's pain complaints will be resolved as indicated by a NPRS score of 0/10 in order to return to work and leisure activities.

Patient will increase muscle strength of abdominal and multifidi muscles to 4+/5 and 5/5 to improve active spinal stabilization.

Patient will be independent on HEP to further improve spinal posture and stabilization to prevent reoccurrence of injury.

PLAN:

Physical therapy treatment twice a week for four weeks, initially consisting of spinal manipulation and myofascial mobilization, patient education regarding condition and prognosis, and HEP consisting of ROM and muscle strengthening exercises, to progress to lumbar stabilization program and postural/ergonomic instruction.

Signature:

Ellen Stevens, FL PT 14723

97001 Initial Evaluation
Time: 10:00am-10:45am

PT TREATMENT NOTE

Name: John Smith   **MR#:** 60759

Date: 10/12/10   **Time:** 10:00 AM-10:58 AM

S: Patient states that "low back pain has decreased to 3/10 overall, maximum pain of 4/10, and less morning pain and stiffness."

O:

97140 Manual Therapy: 16 min: Manual therapy including manipulation of lumbar spine in prone position, and myofascial mobilization of lumbar paravertebral musculature. Mobility improved to 2/6 @ L4-5 and 3/6 (normal) @ L5-S1. Tone of paravertebral mm decreased.

97110 Therapeutic procedure: 28 min: Strengthening exercises for transverse abdominis mm in supine with verbal cueing to facilitate muscle contraction 3×10 reps bilat. Supine trunk rotation exercises in hook-lying position to strengthen oblique abdominal mm, 3×10 reps bilat. Strengthening of bilat. multifidi in prone position using leg lifts with manual resistance 3×10 reps bilat. and leg and opposite arm lifts 3×10 reps in supine. Review of home exercise program including trunk mobility and strengthening exercises. Strength: abdominal mm 3/5, multifidi 4+/5. Patient was able to return demonstrate HEP.

97010 Neuromuscular Reeducation: 14 min: Postural instruction in standing position to decrease lumbar lordosis and increase posterior pelvic tilt. Verbal cuing is required for correction of posture.

A: Patient is progressing toward achievement of all his STGs. He is returning to "light duty" at work next week, with a lifting restriction of 10 lb as ordered by physician. Oswestry disability score decreased to 34/100.

P. Continue per treatment plan 2× a week, including joint/muscle manipulation, trunk strengthening exercises, and postural instruction. Will progress lumbar stabilization exercises next week.

Signature:

Ellen Stevens, PT 14723

97140 Manual Therapy: 16 min, 1 unit
97110 Therapeutic procedure: 28 min, 2 units
97010 Neuromuscular Reeducation: 14 min, 1 unit
Total RX time 58 minutes

PT DISCHARGE SUMMARY/SUMMATION OF CARE

Name: John Smith

DOB: 04-01-1965

Medical Diagnosis: 847.2 Lumbar Sprain

Date: 11/12/10

MR#: 60759

Physician: Frank Green, M.D.

Physical Therapy Diagnosis: Pattern 4F: Impaired Joint Mobility, Motor Function, Muscle Performance, Range of Motion, and Reflex Integrity Associated With Spinal Disorders

Reason for Discharge: Anticipated goals and expected outcomes have been met.

Current Physical/Functional Status: Pain as reported on NPRS has decreased to 0/10. Lumbar spine mobility has normalized, and is symmetrical bilaterally. Abdominal strength has increased to 4+/5. Disability as reported on Oswestry scale has decreased to 5/100, patient has returned to work without restrictions, and has resumed leisure activities.

Goals/Outcomes Achieved:

Patient will have an Oswestry disability score of 10/100 and a reduced FABQ-W score of less than 5 in order to return to work and leisure activities: **MET**

Patient's pain complaints will be resolved as indicated by a NPRS score of 0/10 in order to return to work and leisure activities: **MET**

Patient will increase muscle strength of abdominal and multifidi muscles to 4+/5 and 5/5 to improve active spinal stabilization: **MET**

Patient will be independent on HEP to further improve spinal posture and stabilization to prevent reoccurrence of injury: **MET**

Discharge plan: Patient will continue home exercise program including trunk muscle strengthening and lumbar stabilization program in order to prevent reoccurrence of injury.

Signature:

Ellen Stevens, PT 14723

PT SOAP Daily Note SNF setting

Name: Barbara Hillard   Date: 3/28/2010
Time: 8:00 AM to 9:00 AM

S: Patient stated: "Now able to get a full night's sleep of 8 hours without waking up in pain from hip like before. However, I still feel unsteady when standing up from sitting in a chair without the use of my walker."

O: Precautions: WBAT R LE, R hip precautions

15 minutes: 97116 gait training: contact guard with front wheeled walker (FWW) three-one-point pattern; even surface ×60 feet tile, carpet surfaces 3 times each. Training stairs, 5x up/down; ascended/descended using FWW contact guard with verbal cues for FWW placement, and gait pattern. Decreased R hip flexion when ascending stairs in comparison to L. Tendency to misjudge height of stair with RLE when ascending without verbal cues.

15 minutes: 97110: Therapeutic procedure: Standing within parallel bars: R hip Flex, Ext, Abd, and bilateral mini squats, 10 reps ×2 sets each, 30 sec rest in between sets, while observing R hip precautions. Supine: short-arc quad extensions bilaterally: 10 reps ×2 sets, 30 sec rest in between reps; active R knee extension hamstring stretch ×3, 20 sec hold. Strength: R hip FL, Ext, Abd 3+/5, quads 4/5.

15 minutes: 97112: Neuromuscular reeducation: Balance training: bilateral neutral stance on foam within parallel bars, eyes open with minimal assist for balance, two fingers touching parallel bars bilaterally for balance. Balanced maintained for 20 sec, 5 reps. Progressed to no contact with parallel bars, balance loss after 10 sec, 5 reps. Required use of parallel bars to right self.

15 minutes: 97010: Cold pack R hip pain in L sidelying, pillow between knees for comfort following gait and exercise. Skin on hip intact prior and following application of cold pack, normal response to cold present. Reported pain 1/10 after CP.

A: Progressed from regular walker to front wheeled walker in order to increase mobility on all surfaces, including carpet and outdoor surfaces. Patient shows increased balance during functional activities. Patient progressing towards her established goals of D/C from SNF.

P: Will continue with PT 3×/week for gait training, progressive the ex, neuromuscular reeducation, and cold pack. Plan to educate patient to use cane during gait training for next visit.

Signature:

John Barker, FL PT 000234

15 minutes: 97116: Gait training 1 unit
15 minutes: 97112: Neuromuscular reeducation 1 unit
15 minutes: 97010: Cold pack 1 unit
15 minutes: 97110: Therapeutic procedure 1 unit

Wound care assessment note, SNF setting

Patient: Alexa Smith, chart number 263357, DOB 03/12/1940

Date: 3/28/2010

Time: 8:00 AM to 9:00 AM

Primary Diagnosis: Hemiplegia Dominant Side

Treatment Diagnosis: Muscle Weakness, Difficulty Walking, Full Thickness Non-healing Surgical Wounds

Payor: Medicare Part A

Plan of Treatment: SNF Wound Care

History: Patient sustained a fall on 5/7/10 resulting in a hematoma to the left hip. The hematoma migrated distally in the LLE, resulting in compartment syndrome of the L lower leg. Surgical intervention was indicated and he underwent a fasciotomy to the LLE. Due to decreased mobility the patient developed an unstageable pressure ulcer to the L heel in addition to the non-healing surgical wound.

Patient has a PMH consisting of R posterior-medial frontal lobe CVA which contributes to his anxiety. Due to increases in the patient's pain and poor response to conventional wound treatment, the wound care nurse requested physical therapy intervention for pain management and wound care interventions.

Assessment: Patient presents with three separate LLE wounds: Fasciotomy wounds are located in the left lateral and medial calf region.

Site 1: Left lateral calf surgical; wound measures 18 cm (l) × 4 cm (w) and presents with 40% yellow slough and 60% granular tissue with moderate serosanguinous drainage without apparent odor. Wounds are full thickness with damage to epidermal, dermal, and subcutaneous tissue. No undermining or tunneling: hyper-granulation tissue at 1:00–3:00.

Left medial calf surgical wound measures 15.3 cm (l) × 4.8 cm (w) and presents with 25% yellow slough and 75% granular tissue with copious serosanguinous drainage without odor. Wounds are full thickness with damage to epidermal, dermal, and subcutaneous tissue.

Left heel presents with unstageable pressure ulcer measuring 5.2 cm (l) × 1.2 cm (w) with 90% loosely adherent yellow/brown eschar and 10% granulation tissue with minimal drainage, no tunneling, or undermining present.

Pain: The patient reports pain scale of 10/10 for LLE at worst: 6/10 at best

Short-Term Goals: 2 Weeks

1. Pain: The patient will report decreased pain for LLE grossly to 8/10 through use of therapeutic modalities such as ultrasound and electrical stimulation to increase functional mobility

2. Wound Care: Site 1: Patient will exhibit L lateral calf full thickness surgical improving to 16 cm (l) × 2.5 cm (w) for improved skin integrity to reduce risk of infection. Decrease pain and improve functional mobility. Wound characteristics will improve to 30% slough, 70% granular with minimal serosanguinous drainage

3. Wound Care: Site 2: Patient will exhibit L medial calf full thickness surgical improving to 13 cm (l) × 3.5 cm (w) for improved skin integrity to reduce risk of infection. Decrease pain and improve functional mobility. Wound characteristics will improve to 20% slough, 80% granular with minimal serosanguinous drainage

4. Wound Care: Site 3: Patient will demonstrate healing of left heel unstageable ulcer to measure 4.3 cm (l) × 0.8 cm (w) for improved skin integrity to reduce risk of infection. Decrease pain and improve functional mobility.

Long Term Goals: 90 Days

Patient will demonstrate resolved LLE calf wounds and L heel wound, report decreased pain to 3/10 at worst in order to increase his functional mobility and improve quality of life.

Signature:

Erika Stevens PT, FL PT 14723

SOAP Daily Note Outpatient Orthopedics

Name: Barbara Hillard   **Date:** 3/28/2010

Diagnosis: 726.2 Shoulder Impingement Syndrome

Physical Therapy Diagnosis: Pattern 4D: Impaired Joint Mobility, Motor Function, Muscle Performance, and Range of Motion Associated With Connective Tissue Dysfunction

Time: 11:00 AM to 11:45 AM

S: Patient stated: "Able to reach to high self of kitchen cabinet with a lot less pain."

O: 97140 Manual Therapy 15 min: Manual therapy including mobilization of R GH joint in inferior, posterior, and anterior glide directions grade III/IV. Mobility improved to 2/6 (moderate restriction) in all three directions.

97110 Therapeutic procedure 17 min: in standing: AROM in FF (forward flexion), ABD within painfree range, with verbal cueing to facilitate scapular motion and reduce shoulder hiking. Standing strengthening exercises for rotator cuff mm in ABD, IR and ER using yellow theraband 3×15 reps. Reinforcement of home exercise program including self-mobilization, ROM, and strengthening exercises. Patient needs continued verbal cuing to decrease shoulder hiking. Strength of RC MMT 4−/5. Moderate patient compliance with HEP: completes 50% of prescribed sessions.

97112 Ultrasound 13 min: US 6 minutes, 1 W/cm^2 pulsed 20% duty cycle 1 MHz to R supraspinatus tendon, patient seated with arm behind back. Total setup and cleanup time 13 minutes.

A: Patient is progressing towards achievement of STGs. Functional status is improving as noted by improved overhead activities.

P. Continue per treatment plan 3× a week, including joint mobilization, PREs, and US. Will progress to red theraband next week for PRE.

Signature:

Erika Stevens, FL PT 14723

97140 Manual Therapy: 15 min, 1 unit

97110 Therapeutic procedure: 17 min, 1 unit

97112 Ultrasound: 13 min, 1 unit

Initial Evaluation and Treatment Plan—Shoulder Evaluation

Name: Barbara Hillard

Date of Evaluation: October 8, 2012   **Date of Onset:** July 2012

Diagnosis: Adhesive Capsulitis Right Shoulder

History/Mechanism of Injury: Patient is a 56-year-old male who reports gradual onset of pain beginning in July of this year following repainting two rooms in his house. Initially he reported pain with activity, however the primary complaint at this time is of stiffness and difficulty moving the right arm overhead.

Psychosocial/Functional Deficits: Functionally he is limited in dressing, tucking in his shirt, combing hair, and reaching his wallet. He has been able to continue his daily work routine as an accountant. His job duties are primarily at the computer, but requires free rests.

PMH: Type 1 SM HTN, Hyperlipidemia

Current Medications: Lisinopril, Lipitor, Metformin, Lantos BID

Vitals: BP 130/88, HR 82

Symptomology: Constant___ Intermittent___ Variable__x_ Unchanging ___ Daily
↑ or ↓ symptoms with activities. Pain is increased with any overhead movement or movement away from the body.

Decreased with rest?

Pain Pattern/Intensity (0-10 scale) R shoulder: Rest: 2/10: Activity: 5/10

Hand Dominance   Right

Comments: Holds RUE in protective posture against treat with forearm across abdomen

Observation/Inspection: Forward head posture, mild thoracic kyphoisis

Joint Clearing: Cervical spine: screened and cleared

GH +=pain	AROM L	AROM R	PROM L	PROM R	Strength L	Strength R
Flexion	180	90	180	100	5/5	2/5
Extension	30	20	30	25	5/5	4/5
Abduction	180	90	180	95	5/5	2/5
Internal Rot	70	35	70	40	5/5	2/5
External Rot	85	40	85	42	5/5	2/5

Palpation: Moderate tenderness noted at deltoid

Joint Play Assessment: Inferior glide 1/6: Anterior 3/6: Posterior: 2/6

Special Tests: + Hawkins, + Neer, −Speeds, −Drop arm, −Load shift

ASSESSMENT: Signs and symptoms consistent with impingement syndrome and adhesive capsulitis: patient has good prognosis for recovery of motion and functional use of RUE

Problems/Physical Findings: Limited functional use of RUE for ADLs.: Decreased active and passive ROM of the right shoulder

(*continued*)

TREATMENT PLAN:

Patient will be seen 2×/week for 3 weeks

GOALS

STG	To be completed in 2 weeks	
1	Increase ROM in all right shoulder motions by from 90° to 100° to improve ability to perform ADLs	
2	Decrease pain in right shoulder to 1/10 at rest to improve ability to perform ADLs and 3/10 during activity	
3	Increase strength of right shoulder musculature by ½ MMT grade to improve ability to perform ADLs	
LTG	To be completed in 4 weeks	
1	Increase ROM of all right shoulder motions by 15 degrees to improve functional mobility with dressing and grooming	
2	Increase strength of right shoulder musculature to 4/5 to improve ability to perform overhead reaching tasks	
3	Decrease pain of right shoulder to 1/10 with activity to allow for return to recreational activities	

Uninterrupted work

Barriers to achieving treatment goals?   ☐ Yes   × No

Family/patient involved in and verbalized understanding of goals?   × Yes   ☐ No

Patient was instructed in shoulder as it pertains to the injury?   × Yes   ☐ No

Clinician: Kathy Swiss, PT,DPT, OCS   **License: NE PT 04569**

Therapies Summary

Admitting Dr. Grant

Ordering Dr. *Same as admitting*

Order *PT/OT Consults*

Operative Procedure

Admitting Diagnosis *EMS/SOB DUE TO TRAUMATIC   Y*

Current Diagnosis *SOB, S/P FALL, RIB FRACTURES*

Order Date *10/04/10*   Age *74*

Current Med. Hx. *PATIENT ADMITTED APPROX 5 DAYS S/P FALL SUSTAINING MULTIPLE RIB FRACTURES, POSSIBLE LEFT PATELLA FRACTURE (AWAITING XRAYS) ADMITTED WITH BILATERAL PNEUMONIA*

Past Medical History *HTN, END STAGE RENAL DISEASE, CURRENTLY RECEIVING HEMODIALYSIS, AAA, CARDIOMYOPATHY, AICD PLACEMENT*

Precautions *Cardiac Falls*

Clinical Observations *IV'S, Foley, 02, Telemetry, Pulse ox.,*

Pain   Yes × No   Scale *4/1*   Nrsg Notified   Yes × No
                                    0

Location *RIBS* Fx   Interference w/ Tx *NO*

#1 Test *See chart*   Date Done   Clinical Impression

Pts   Learning Style *Verbal Visual Demo*   Barriers to learning *None*

Permission given by patient to discuss/display pertinent information.   Yes × No

Comments *PLOF PATIENT WAS INDEPENDENT IN MOBILITY WITHOUT USE OF ASSISTIVE DEVICE*

– Social History –

Lives with *Alone*   Living Arrangement *Home*

Stairs/Steps in Home   Yes   No ×

Threshold Step   Who will be helping you at home?   *Children*

– Evaluation –

× General Evaluation   Ortho Evaluation

PROM

See Rehab Flowsheet   within fuctional limits: ×   Within fuctional limits except:

Shoulder   Elbow   Wriest   Hip   Knee   Ankle   All Ext   ×   Other

Other   Comment   *POSSIBLE LEFT PATELIA FRACTURE: AWAITING XRAY RESULTS*

Strength

Within functional limits: ×   Within functional limits except:

Shoulder   Elbow   Wrist   Hip   Knee   Ankle   All Ext   ×   Other

Other   Comment   *GROSS STRENGTH BUE / LE IS 4–/5. AROM/STRENGTH WFL IN BUE WITH ADL'S AND SIT TO STAND.*

× *Mobility*

Rolling *Min Assist/Contact Guard*   Supine to Sit *Mod Assist*

Scooting *Mod Assist*   Sit to Stand *Not Tested*

Basic Transfer *Not tested*

	Static	Dynamic
Balance		
Sit	Good	Good
Stand	Not tested	Not tested

Ambulatory Status *Not tested*   Distance (ft)

(continued)

× **Coordination**   (Movement, Quality)   *Gross Intact, GROSS/FINE INTACT IN BU E*

× **Motor Control**   *Normotonic, NORMOTONIC BUE*

× **Sensation**   Intact throughout   Intact throughout except: × Not tested

× **ADL's**

Feeding *Setup/Indep-*   Grooming *Setup/Indep-*   Bathing *UE Min Assist,*   Dressing *UE Supervision,*
           endent   *endent*   *LE Mod Assist*   *LE Max Assist*

Comments:

× **Cognition**

Orientation   *Alert and Oriented to person,*   Attention   *Fair*
                    place time

Insight into Disability   *Good*   Memory   *Good*

Problem Solving   *Good*   Follows Directions   *Multiple*

Sequencing   *Impaired-required verbal cues for*   Safety   *Impaired*
                  handplacement and sequencing with
                  Transfers

Hearing   *Intact*

Comments:

× **Visual Status**   Intact   Impaired

Ocular Pursuits

Visual Fields

Depth Perception

Figure-Ground

R/L Discrimination

Body Scheme

Comments   *Visual Status Grossly Intact for age, wears glasses for reading and reports*
                 Bilateral Cataract Sx.

  Wound Evaluation

  FIMI

Bed Mobility	3	1 – Dependent
		2 – Max Assist
		3 – Mod Assist
		4 – Min Assist/Contact Guard
		5 – Supervision/Stand-By Guard
Basic Transfers	8	6 – Modified Independent w/Asst Device
		7 – Independent
		8 – Not Tested
		9 – Not Applicable
Basic Ambulation	8	
Step Ambulation		
Car Transfers		
Toilet Transfer	4	
Cognition	5	
Feeding	6	
Bathing	4/3	
Dressing	4/2	
Grooming	6	

(*continued...*)

(*continued...*)

Wheelchair Propulsion	**8**
Wheelchair Management	**8**

– Assessment –

Rehab Problems	***Decreased endurance. Decreased ROM/Strength. Impaired functional mobility, Decreased independence in ADL's.***
Rehab Potential	***Good***

Anticipated PT/OT discharge needs   ***DC NEEDS UNDETERMINED AT THIS TIME: DC HOME WITH HEALTH VS SHORT TERM REHAB STAY***

#1 STG (1–3 visits)   ***Minimal/Contact Guard Assist Bed Bobility***

#2 STG (1–3 visits)   ***Minimal/Contact Guard Assist Transfers***

#3 STG (1–3 visits)   ***Minimal/Contact Guard Assist Ambulation***

#4 STG (1–3 visits)   ***SETUP/MIN ASSIST WITH LE BATHING WITH A. E.***

#5 STG (1–3 visits)   ***SETUP/MOD ASSIST WITH LE DRESSING WITH A. E.***

#6 STG (1–3 visits)   ***CGA WITH TOILET TRANSFERS WITH A. E.***

#1 LTG (3–5 visits)   ***To be determined.***

Wound Care Goals

Plan   (Frequency and Focus)   ***PT 4–6 times a week Strengthening ROM Bed mobility Transfers Gait ADL's Pt/Family Education & Teaching, OT 3–5X/WK FOR ADL'S, A. E., BASIC/BATHROOM TRANSFERS, FUNCTIONAL, MOBILITY SAFETY, ENDURANCE ACTIVITIES, AND PATIENT/CAREGIVER EDUCATION AND TRAINING***

Patient/Family Goals   ***Return to independent lifestyle.***

Goals and plan mutually set   Yes   ×   No

Miscellaneous Charges

PT Evaluation   ***1 PT***   OT Evaluation   ***1 EVAL***

Discharge Summary

PT: Gabby Smith	Therapies Summary

Admitting Dr. Alexa   Admitting Diagnosis   **PNEUMONIA, RESPIRATORY FAILURE**

Ordering Dr. **Same as admitting**   Current Diagnosis   **PNEUMONIA, RESPIRATORY INSUFFICENCY**

Order **PT/OT Consults**   Order Date **10/08/2010**   Age **75**

Operative Precedure   Current Med. Hx.   **PATIENT WAS GETTING RADIATION AND XELODA CHEMOTHERAPY. DEVELOPED PROGRESSIVE WEAKNESS AND COUGH. BROUGHT TO THE ER BY EMS AND PLACED ON BIPAP. CHEST X-RAY SHOWED LOWER LOBE PHEUMONIA. GIVEN IV ANTIBIOTICS AND ADMITTED TO THE MICU.**

Past Medical History   **ESOPHAGEAL CA, S/P TOTAL ESOPHAGECTOMY, A-FIB, MITRAL REGURGITATION, BPH, DYSLIPIDEMIA, PNEUMONIA, LEFT PNEUMOTHORAX, POSTOPERATIVE RESPIRATORY FAILURE, AND CHEMO/RADIATION THERAPY**   Precautions **Falls**

Clinical Observations   **IV's, 02, Telemetry, Pulse Ox.,**

Pain   Yes   No ×

#1   Test **See chart**   Date Done   Clinical Impression

Pts Learning Style **Verbal Visual Verbal Visiual Demo**   Barriers to learning **None**

Permission given by patient to discuss/display pertinent information.   Yes × No

Comments **PLOF PATIENT WAS USING A WALKER AT HOME FOR MOBILITY**

– Social History –

Lives with **Spouse**   Living Arrangement **Home**

Stairs/Steps in Home   Yes × No   Number **1**   Side bannister is on   up going side.

Threshold Step   Who will be helping you at home?   **Spouse**

– Evaluation –

× General Evaluation   Ortho Evaluation

PROM

See Rehab Flowsheet   × Within functional limits: Within fuctional limits except:

Strength

Within functional limits: × Within functional limits except:

Shoulder   Elbow   Wrist   Hip   Knee   Ankle   All Ext ×   Other

Other **BUE** Comment **AROM WFL IN BUE, PATIENT WITH SIGNIFICANT DECONDITIONING AND WEAKNESS. BUE STRENGTH NOT FORMALLY TESTED HOWEVER ESTIMATE BUE STRENGTH AT 3+/5. GROSS STRENGTH OF BLE IS ESTIMATED AT 3/5**

× **Mobility**

Rolling **Min Assist/Contact Guard**   Supine to Sit **Mod Assist**

Scooting **Min Assist/Contact Guard**   Sit to Stand **Mod Assist**

Basic Transfer **Mod Assist**

(continued)

Balance	Static	Dynamic
Sit	*Fair +*	*Poor*
Stand	*Fair +*	*Fair +*

Ambulatory Status   *Mod Assist Two Wheeled Walker*   Distance (ft) *STEPS*

× **Coordination** (Movement, Quality) *GROSS WFL, RESTING AND INTENTION TREMORS NOTED IN BUE*

× **Motor Control**   *LOW TONE IN TRUNK AND BUE*

× **Sensation**   Intact throughout   Intact throughout except: × Not tested

× **ADL's**

Feeding *Dependent*	Grooming *Min Assist/Contact act Guard*	Bathing *Mod Assist with UE Bathing, Max Assist with LE Bathing*	Dressing *Min Assist with UE Dressing, Dependent with LE Dressing*

Comment: *CURRENTLY ON TPN, SCORES FOR GROOMING, BATHING, AND DRESSING ARE ESTIMATED BASED ON ASSISTANCE WITH MOBILITY.*

× **Cognition**

Orientation *Alert and oriented to person*	Attention *Fair*
Insight into Disability *Fair*	Memory
Problem Solving *Fair*	Follows Directions *Two Step*
Sequencing *Impaired*	Safety *Impaired*
Hearing *Intact*	

Comments:

× **Visual Status**   Intact   Impaired

Ocular Pursuits

Visual Fields

Depth Perception

Figure-Ground

R/L Discrimination

Body Scheme

Comments *Visual Testing deferred at this time secondary to fatigue. Will assess when appropriate.*

Wound Evaluation

FIMI

Bed Mobility	*2*	1 – Dependent
		2 – Max Assist
		3 – Mod Assist
		4 – Min Assist/Contact Guard
		5 – Supervision/Stand-By Guard
Basic Transfers	*2*	6 – Modified Independent w/Asst Device
		7 – Independent
		8 – Not Tested
		9 – Not Applicable
Basic Ambulation		
Step Ambulation		
Car Transfers		
Toilet Transfer	*8*	

(*continued*)

Cognition	4
Feeding	1
Bathing	3/2
Dressing	4/1
Grooming	4
Wheelchair Propulsion	8
Wheelchair Management	8

– Assessment –

Rehab Problems   *Decreased endurance. Decreased ROM/*   Rehab Potential   *Guarded*
Strength. Impaired functional mobility.
Decreased independence in ADL's.
Impaired balance

Anticipated PT/OT discharge needs   *SNF VERUS HOSPICE CONSULT*

#1 STG (1-3 visits)   *DAILY ROM TO BUE FOR INCREASED INDEPENDENCE WITH ADL'S*
AND MOBILITY

#2 STG (1-3 visits)   *MAX ASSIST WITH LE DRESSING TO DOFF/DON BOOTIES WHILE SITTING*
UP IN CHAIR

#3 STG (1-3 visits)   *ASSESS BEDSIDE COMMODE TRANSFERS*

#4 STG (1-3 visits)   *Minimal/Contact Guard Assist Bed Mobility*

#5 STG (1-3 visits)   *Minimal/Contact Guard Assist Transfers*

#6 STG (1-3 visits)   *Minimal/Contact Guard Assist Ambulation*

#1 LTG (3-5 visits)   *To be determined.*

    Wound Care Goals

Plan   (Frequency and Focus)   *OT 3–5X/WK FOR ROM TO BUE, ADL'S, BEDSIDE COMMODE*
TRANSFERS, ENDURANCE ACTIVITIES, SAFETY, AND PATIENT/
CAREGIVER EDUCATION AND TRANING PT 4–6 times a week
Strengthening ROM Bed mobility Transfers Gait ADL's
Pt/Family Education & Teaching

Patient/Family Goals   *Return to previous lifestyle.*

Goals and plan mutually set   Yes   ×   No

    Miscellaneous Charges

PT Evaluation   *1 PT*   OT Evaluation   *1 OT*

    Discharge Summary

PT Initial Note: Patient with Rheumatoid Arthritis

Name: Joan Smith
DOB: 04-01-1965
Medical Diagnosis: Rheumatoid arthritis

Date: 11/12/10
MR#: 60759
Physician: Frank Green, M.D.

Problem List:
- Reduced ROM
- Joint pain
- Joint swelling/stiffness

Subjective (S):
- Female—48 years old
- Complaints of swollen and painful joints
  - Hands (All PIP's, right: MCP's 2-5, left: MCP's 2-4)
  - Both wrists
  - Both knees
  - Feet (MTP's)
- Complaints of inability to wear rings
- Experiences morning stiffness for 1 hour
- Reports that these symptoms have been ongoing for 3 months and are getting worse despite of the NSAIDS but have recently improved with the use of Entrel.
- Complaints that pain prevents her from grocery shopping (too much walking)
- Reports feeling depressed
- Patient presented to the clinic with the following lab values from her doctor:
  - Anemia (Hgb 10.5 HCT 32)
  - ESR 45 (moderately elevated)
  - WBC 12,500 (slightly elevated)
  - Plts 550,000 (elevated)
  - Total protein is elevated
  - Albumin is decreased
  - Rheumatoid factor 58 (elevated)
  - ANA 1:160 H (elevated)
  - Uric acid 5.3 (normal)
- Patient presented to the clinic with the following radiographic findings from her doctor:
  - Soft tissue swelling visible in the hands around the involved joints
  - Juxta-articular osteopenia

Objective (O):
- 2 + swelling and 2 + tenderness all MCPs and PIPs—joints soft and spongy to palpation
- Fist closure 50 % of normal
- Wrists 2 + swollen and warm to touch, ROM 30% of normal in any direction
- Linear area of swelling 1 cm wide and 4 cm long on dorsum of right carpals
- Knees: 3 + swelling right; 2 + swelling left
- MTPs: 2 + swelling #2 and #3 right; and left and right all 2 + tender
- Patient complains of pain with moving involved joints for examination

(*continued*)

Assessment (A):

- Signs and symptoms are consistent with rheumatoid arthritis (RA) affecting numerous joints
- This patient will benefit from physical therapy to reduce joint pain and swelling and to increase ROM in order to improve functional ability to perform ADLs.

Plan (P):

- Short-term goals (2 weeks)
  - Patient will have deceased swelling by measure of 1+ in all affected joints to increase functional ability to perform ADLs.
  - Patient will have increased grip closure of 60% of normal to increase functional use of the hands.
  - Patient will have decreased pain levels by 2/10 on pain scale to improve patient comfort and increase functional ability to perform ADL's.
- Long-term goals (4 weeks)
  - Patient will have minimal swelling (1+ or less) in affected joints in order to increase functional ability to complete daily household chores
  - Patient will have increased grip closure of 80% of normal to increase functional use of the hands for meal preparation.
  - Patient will have minimal pain levels (2/10 maximal) to improve patient comfort and increase functional ability to participate in volunteering at her children's school.
- Interventions
  - Cryotherapy (ice packs/baths) to control swelling in affected joints
  - Joint mobilizations (Grade 1) to reduce pain in affected joints (pain gating)
  - Aquatic therapy to begin initial ROM and strengthening exercises
  - Patient education on:
    - Joint protection—splinting/braces, adaptive equipment, activities to avoid
    - Gait training—proper use of appropriate assistive device
    - Home exercise program—ROM, strength, cryotherapy

Clinician: Kathy Swiss, PT, DPT, OCS   **License: NE PT 04569**

REFERENCES

1. www.apta.org. APTA Guide to Practice.

2. www.cms.gov/transmittals/downloads/R52BP.pdf

ADDITIONAL REFERENCES

Steiner WA, Ryser L, Huber E, Uebelhart D, Aeschlimann A, Stucki G. Use of the ICF Model as a Clinical Problem-Solving Tool in Physical Therapy and Rehabilitation Medicine. *Phys Ther* 2002;82(11):1098–1107.

Rundell SD, Davenport TE, Wagner T. Physical Therapist Management of Acute and Chronic Low Back Pain Using the World Health Organization's International Classification of Functioning, Disability and Health. *Phys Ther* 2009;89(1):82–90.

Escorpizo R, Stucki G, Cieza A, Davis K, Stumbo T, Riddle DL. Creating an Interface between the International Classification of Functioning, Disability and Health and Physical Therapist Practice. *Phys Ther* 2010;90(7):1053–1063.

Helgeson K, Russell-Smith A. Process for Applying the International Classification of Functioning, Disability and Health Model to a Patient with Patellar Dislocation. *Phys Ther* 2008;88(8): 956–964.

www.apta.org. Defensible Documentation.

www.cms.gov

www.cms.gov/ElectronicBillingEDITrans/15_1450

CHAPTER 9 REVIEW QUESTIONS

1. What is the difference between the CMS 700 form and the CMS 1500 form?

2. What activities should tests and measures focus on in the initial examination?

3. Why might it be preferable to use the 700 form for a MAC that requires it or a reasonable facsimile?

4. Explain why strength and range of motion are best described in numbers as fractions, but tone, which can also be described in fractions, is preferably described in verbiage?

5. Explain rehabilitation potential in the context of physical therapy.

6. Identify two components included in muscle performance and provide an example for each.

7. Explain the relationship between safety/risk reduction and strength.

8. Explain why precautions and contraindications are necessary relative to PT intervention and their relationship to medical necessity.

9. A patient/client is referred to PT with a primary complaint of pair. The PT is unable to evoke pair symptoms during the initial examinations. Does this patient qualify for PT? Defend your answer?

10. Provide an example of objective descriptions of:

    a. Gait

    b. ROM

    c. Balance

    d. Strength

    e. WC mobility

    f. Motor control

11. Why is CPT code verbiage necessary when documenting PT?

12. Why should the term walking or walked not be used for skilled PT documentation?

10 Pediatric Documentation

Documentation and reimbursement for physical therapy services when working with the pediatric population present some unique challenges. This section will address the nuances of documentation, billing, and reimbursement issues in the context of documentation, specific to pediatric physical therapy. However, the basic contextual guidelines are applicable to the adult population as well.

I. Initial Examination

Many of the major categories for examination of the pediatric patient are the same as for the adult patient. In general, physical therapists must examine range of motion (ROM), muscle tone, muscle performance/strength, sensation, posture, and function regardless of whether the child has a musculoskeletal or neurological/neuromuscular pathology. However, the focus and content of each of these categories is unique for the child who has a neurological impairment. In particular, young children require increased emphasis on assessment of their developmental motor skills. This section will focus primarily on conducting and documenting the content for a developmental evaluation of an infant or young child. Pediatric clients with specific diagnoses such as spina bifida warrant a more directed examination. However, the major categories described in this chapter will serve the physical therapist well for the general pediatric population.

During the initial examination and evaluation, recording by videotaping/CD or digital recording can be beneficial both to the physical therapist as well as to the child's parent or guardian. For the therapist, reviewing the recording may allow examination of the child's movement at a pace more conducive to reflective observation. For the parent or guardian, the videotape/CD/digital recording may be a helpful reminder of the progress a child has made, which may be difficult to appreciate otherwise. Before recording a session, the therapist should obtain express written permission from the caregiver. From a risk management perspective, the videotape becomes a part of the medical record and must be afforded the same confidentiality as dictated by HIPAA.

A. History

As with any patient/client, the history should be the first assessment. The most efficient way to obtain a history is with a form developed specifically for the parent/caregiver or legal guardian to complete prior to the first session. The therapist can then use the information to obtain clarification during initial session. If there is a medical record available, the information included could be useful and may indicate information that might otherwise be difficult to obtain, such as whether there is any history of maternal drug or alcohol abuse. However, when a medical record is not available, it may not be advisable to question a parent about this history because of the degree of parental guilt that will be associated with the questions. Although the question is included in the history prototype form included for reference, the information in the history is the discretion of the facility (see Table 10-1).

TABLE 10-1 · Pediatric History

Pediatric History

Child's:

Last name: **First name:**   **Middle initial:**   **DOB:**   **Age:**

Gestational age: _____ **Gender:** ___female ___male

                Tel#:   **Address:**

City: **State:**   **Zip:**

Name of parent or responsible party:

Telephone and address if different than child's: **Primary language:** _____

      Second language: _____

Social : Parents are: ___married ___separated ___divorced ___single

Child lives with: _____

Does the child have siblings? _____no _____yes If yes, number and ages _____
Was this child one of a multiple birth? _____no _____yes If yes, please indicate: ___twins ___triplets ___quads ___quints

Is primary caregiver responsible for the care of others in the home? ___no ___yes Explain:

Dwelling: Do you have to negotiate stairs into or inside your home? ___ no ___yes

Do you have transportation available? _____ yes _____no

Reason for PT:

Please indicate if birth mother had any of the following problems during the pregnancy:

____pre-eclampsia

____diabetes

____thyroid problems

How many pregnancies did the birth mother have? _____   **How many live births?** _____

TABLE 10-1 · (Continued)

17

CHAPTER 10 Pediatric Documentation

Does the child have any vision problems? _____no _____yes If yes, describe: _____

Does the child have any hearing problems? _____no _____yes If yes, describe: _____

Family history: Are there any other family members with similar problems? _____yes _____no

If yes, please describe:

Please check as appropriate for each category:

Type of delivery: _____vaginal _____C- section   Did the baby present breech? _____yes _____no

Were forceps used? _____yes _____no   Was vacuum extraction used? _____yes _____no

What was the baby's birth weight?_____	What was the baby's APGAR score? Did the baby need ventilator support?_____yes _____no	How long was the baby in the hospital? Was the baby in the NICU?

Please indicate any diagnostic tests the baby/child has had:

Please check as applicable	No	Yes	Describe
Respiratory Problems			
Seizures			
Head injury			
Falls			
Heart problems			
Shunt placement			
Abnormal bleeding &/or bruising			
Abnormal growth			
Diabetes			
Gastrointestinal			
HIV			

TABLE 10-1 · Pediatric History (Continued)

Wheezing, coughing during or after activity			
Allergies			
Other			

Medications: Prescription:

   Over the counter:

General nutrition: Is the child breastfed: now ____yes _____no   **Was the child breastfed?** _____yes ____no   **How long?**____

Is the child bottle fed now? ____yes ____no   **Combination breast/bottle:** _____yes _____no

Please indicate any other information that may be important or you wish to discuss:

The above information is accurate and true to the best of my knowledge, and I give my consent for the evaluation to be performed.

Signature of responsible party: _____**Date:** _____

Printed Name: **Relationship to the child:**

B. Observation

Before conducting the objective tests, the therapist should allow the child to play independently without assistance, if the child has the ability to engage in play. This provides the therapist with the opportunity to observe how the child moves and what the child is able and unable to accomplish motorically. In addition, it allows the child time to warm to the therapist. While observing, general comments about motor control and movement patterns can be recorded as observed in a designated section on an evaluation form. As with adults, general observations regarding movement as well as the history drive the decision making for performance of specific tests and measures. If the child is too young to engage in play or too involved to engage in play, the therapist should engage in a communication/warm-up process consistent with the child's abilities.

C. Objective Data

Information gathered while observing the infant or child move independently and while taking the history from the parent or guardian will help narrow the focus of the objective assessment. For example, if the therapist notices that the child tends to scissor (cross) the legs when crawling on the floor, the therapist will want to assess hip adductor tone for possible spasticity. Recommendations for categories of objective assessment are provided in the following sections. However, specific categories may be more indicated in a child with a neuromuscular disorder than a musculoskeletal disorder. Examination and evaluation of a child with an acute musculoskeletal pathology, such as post-fracture or surgery, may more resemble that of an adult.

State of Alertness. Record in the appropriate section on the form if the infant or child is awake, happy, angry, agitated, or drowsy, or exhibits stranger anxiety or separation anxiety, with specific descriptions of the behaviors, e.g., smiling, crying, hiding face. Because the behavioral or emotional states of the infant/child will affect the muscle tone and motor activity exhibited, it is important to note these levels of alertness.

Asymmetries Related to Movement. To record any asymmetry, document in the appropriate section if the infant or child prefers to weight bear on one side or prefers to reach with one arm more than the other, if the child shifts weight better to one side than the other, and if the child primarily transitions (changes position) only in one direction.

Postural Alignment. Recording postural alignment in a child includes documenting the presence of orthopedic deformities, rib flaring, scapular winging, cortical thumb posture, frog leg posturing, opisthotonus, ankle pronation or supination in standing, genu valgus, genu varus, genu recurvatum, hip subluxation or dislocation, scoliosis, or leg length discrepancy.

Muscle Tone. Assess and document muscle tone during active and passive movement. Describe the muscle tone according to location. For example, is there a difference between trunk tone and lower extremity tone? If so, indicate which may be low tone compared to high tone. Document if the muscle tone is different distally compared to proximally. Muscle tone should also be quantified either using a standardized scale, such as the Ashworth or modified Ashworth scale, or with more generic terms such as mild, moderate, or severe increased or decreased muscle tone. Position of assessment is also critical as tone may fluctuate with position changes, e.g., sitting versus standing; versus spine.

Modified Ashworth Scale.

5/5: Normal tone: no increase or decrease

4/5: Slight tone increase, catch and release, or minimal resistance at end of range

3/5: Slight increase in tone manifested by catch, followed by minimal resistance

2/5: More marked tone through most of the ROM but affected part(s) easily moved

1/5: Considerable increase in muscle tone, passive movement is difficult
0/5: Affected part(s) rigid in flexion or extension

> **Author's Note:** Although the Modified Ashworth includes fractions from 0/5 to 5/5, the numbers alone should be avoided since they may be confused for strength. They should be accompanied by the appropriate verbiage.

Range of Motion (ROM). Both passive and active ROM should be assessed and documented objectively. The ranges should be expressed as fractions, i.e., passive hip flexion 100/140 in which the finding is documented over the "normal" range of a joint. In addition, goniometric measurements of contractures should be documented. Flexibility should be assessed for the following muscles in particular: hip flexors, hip internal and external rotators, hip abductors and adductors, hamstrings, sartorius, plantarflexors, shoulder girdle musculature, and forearm pronators and supinators.

Muscle Performance/Strength. Although standard muscle testing cannot be performed in infants and young children, inferences regarding strength may be made based on the child's ability to move against gravity. For example, a child who has difficulty walking downstairs may have eccentric quadriceps femoris weakness. In addition, inferences regarding adequacy of muscle strength can be made based on postural alignment. For example, a child who displays rib flaring often has weakness of the oblique abdominal muscles. Pediatric patients may present with difficult "grading" muscle movements as well. For example, assessment must be made whether the child exhibits a burst of energy to accomplish a motor task but is unable to perform the task slowly and under more control. Therefore, functional strength assessment or muscle performance may be the most appropriate to describe.

Sensation and Perception.

Assess and document how the infant or child responds to touch and if any self-calming techniques are used. Also observe whether the child exhibits a strong startle response that interferes with functional skills, such as sitting independently, and if the child displays any evidence of tactile defensiveness. For example, determine from the child's parents/caretakers if the child dislikes walking on the grass or dislikes certain textures of food. Visual tracking and hearing should also be screened and described in the documentation.

Skin Integrity.

Assess and document if the child has any scars, pressure sores, unusual temperature of the skin and extremities, circulation problems with the fingers and toes, or discoloration on the skin or mottling. Also check the child for the presence of birth marks or any bite marks, burn marks, or bruising that may be evidence of child abuse or neglect.

Author's Note: If abuse or neglect is suspected, the therapist should report it to authorities in a manner consistent with state law.

Cardiopulmonary Status.

Determine and document if the infant or child has any unrepaired heart defects or cardiopulmonary pathology, precautions or contraindications. Indicate if the child requires oxygen or ventilator support and note the child's aerobic capacity/endurance, including any shortness of breath observed. Also indicate if the child requires monitoring, vital signs should be assessed.

Reflexes and Reactions.

Assessment and documentation of the following reflexes or reactions are of particular importance with regard to functional ability: asymmetric tonic neck reflex (ATNR) and equilibrium or protective reactions in sitting and standing. The presence of any tremors or clonus should also be noted. Clonus is considered significant if it lasts for more than four beats. The muscle group exhibiting clonus should be documented. In addition to developmental reflexes, deep tendon reflex assessment may, in some cases, be indicated and require documentation.

Gross Motor Development.

Infants and toddlers should be assessed for the presence of motor milestones in supine, prone, sitting, and standing. In addition, an infant's ability to roll, commando crawl, creep on hands and knees, and transition in and out of positions should be assessed and documented. The therapist should note whether the infant or young child can perform gross motor milestones (which are standard and found easily in the literature) as well as the quality of the movement used when performing the milestones. In addition, each of the following should be assessed and documented as age and development appropriate: head control, quadruped, gait, stair climbing, primary method of mobility, balance in all positions, length of time able to maintain standing on one leg, running, jumping, hopping, skipping, kicking a ball, catching a ball, and use of assistive devices or orthotics.

In addition to assessing these gross motor skills, evaluating the child for patterns or trends in movement can be helpful. For example, indicate if the child exhibits difficulty initiating, sustaining, or terminating movement as an adult with Parkinson's disease might, or if the infant tends to only use the extensor muscle for moving rather than balance between the flexors and the extensors. Determine and document if there are any stereotypical movement patterns, such as scissoring gait or posturing of the arms into shoulder flexion with internal rotation, forearm pronation, and wrist and finger flexion. Standardized pediatric assessment/tools are recommended.

The physical therapist who works with occupational therapists (OT) and speech therapists/speech language pathologists (SLP) or any interprofessional team also needs to screen the infant or child for difficulty with fine motor or oral motor skills in order to refer the patient for services that may be indicated but have not yet been consulted. The following sections provide suggestions for screening and documenting fine motor and oral motor development.

Fine motor development. Assess and document if the infant or child is able to reach, grasp, play at midline, cross midline, or transfer an object hand to hand.

Oral motor development. Indicate and document if the infant makes any vocalizations, if the parent or guardian is having any difficulty feeding the child (i.e., if the child gags or chokes when feeding). Determine if the young child is eating age-appropriate food, such as baby food or table food, and if there are any foods the child refuses to eat. Also determine if the child drools often or regurgitates. In infants, note if the sucking reflex is absent or weak.

II. Assessment

A. Summary Statement

After gathering the subjective and objective components of the evaluation, the physical therapist should develop a summary statement of the patient's status in order to establish functionally oriented goals. One strategy for beginning the assessment portion of an evaluation is to begin with a one-sentence summary of the therapist's findings. For example, "a 9-month-old male born at 27-week gestational age with history of Grade IV intraventricular hemorrhage recently diagnosed with cerebral palsy." This provides the reader a brief overview of the significance of the patient's possible impairments and functional limitations.

> **Author's Note:** The beginning summary statement example may also be the way the patient/client history is presented in the report, as in adult documentation.

B. Problem List

Many healthcare settings also require a "problem list," which may, in actuality, be the summary statement in some organizations. In the functional outcome record, identification of the problems assists all that need access to the record by providing a clear indication of what the challenges are. In the second edition of the American Physical Therapy Association's (APTA) *Guide to Physical Therapist Practice*,[1] the Nagi Disablement Model was used to categorize the summary into pathology, impairment, functional limitations, and disabilities. Recently the APTA has adopted, the International Classification of Disease, Disability, and Function (ICF) Model to categorize the summary into body structure and function, activities, and participation. Each category in the body of the evaluation documentation will contain the objective assessment. The problem need not repeat the details but should contain the problems in a summative manner. The following is an example of a general problem list:

- Moderate increased tone in plantar flexors, hamstrings, hip adductors
- Decreased strength in abdominals
- Decreased active & passive dorsiflexion ROM bilaterally
- Requirement of moderate assistance with posterior walker, nonfunctional distance
- Dependent for transfers

See Example 1

The following are some examples of goals for the child described in the above problem list:

■ Example 1

Short-term goals (to be achieved in 1 month): The child will be able to:

1. stand with support of walker and minimal assistance with feet flat (addresses dorsiflexion ROM);

2. ambulate or achieve gait, 25' with posterior walker, minimal assist of 25% (also describe pattern).

Long-term goals (to be achieved in 3–6 months): The child will be able to:

1. assume a deep squat position with moderate assistance for 60 seconds (addresses dorsiflexion ROM) to engage in play;

2. ambulate or achieve gait, 100' with posterior walker and contact guard assistance with directional changes on even surface.

C. Rehabilitation Potential/Prognosis

As with adults, a statement regarding the infant or child's rehabilitation potential should be included. Rehabilitation potential refers to the length of stay (LOS) or the specific period of time the child is being treated in the facility/organization. Prognosis, as described in the *Guide to Physical Therapist Practice*, refers to a more long-term determination of progress, and is not usually required in documentation unless specifically requested by a payer source.

When rating a pediatric patient's rehabilitation potential, it is helpful to include a rationale for the rating: for example, "good rehabilitation potential as evidenced by ability to achieve quadruped with facilitation today." The statement may also include a reference to the child's level of motivation, including an example: for example, "good rehabilitation potential as evidenced by the child's strong desire to interact with environment while observed reaching for objects and babbling to therapist" or " good rehabilitation potential based on established goals."

Patients who are rated as having either "excellent" or "poor" rehabilitation potential may a challenge with reimbursement for physical therapy services. This results from the belief that patients with "excellent" rehabilitation potential can get better without physical therapy. In contrast, patients with "poor" rehabilitation potential are viewed as receiving very little benefit from therapy services and, therefore, declared ineligible. If the PT is setting the goals with the parents or responsible party, and has considered all relevant information, the rehabilitation potential should be successful.

D. Goals/Functional Outcomes

From a reimbursement perspective, perhaps the most important component of the evaluation process is the goals section. In pediatrics, many outpatient physical therapy settings will develop specific, measurable, short-term goals and less specific or objective long-term goals. Short-term goals may be designed to be achieved in 1 month, whereas long-term goals are designed to be achieved in 3–6 months, although the time frame should be designated.

Regardless of the time frame preferred in the pediatric practice setting, goals should be documented in the same fashion as physical therapy goals for adults. Goals should include what is to be achieved, the time frame for achieving it, and under what conditions or criteria. Similar to goals for adult patients with neurologic disorders, goals for pediatric patients should be listed in functional terms and should include what goals the parent/caretaker or guardian has for the child. This may mean listing the parent's goal as a long-term goal and using the short-term goal as components necessary to achieve the parent's goal. For example, parents of infants often state they want their child to be able to walk. This can be listed as the long-term goal, and the therapist can use this as a "teachable moment" for helping the parents understand what component skills the child needs before being able to walk. At times, this may mean discussing that ambulating with an assistive device qualifies as "walking."

> **Author's Note:** As walking is not considered a skilled term and does not correspond to a current procedural terminology (CPT) code, the terms "walk or walking" should only be used when quoting the parents/caretakers or guardian. The PT should, for interventions in the plan of care and other documentation, use the terms gait training, as it corresponds to the CPT billing code, or ambulation training.

Regardless of whether a therapist is writing goals for a child or an adult, the word "maintain" should not be used. Third-party payers will not reimburse for therapy services designed to assist a patient in "maintaining" a certain skill or ability. It is believed that "maintenance" activities do not require the skills of a physical therapist or physical therapist assistant. Instead, the therapist should write goals to indicate what the child will be able to do as a result of physical therapy and why they need to have that specific skill.

III. Plan/Plan of Care

When compiling the findings, the therapist should consider the techniques that can be used to help the child achieve the established goals. The "plan" portion of the evaluation should include the frequency and duration the child will be treated; any recommendations for additional consultations, such as referral to OT, speech language pathology, or an orthotist; what treatment methods will be used; and how the findings and plan will be communicated to the referring physician (as indicated).

Regarding treatment methods, general references indicating the focus of therapy are usually sufficient. For example, "therapeutic exercise: instruction to parents of home exercise program and strengthening, and functional activities: developmental activities, gait training," indicates what the focus of the therapy session will be. The setting for physical therapy may need to be stated as well. Indicate where the child will receive physical therapy (i.e., in the home setting, in an outpatient clinic, at day care, or at school). As with adults, the interventions should be identified using the CPT code verbiage, i.e., therapeutic exercise, neuromuscular reeducation, therapeutic activities, gait training, etc., before listing specifics in each category. This will help ensure that when billing for services, the codes and verbiage match the information for each treatment session.

> **Author's Note:** The therapist should know, based on payer source, what codes may not be covered for PT or need to be bundled.

IV. Documentation of the Continuation of Care

Requirements for documentation of treatment sessions, treatment notes, progress notes, and progress reports vary between facilities. While some facilities require a complete note for the treatment session, other facilities may utilize a flow sheet method of recording attendance, treatment goals for the day, and significant findings for each therapy session. Inpatient rehabilitation facilities for children may only require weekly documentation. However, from a health information perspective and medical record "rules," entries should be made for each visit. Failure to do so may result in denial of payment. As a result, it is prudent for each physical therapy practitioner to be aware of the facility's requirements as well as the requirements of the reimbursing agency. The format of the entry, e.g., SOAP, narrative, or other, manual or electronic, should be consistent throughout the organization. Payer sources do not usually dictate format unless there are specific forms that are required. It is the therapist's responsibility to know if a payer does have specific requirements.

In general, treatment notes/reports should contain the following:

- Childs full legal name
- Date of the treatment
- Number of units or time
- Specifics regarding the treatment that was provided, including any parent education or home exercise instruction that was provided in skilled terms, stressing training and CPT codeable verbiage
- Child's response to treatment (was the child able to complete the task with assistance or was the child still unable to complete the task even with the skill of the therapist or assistant?)
- Length of the session

Progress notes would include all of the components listed in addition to the progress made relative to a prior report; the initial examination/evaluation or previous progress note or report, goals for upcoming session and plan for next visit(s).

- Goals of the session
- Plan for the next visit

Regardless of the frequency of documentation, physical therapists should provide regular written updates to the referring physician indicating the child's progress and the treatment plan. Similar to the initial examination, the treatment plan should include the frequency and duration of physical therapy services, the type of treatment, the treatment setting, and any recommendations for additional services or consultations. As indicated in the reimbursement section, written physician authorization may be necessary to continue therapy services depending in the payer source.

V. Discharge Summary/Documentation of Summation of Care

When a child has achieved maximal outcome for a specified time, has completed a pre-authorized number of visits, or is no longer receiving services for any reason and is being discharged from physical therapy, a discharge summary or documentation of the summation of the episode of care must be completed. Ideally, a discharge summary contains a statement of all the changes and significant findings addressed in the initial evaluation. The current functional status, method of mobility, and adaptive equipment should be addressed. A statement regarding progress toward the short- and long-term goals and whether or not the goals were achieved should be included. If some goals were not achieved, reasons for modifying or not achieving the goals should be stated. A plan should also be included such as "Parent will continue with home exercises as instructed and will call if they have any questions." The discharge summary is particularly valuable if the child requires additional services in the future as the summary serves as a record of progress gained and function that may have been lost. A copy of the discharge summary should be sent to the referring physician as well (see Appendix E for documentation guidelines).

VI. Reimbursement

Pediatric physical therapy providers have several primary methods for obtaining reimbursement: through federal regulations under the Individuals with Disabilities Education Act (IDEA), including Early Intervention under Part C, school-based services under Part B, state Medicaid , private insurance, cash payments, and philanthropic and professional organizations. A description of each of these methods of funding is provided in the following sections. Qualifications for providers, requirements for the provision of services, and procedures for reimbursement are also discussed. Table 10-2 contains a summary of the requirements for provider eligibility for each of the funding agencies.

TABLE 10-2 • Provider Eligibility Requirements

Requirements	IDEA Part C	IDEA Part B	Medicaid	Insurance
Current state license	Yes	Yes	Yes	Yes
Provider application	Yes	Local education agency specific	Yes	Only for network providers
Specific provider number	Depends on State	No	Yes	Depends on Insurance company
Resume	Yes	Depends on local education agency	Yes	Depends on Insurance company
Background check	Depends on State	Depends on state and local education agency	Yes	No
Occupational license	Depends on State	No	Depends on State	Depends on Insurance company
Liability insurance	Yes	Yes	Yes	Yes
Specific pediatric training	State-specific training modules	Local education agency specific	No	No
Contract	Yes	Local education agency specific	Yes	Yes, for network providers
National Provider Identification number	Yes	No	Yes	Yes or social security number
Federal identification number	Yes	Depends on local education agency	Yes	Yes or social security number for individual provider

Individuals with Disabilities Education Act (IDEA)

A. Early Intervention—Part C

The Individual with Disabilities Education Act (IDEA) was originally adopted in 1991, reauthorized in 1997. In 2004, it was authorized again and changed to the Individuals with Disabilities Education Improvement Act (IDEIA). IDEA federally mandated requirements for the provision of early intervention services (also known as Early Steps in some states) for children with disabilities between the ages of 0 and 3 years old. Part C, previously referred to as Part H, is a federal grant program that assists and allows each state to develop its own guidelines for eligibility criteria and procedures for providing early intervention services. Each state designates a lead agency for coordination and funding of early intervention services. Annual funding is based upon census figures of the number of children, birth through 36 months of age. Many states utilize the following criteria to determine if a child qualifies for early intervention services:

1. The child must exhibit certain percentage of delays (as specified by each state) in one or more of the following developmental areas:
   - Physical: health, hearing, or vision
   - Cognitive: thinking, learning, or problem solving
   - Gross or fine motor skills: moving, grasping, or coordination
   - Communication: language, speech, or conversation
   - Social and emotional: playing or interacting with others
   - Adaptive development: self-help skills such as feeding, toileting, or dressing
2. The child has an established medical condition such as Down syndrome or spina bifida that will result in developmental delay.
3. The child is at risk for developmental delay due to state-specified factors, such as prematurity, or a congenital cardiac condition.

Qualification for this program does not depend on the family's income. Early intervention services are available for any child who meets the eligibility requirements up until the child's third birthday. To determine eligibility of children, the lead agency for each state establishes a team of professionals to screen birth to 3-year-old children who have been identified as possibly needing early intervention services. The team consists of the family in conjunction with some combination of the following professionals: psychologist, nurse, physician, physical therapist, occupational therapist, or speech language pathologist/speech therapist. A service coordinator from the team is designated and assigned to the family and child to assist with the provision of services as determined by the team. Ultimately, the family makes the final decision regarding recommendations that will affect their child.

The team of professionals that evaluates the child often uses a standardized assessment tool to determine the presence and severity of developmental delay and to determine eligibility for services under Part C. There are a variety of evaluation tools that compare the child's performance with other typically developing children. Two commonly used standardized assessment tools are the Bayley Scales of Infant Development II and the Peabody Development Motor Scales. However, specific tests or standardized assessments are not required to determine eligibility. An objective narrative therapy assessment addressing delays is acceptable for documenting a child's developmental needs, but as in adults standardized tests and measures are preferable.

Following the developmental evaluation, an Individual Family Support Plan (IFSP) is written to document the treatment plan based on the results of the team assessment and family input. This plan identifies specific concerns, priorities, and resources available to the families. The plan must be reviewed every 6 months in addition to an annual IFSP meeting to determine what services are still needed.

IDEA mandates that therapy services must be provided in the natural environment for the child. A "natural" environment for a child may be the child's home, day care, or other community settings.

Qualifications for Providers.
Table 10-2 outlines the requirements for providers of early intervention physical therapy services. In order to provide therapy services for children and families covered by Part C, professionals must have the following:

1. Current state license
2. Occupational license
3. State Medicaid provider number
4. Resume
5. Liability insurance
6. National Provider Identification number (NPI)

Additional requirements may include the following:

1. One year of post-degree professional experience
2. Level II Background Screening (including finger printing)
3. Early Intervention specific Continuing Education Units (CEU)
4. Current certifications in area of practice
5. Completion of orientation and training modules covering such topics as:
   a. The family-centered philosophy
   b. An introduction to service coordination
   c. Transitioning the child from Early Intervention to public school
   d. Individualized Family Support Plan (IFSP)

Professionals must agree to sign a contract to provide services to Part C clients. This contract may include a procedural safeguards statement and a memorandum describing services and methods for reimbursement. However, having appropriate credentials does not guarantee approval as a provider. Some states may require a renewal procedure for the provider to continue to offer services to Part C clients.

Requirements for Providing Services.
Once the professional has met all of the qualifications to provide therapy services, the therapist must obtain a referral from the Developmental Evaluation Intervention Team, a current IFSP, and a physician's referral for physical therapy services. Therapy services may then be provided in the

natural environment consistent with that particular state's provisions. When the IFSP is updated, a recommendation for continuation of therapy services must be provided. Any changes in the services must be cleared through the service coordinator.

Procedures for Reimbursement. In order to receive reimbursement for therapy services through Part C, the therapist must first bill the family's primary funding source. The family may have to assume responsibility for applicable co-payments and deductibles. For example, if there is private insurance, the private insurance agency must be billed first. If services are not covered by the family's insurance company, the services may be covered by Part C. The services would have to be documented as medically necessary and approved by the local agency that manages Part C.

Similarly, if the family has Medicaid, the therapist must first bill Medicaid for therapy services. If the services are not covered by Medicaid, then they may be provided with approval from the local Part C agency. Services must also be deemed medically necessary with submission of required documentation. Co-payments and deductibles may not apply to these recipients.

Part C is considered the payer of last resort in relationship to all other third-party payers. Reimbursement rates and claim submission time frames are determined by each state agency. After receiving reimbursement from the family's insurer, the therapist can then bill Part C for the remaining balance up to the allowable state Medicaid rates or the agreed-upon allowable rate as determined by each state. When the Part C funding for a service is accepted, this reimbursement must be considered as the full payment for the services and the provider may not bill the balance of services to the family nor third-party payers. Progress notes and recommendations must be submitted when billing Part C. Providers are required to maintain records and information related to the provision of covered services, the cost of the services and the payments received by the provider on behalf of the client. Table 10-3 contains a summary of requirements for reimbursement for each of the three major types of funding sources.

B. IDEA—Part B

The provision of therapy services to children ages 3–21 is covered by Part B of IDEA. The federal legislation stipulates that all children deserve a quality education alongside their peers. The legislation allows for all children and youth in this country the right to a Free and Appropriate Education (FAPE) in the Least Restrictive Environment (LRE).

Under IDEA, planning and service delivery must be provided by a multidisciplinary team of professionals that must include a standard classroom teacher, a special education teacher, a representative of the local education agency (LEA), and

---

TABLE 10-3 • Reimbursement Requirements

Requirements	Part C	Medicaid	Private Insurance
Physician referral	Required or from IEP team	Required	Depends on state practice act and/or insurance company
Medically necessary	Yes	Yes	Yes, for continued service
Assessment	Provided by team	Yes	Often required
Plan of Care	Yes	Yes	Often required
Progress notes	Yes	To be on file	Often required
Renewal of prescription	Annually	Every 6 months	Dictated by insurance company and/or state practice act
Reassessment	Annually	Every 6 months	Depends on insurance company and/or as condition changes, i.e., surgery
Billing forms	CMS 1500	CMS 1500	CMS 1500

the parents or guardian of the child. At the discretion of the parents or guardian and LEA representative, other individuals who have knowledge or special expertise regarding the child may also be included, such as physical, occupational, or speech therapists. Every child receiving special education must receive an Individualized Education Program (IEP) that is developed by this multidisciplinary/interprofessional team.

A parent or guardian, state agency, or local educational agency can refer a child for evaluation to determine if the child has a disability as defined under IDEA. The referral for a related service, such as physical therapy, can be initiated by anyone on the team for a child who has an IEP in place. The IEP team decides if the goals they developed need the support of a related service. Physical therapists may screen a child before a referral is made by the IEP team. In states where the practice act for physical therapy requires physician referral, it must be obtained to perform the evaluation. In states where there is direct access, the physical referral may not be necessary unless required by third-party payers. In all cases, a physical referral is recommended in order to maintain communication with others outside the educational environment who are involved in the child's care.

Once a referral is made to determine if the child has a disability, a full and individualized initial evaluation must be performed. This evaluation requires parental consent and must be completed within 60 student attendance days. The physical therapy evaluation can be part of the initial evaluation to determine eligibility for special education or can be performed after eligibility has been established.

Reimbursements for Providing Services.
IDEA statutes and regulations mandate FAPE to eligible individuals with disabilities. There are specific formulas for the grants awarded to each state that depend on the number of children who receive special education and related services. School districts in each state may have specific funding criteria for the allocation of those funds. Physical therapists do not directly bill for the provision of services rendered under Part B of IDEA. However, school districts may enroll as providers of Medicaid services and receive the federal share of Medicaid payments for providing Medicaid covered services, such as physical therapy, to Medicaid recipients. Medicaid will be discussed further in the next section.

C. Medicaid

Medicaid is a dual funded system, based on federal and state monies, with the individual administrating and states reserving the right to determine service reimbursement. This program is considered a state-funded health insurance plan designed for children from 0 to 21 years of age who meet certain income and disability criteria. Each state appoints a lead agency to manage Medicaid funding and contracts a fiscal agent to handle provider reimbursement. Medicaid will reimburse for physical therapy services at the maximal Medicaid fee or the provider's customary fee, whichever is less.

Qualifications for Providers for Medicaid.
The qualifications for providers of Medicaid are specific to each state. In general, in order to provide therapy services for children and families covered by Medicaid, professionals must:

1. apply for provider status;
2. be fingerprinted for a criminal background check;
3. provide a federal identification number (FIN) for businesses;
4. provide the social security number (SSN) for individual providers;
5. maintain a current state professional license;
6. obtain an occupational license (where applicable);
7. purchase liability insurance;
8. obtain a business license (where applicable);
9. have the billing agent sign the provider agreement;
10. obtain a group Medicaid number if two or more providers are practicing together. Each member of the group must also enroll as an individual provider within the group.

> **Author's Note:** In order to provide services to adults under Medicare, a PT or facility must also obtain a Medicare provider number.

Requirements for Providing Services. After meeting all of the qualifications to provide therapy services, the therapist must obtain a physician's referral before evaluating a child. The physician's referral should include the recipient's diagnosis, type of evaluation and service requested, the duration and frequency of treatment, and the physician's authorization number (if applicable). After completing the initial examination, the therapist must submit a copy of the evaluation and plan of care to the referring physician for signature and authorization for treatment. Treatment may not begin until the physician's authorization is received.

Each state establishes guidelines regarding the frequency and duration of therapy services. In some states, visits are approved for 6 months, and then the patient must be reassessed with the plan of care and frequency of therapy again submitted to the physician for authorization prior to the continuation of therapy services.

Each plan of care must include, but is not limited to, the following:

> **Author's Note:** The information required is the same as that included in any PT treatment plan/POC.

- Child's name
- Child's date of birth
- Child's diagnosis medical diagnosis and treatment diagnosis
- Child's Medicaid ID number
- Diagnosis code (currently ICD-9)
- Name of referring physician
- Date of evaluation–stand of case (SOC)
- Requested period for treatment
- Examination/assessment
- Recommendations including frequency and duration
- Achievable, measurable short- and long-term goals
- Physician's signature and authorization number
- Provider's signature and provider number

Procedures for Reimbursement. Many states provide software programs for electronic billing and electronic transfer of funds. Health insurance claim forms developed by the Center for Medicare and Medicaid (CMS), referred to as CMS 1500 (see Appendix C) forms, are required (as for most adult PT reimbursement). These claim forms speed optical scanning for quicker turnaround in processing and reimbursement. As outlined by each state, the CPT codes must be used for billing. The physician's authorization number may be needed for billing purposes. Accuracy in completion of the form improves efficiency in reimbursement. If the form is not completed accurately, it could result in a technical denial requiring resubmission.

As with all physical therapy services, only services deemed medically necessary, according to each individual state, will be reimbursable. Depending on the state, covered services often include physical therapy, occupational therapy, speech and language therapy, and early intervention. In certain states, Medicaid may also reimburse wheelchair evaluations and fittings to recipients age 21 and older. Justification for wheelchairs often require lengthy documentation specific to the child's need for the chair and the adaptations or type of chair needed.

For children covered by private insurance, the private insurance agency must be billed before submitting for reimbursement through Medicaid. Medicaid can then be billed for deductibles, the remaining balance (up to the Medicaid rate), or claims that were denied.

In many states, public schools are allowed to bill Medicaid for therapy services provided at the school. All requirements for providing services and reimbursement apply. Medical necessity in an educational environment must be determined by the school district.

D. Insurance

Private insurance companies are governed by a state insurance commissioner. Each health insurance company outlines which therapy services are covered as stated in the individual subscriber's policies. Specific regulations contained in a subscriber's policy may include:

- pre-existing conditions (with the "new" healthcare legislation passed in March 2010, a payer will no longer be able to deny a child coverage based on preexisting conditions);
- waiting periods;
- deductibles;
- allowable charges;
- percent of allowable charge covered;
- co-payment;
- documentation required from the service provider.

Some insurance companies payers require therapy providers to have company-specific provider numbers. Other companies require that therapy providers apply to become part of their "network" of providers. This is especially true in managed care organizations such as HMOs, point of service (POS) plans, and preferred provider organizations (PPOs).

> **Author's Note:** Some HMO's now have an "any willing provider" clause. This means that a provider need not be a HMO designated provider, but must accept the HMO rate of payment.

Private insurance companies may also use national credentialing agencies where the therapy provider completes one application for multiple insurance companies. Therapy services that are part of a network must agree to accept a set fee or capitation as the maximum allowable charge for services rendered. This type of insurance appeals to subscribers since there is either low or no deductibles and reduced co-pay. However, if the subscriber wishes to utilize an out-of-network provider, there is often an increased deductible, increased co-payment, co-insurance, or special permission required.

Requirements for Providing Services.
To provide services for private insurance companies, therapists must have a current professional license for that state. To apply to be a network provider, the therapist must have current liability insurance, an occupational license, and must submit a resume. A provider with one type of insurance with an insurer does not necessarily entitle the PT to bill for services for that company. Insurance companies may have additional requirements.

Procedures for Reimbursement.
Most private insurance companies require a referral from a physician in order to reimburse for therapy services, even in direct access states. Some companies require an updated physician referral on a monthly basis; others require the referral be updated annually. A copy of the therapy examination may be required in addition to results of a standardized developmental assessment; written narrative addressing prognosis, short-term goals, and long-term

goals; and the frequency and duration of therapy sessions. Interim progress notes and recommendations may also be required. Following major surgeries or changes in the child's condition, an updated physician referral and evaluation may be required.

For many insurance companies, CMS 1500 form is the standard requirement. These form must include the following information:

- Signature of the subscriber on file
- Signed assignment of benefits form on file
- Name and date of birth of the child
- Child's diagnosis
- Place of service
- Subscriber's policy and/or group number
- Therapy provider's identification number (if applicable)
- Business tax identification number or provider number and/or National Provider Identification number
- Address of provider
- Signature of provider or assigned designee and date of services
- Appropriate CPT codes for services rendered
- Inclusion of appropriate modifiers to identify each discipline and for coding edit requirements, e.g., GP for services delivered under an outpatient physical therapy plan of care, GN for services delivered under an outpatient speech therapy plan of care, and GO for services delivered under an outpatient occupational therapy plan of care, -59 if two services are rendered that require clarification in order to be reimbursed as separate services/interventions[2]
- Units of service provided

Schools/school-based therapy providers may also bill private insurance for reimbursement of therapy services but must have the permission of the child's family to do so. If the family refuses, the school must still provide therapy services deemed medically necessary in an educational environment.

Cash Payments

In today's practice, more PTs are moving toward accepting cash payments. Fees for the services should be reasonable and consider the setting where they are performed. Providers must adhere to state practice acts and should carry liability insurance. Upon accepting the patient for services, the examination, evaluation, and diagnosis must be made. Completion of documentation of services provided should be maintained. Where reimbursement is available, it would be unethical for a PT to charge cash only.

Pro Bono/Philanthropic

Principle 10 of the APTA's *Guide for Professional Conduct*[3] states: "A physical therapist shall endeavor to address the health needs of society." Therapist provision of services at a reduced or at no cost should be rendered to those lacking the ability to pay for services within reason. Philanthropic organizations exist that will provide pro bono durable medical equipment or therapy services when not covered by other means. There are organizations at the national, state, and local levels. Examples of such organizations are United Cerebral Palsy, Juvenile Arthritis Association, or local charities and churches. Therapists should be knowledgeable and able to provide families with information about such organizations.

Summary

The length of time the medical record for a child should be kept differs from that of an adult. As litigation may be involved with a child who has a disability, the PT must know the regulations regarding the time period required for retaining records (see Chapter 7). In some cases it may be as long as 21 years.

Although there are some differences between pediatric and adult documentation, the same basic components are required. There must be medical necessity with the need for skilled physical therapy evident in the documentation. Emphasis must be on functionally oriented goals, with justification as to why the child needs the skill if the child never developed it or why the child needs to relearn the skill if it was lost secondary to a new injury. Involvement and instruction to the caregivers must also be included. If equipment or adaptive devices are required for the child, it is the responsibility of the PT to determine if payment is available. If it is, the PT must then justify why the device is necessary through appropriate documentation.

REFERENCES

1. APTA. *Guide to Physical Therapist Practice*, 2nd ed. American Physical Therapy Association, 2003.

2. http://www.wpsmedicare.com/j5macpartb/resources/modifiers/modifiers59and76.shtml. Accessed April 6, 2011.

3. APTA Guide for Professional Conduct http://www.apta.org/uploadedFiles/APTAorg/About_Us/Policies/Bylaws_and_Rules/GuideforProfessionalConduct.pdf#search=%22APTA Guide for Professional Conduct%22. Accessed April 10, 2011.

ADDITIONAL REFERENCES

Bayley N. *Bayley Scales of Infant Development*, 2nd ed. San Antonio, TX, Psychological Corporation, 1993.

Blue Cross/Blue Shield of Florida: www.bcbsfl.com

Chandler LS, Andrews MS, Swanson MW. *Movement Assessment of Infants*. Rolling Bay, WA, Infant Movement Research, 1980.

Folio RM, Fewell R. *Peabody Developmental Motor Scales and Activity Cards*. Chicago, IL, Riverside Publishing, 1983.

Individuals with Disabilities Education Act of 1990, 20 USC s1401.

McEwen I, ed. *Providing Physical Therapy Services*, Section on Pediatrics, APTA, 2000.

Newborg J, Stock JR, Wnek L, Guidubaldi J, Svinicke J. *Battelle Developmental Inventory*. Chicago, IL, Riverside Publishing, 1984.

Piper MC, Darrah J. *Alberta Infant Motor Scale (AIMS)*. Philadelphia, PA, WB Saunders, 1994.

Russell D, Rosenbaum P, Avery L, Kane M. *Gross Motor Function Measure (GMFM-66 and GMFM-88) User's Manual*. Toronto, Ontario, Canada, Blackwell Publishing, 2002.

CHAPTER 10 REVIEW QUESTIONS

1. Compare and contrast pediatric and adult documentation.

2. What information should a treatment plan for a child include?

3. What is Part C? How does a child qualify for Part C funding? Explain the role of documentation.

4. In pediatrics, what is the relationship between observation, assessment, and documentation?

5. Give five examples of behaviors/activities that should be assessed and documented in pediatrics, as age and developmentally appropriate.

6. Explain the concept of rehabilitation potential. Why is it better to use "good" rather than "excellent"? Why is it recommended not to use "poor" to rate rehabilitation potential?

7. What are the basic elements of a progress report?

8. Describe the most efficient way to obtain a history for a child. What is the purpose of the history and how does it relate to the decision-making process for the initial examination session?

9. What aged children are eligible for Medicaid funding? What is the funding source for Medicaid?

10. What is the role of the problem list in the initial examination? How much detail needs to be documented in it?

11. Are specific documentation formats required for most payers? What is required in pediatric documentation for all payers sources.

12. Explain the difference between rehabilitation potential and prognosis

11 The Electronic Medical Record

Stephen M. Levine, PT, DPT, MSHA and Helene M. Fearon, PT

The implementation and use of electronic medical records (EMRs) is now one of the highest priorities for healthcare providers, organizations, and government agencies in the United States. An EMR can provide many benefits for providers and their patients, and can improve care by enabling functions that paper medical records cannot deliver:

- **Complete and accurate information.** An EMR allows healthcare professionals to have the information they need in a timely fashion in order to provide the best possible care, at the best possible time. The ability to access the patient's complete health history before beginning the evaluation and treatment processes affords additional support for the provider's clinical decision-making process as well as facilitating the patient's involvement in their own healthcare. Use of an EMR has the impact of bringing an individual's complete health information picture into the process of getting appropriate care earlier rather than later. The use of this technology results in better healthcare decision making, and more coordinated care.

- **Better access to information.** EMRs facilitate greater access to the information healthcare providers need to support high-quality and efficient care and improve the health outcomes of their patients. EMRs also allow information to be shared more easily among physician, therapist, and other healthcare provider offices, hospitals, and health systems, leading to better coordination of care.

- **Patient empowerment.** Use of EMRs empowers individuals to take a more active role in their health and in the health of others for whom they have responsibility. Patients can receive electronic copies of their medical records and share their health information securely over the Internet with whomever they choose. EMRs can support better follow-up information for patients—for example, after a clinical visit or hospital stay, instructions and information for the patient can be effortlessly provided, and reminders for other follow-up care can be sent easily or even automatically to the patient.

Currently, a majority of healthcare providers still use medical record systems based on paper, yet this is generally the most inefficient and time-consuming manner in which to document, especially if the required or desired elements are to be documented correctly. With the ongoing political and economic pressure to incorporate health information technology into practice, it is essential for physical therapists, and other healthcare providers, to understand the benefits and barriers to adoption of electronic documentation, the potential effects of introducing point-of-care (PoC) documentation into the therapist–patient relationship, and key points to consider prior to the lease or purchase of a system in order to effectively prepare for the successful transition to an EMR.

I. THE PUSH TOWARD ELECTRONIC MEDICAL RECORDS: UNDERSTANDING THE CURRENT ENVIRONMENT

Health Information Technology (HIT) is changing rapidly in the United States. The goal at the federal level is to have EMR systems in use across the country, in all provider settings, by 2014. A 2008 study published in the *New England Journal of Medicine* found that only 4% of doctors nationwide used a fully functioning EMR system, while only and additional 13% said they had a basic system.[1] Other studies have confirmed this, indicating that only 17–25% of office-based physicians use EMR systems. Although there have been no published studies on physical therapists' use of EMRs, anecdotal evidence suggests only 13–15% of physical therapists use an EMR, and most of these cases appear to be in the inpatient environment. At the current rate of adoption, it is predicted that EMR systems will reach maximum penetration by 2024, 10 years beyond the federal goal.[2] Reasons for lack of adoption are not fully understood, but published studies and articles related to the use of EMRs are increasing significantly.

The idea of an EMR is not new. In 1991, the Institute of Medicine (IOM) organized a task force that examined issues of medical record systems. In conclusion of the examination, the IOM reported the computer-based record was an "essential technology for healthcare."[3] In 1997, the IOM conducted a follow-up report that identified steady progress toward developing computerized health systems, but noted no system supported all the features of a comprehensive system.

Author's Note It is common to use the terms electronic medical record (EMR) and electronic health record (EHR) interchangeably in some of the federal government's applications and initiatives as well as during discussions of the technology, but it is important to understand that there is a significant difference. While the EMR is used by clinicians and staff within one healthcare organization, the EHR conforms to nationally recognized interoperability standards and can be created, managed, and consulted by authorized clinicians and staff across more than one healthcare organization. For purposes of this chapter, the term EMR will be used, but should be recognized to include EHR, as well.

By 2003, the United States Department of Health and Human Services (DHHS) began promoting widespread use of modern information technology (IT). The DHHS asked the IOM to identify core health delivery-related functionalities, including an electronic health record (EHR) functional model. Following the proposal, in 2004 the Bush administration made HIT one of the nation's top priorities. The DHHS launched the "Decade of Health Information Technology" with goals for EHR's for most Americans in 10 years. An initiative of the DHHS' National Health Information Infrastructure is to "enable regional information sharing throughout the continuum of care by establishing healthcare policies and promoting effective use of data and vocabulary standards."[3]

As the country slowly but steadily has become more aware and accepting of EMRs over the past 20 years, the time was right for the next major step in this initiative. That step occurred when President Obama signed into law the American Recovery and Reinvestment Act of 2009 (ARRA) on February 17, 2009. This law provides for the Office of the National Coordinator for Health Information Technology (ONCHIT) to promote the development of a nationwide interoperable HIT infrastructure. HIT Policy and Standards Committees established and comprised of public and private stakeholders (e.g., physicians), were created to provide recommendations on the HIT policy framework, standards, implementation specifications, and certification criteria for electronic exchange and use of health information. The DHHS goal was to adopt an initial set of standards, implementation specifications, and certification criteria by December 31, 2009.

19

The ARRA provides financial incentives through the Medicare program to encourage physicians and hospitals to adopt and use *qualified electronic medical records* (EMR) in a *meaningful way* (as defined by the Secretary of Health and Human Services). As defined in the legislation, a qualified EMR system is one that "includes patient demographic and clinical health information, such as medical history and problem lists, and has the capacity to (i) provide clinical decision support; (ii) support physician order entry; (iii) capture and query information relevant to healthcare quality; and (iv) exchange electronic health information with, and integrate such information from, other sources."

The ONCHIT was authorized to provide competitive grants to states for providers who become early adopters of qualified EMRs. Medicare incentive payments were designed based on an amount equal to 75% of the secretary's estimate of allowable charges. Incentive payments made to users of the qualified EMR are intended to be reduced in subsequent years through 2015. Early adopters of HIT, whose first payment year is 2011 or 2012, are eligible for additional incentives. Physicians who do not adopt/use a certified HIT system will face reduction in their Medicare fee schedule of −1% in 2015, −2% in 2016, and −3% in 2017 and beyond. E-prescribing penalties would sunset after 2014. The ARRA allows the HHS to increase penalties beginning in 2019, but penalties cannot exceed −5%. Exceptions would be made on a case-by-case basis for significant hardships (e.g., rural areas without sufficient Internet access).

II. WHAT IS "MEANINGFUL USE"?

In the context of the EMR incentive programs, "demonstrating meaningful use" is the key to receiving the incentive payments from the government to assist with the costs associated with transitioning to an EMR. Adopting an EMR means more than using a simple electronic documentation program as a depository of data in a word processor. "Meaningful use" is defined as meeting a series of objectives that make use of EMRs' potential to have an impact on the improvement of quality, efficiency, and patient safety in the healthcare system through the use of certified EMR technology.

On December 30, 2009, The Centers for Medicare and Medicaid Services (CMS) published the proposed rule on "meaningful use" of certified EHR technology. The rule is divided into three stages of focus:

- Stage 1 Focus:
  - Electronic capture of health information in a coded format
  - Using that information to track key clinical conditions
  - Communicating that information for care coordination purposes
  - Initiating and reporting of clinical quality measures and public health information
  - Developing criteria based on objectives tied to proposed measures that must be met in order to demonstrate meaningful use
- Stage 2 Focus: *Expansion of Stage 1 criteria in areas of*:
  - Disease management
  - Medication management
  - Support for patient access to their health information
  - Transitions in care
  - Quality measurement and research
  - Bidirectional communication with public health agencies
- Stage 3 Focus:
  - Achieving improvements in quality, safety, and efficiency
  - Focusing on *decision support* for national high-priority conditions
  - Patient access to self-management tools

- Access to comprehensive patient data
- Improving population health outcomes

In July, 2010, CMS announced its final regulations to specify the objectives that providers must achieve in payment years 2011 and 2012 to qualify for incentive payments. At the same time, the ONC regulations specify the technical capabilities that EMR technology must have to be certified and to support providers in achieving the "meaningful use" objectives. Enacted as part of the ARRA, the Health Information Technology for Economic and Clinical Health (HITECH) Act supports the adoption of EMRs by providing financial incentives under Medicare and Medicaid to hospitals and eligible professionals who implement and demonstrate "meaningful use" certified EMR technology.

The CMS final regulations:

- Specifies initial criteria that eligible professionals (EPs), eligible hospitals, and critical access hospitals (CAHs) must meet to demonstrate meaningful use and qualify for incentive payments.
- Includes both "core" criteria that all providers must meet to qualify for payments, while also allowing provider choice among a "menu set" of additional criteria.
- Outlines a phased approach to implement the requirements for demonstrating meaningful use. This approach initially establishes criteria for meaningful use based on currently available technological capabilities and providers' practice experience. CMS will establish graduated criteria for demonstrating meaningful use through future rulemaking, consistent with anticipated developments in technology and providers' capabilities.

At the same time, the ONC final regulations were published, which:

- Sets initial standards, implementation specifications, and certification criteria for EHR technology under the incentive program;
- Coordinates the standards required of EHR systems with the meaningful use requirements for eligible professionals and hospitals.

With these standards in place, providers can be assured that the certified EHR technology they adopt is capable of performing the required functions to comply with CMS' meaningful use requirements and other administrative requirements of the Medicare and Medicaid EHR incentive programs.

By focusing on the effective use of EHRs with certain capabilities (note the ONC regulations are focused on aspects of HIT that relate more to an EHR than an EMR), the HITECH Act makes clear that the adoption of records is not a goal in itself: it is the use of EHRs to achieve health and efficiency goals that matters. HITECH's incentives and assistance programs seek to improve the health of Americans and the performance of their healthcare system through "meaningful use" of EHRs to achieve five healthcare goals:

- To improve the quality, safety, and efficiency of care while reducing disparities
- To engage patients and families in their care
- To promote public and population health
- To improve care coordination
- To promote the privacy and security of EMRs

It is all but inevitable that the definition of "meaningful use" will continue to evolve within the boundaries of what is reasonably possible using technology available today. Both the ONC and CMS realize that with the extent of fragmentation in the EMR market, achieving meaningful use will not be easy. However, it is something that needs to happen if improvement in patient care is the overriding objective of healthcare reform. The onus will be on the vendors of EMR products to ensure that their products can be "meaningfully used" by the users in line with what is included by CMS in its regulation guiding the incentive payment.

Healthcare providers who are in the process of selecting and implementing EMR software would be advised to include in their contracts that the vendor's product would not only be qualified, but the vendor would incorporate features that will make it possible for them to demonstrate "meaningful use." Even after that, it may not be enough to install and implement a qualified EMR system. The burden of demonstrating that the system is being put to "meaningful use" will be on the physician or other healthcare providers. However, the vendor must make that process easier.

Although the enacting legislation does not identify physical therapists as eligible providers (EPs) for the purposes of receiving the grant funds allocated in the ARRA, it is nonetheless critical for physical therapists and others who are not included in the initial legislation to understand the final published requirements and plan to transition to programs that incorporate as many of these components as possible in order to effectively implement EMRs that will be consistent with future government standards and allow for the achievement of the goals of EMR and, ultimately, EHR adoption.

Professional organizations have also weighed in on the adoption of EMRs/EHRs. The American Medical Association (AMA) is committed to EHR adoption that streamlines the clinical and business functions of a physician office and helps physicians provide high-quality care to patients. The American Physical Therapy Association (APTA) position in regards to the use of electronic records is favorable: the APTA "supports the use of electronic health record systems (EHRs) and promotes the widespread adoption of interoperable EHRs in all physical therapy practice settings."[4]

Clearly the current healthcare environment has created a road map to HIT adoption, and the APTA, through its highest policy-making body, the House of Delegates, has focused the profession on this goal. However, before making the transition to an EMR, physical therapists must have a clear understanding of the terminology used in the HIT environment, the benefits, barriers, and pitfalls of adopting EMRs, be aware of the cultural evolution required for successful implementation, understand how best to prepare for this transition, and know what features and criteria should be reviewed before making a decision on what system is right, both for immediately identified needs as well as for long-term successful implementation and use.

III. DEFINING KEY TERMS

The National Alliance for Health Information Technology (NAHIT) was hired by the ONCHIT to create key health IT definitions, which were released in a report in April of 2008. The executive summary of the report explains why defined terms are needed:

> The ambiguity of meaning created by not having a shared understanding of what these key terms signify becomes an obstacle to progress in health IT adoption when questions about a term's definition and application complicate important policy expectations or directives, contractual matters, and product features. Differences in how a term is used can cause confusion and misunderstanding about what is being purchased, considered in proposed legislation, or included in current applicable policies and regulations.[5]

The following list is not exhaustive, but meant to provide short definitions of key terms that healthcare providers should understand as HIT literacy is enhanced:

- **Electronic medical record (EMR):** An electronic record of health-related information on an individual that can be created, gathered, managed, and consulted by authorized clinicians and staff *within one healthcare organization.*
- **Electronic health record (EHR):** An electronic record of health-related information on an individual that conforms to nationally recognized interoperability standards and that can be created, managed, and consulted by authorized clinicians and staff *across more than one healthcare organization.*

> **Author's Note** It should be restated again here that the terms EMR and EHR are often used interchangeably, despite the significant difference. For the purposes of efficiency, the term EMR will be used throughout this chapter to identify both EMR and EHR, unless otherwise stated.

- **Personal health record (PHR).** An electronic record of health-related information on an individual that conforms to nationally recognized interoperability standards and that can be drawn from multiple sources while being managed, shared, and controlled by the individual.

- **Health information exchange (HIE).** The electronic movement of health-related information among organizations according to nationally recognized standards.

- **Health information organization (HIO).** An organization that oversees and governs the exchange of health-related information among organizations according to nationally recognized standards.

- **Regional health information organization (RHIO).** A health information organization that brings together healthcare stakeholders within a defined geographic area and governs health information exchange among them for the purpose of improving health and care in that community.

- **Clinical decision support (CDS).** Consists of programs designed to assist health professionals with decision-making tasks, linking health observations (signs and symptoms) with health knowledge (best practices and current research) to influence choices made by clinicians to improve care (see the section *Determining the Right EMR: Criteria for Consideration* for additional information).

- **Client/server application.** EMRs reside on a hard drive or a server. The client/server application describes the relationship between two computer programs in which one program, the client, makes a service request from another program, the server, which fulfills the request. In this environment, a facility will view and document in a medical record while it resides on the hard drive or server located within that facility or a facility-owned network (see the section *Determining the Right EMR: Criteria for Consideration* for additional information).

- **Application service provider (ASP).** ASP is a business that deploys, hosts, and manages access to software applications for multiple parties from a central location. The ASP charges a subscription fee to users of the applications, which are delivered over the Internet or other public or private networks. The application software resides on the vendor's system and is accessed by users through a Web browser or by special-purpose client software provided by the vendor (see the section *Determining the Right EMR: Criteria for Consideration* for additional information).

- **Integrated (end-to-end) EMR.** An integrated practice management and EMR system (often heard discussed as an "end-to-end" system) refers to applications that are developed by the same vendor, share a single database or development platform, and are designed to share complex data between applications.

- **Interoperability.** Provides the ability of software and hardware on multiple pieces of equipment made by different companies or manufacturers to communicate and work together. This need is essential for sharing of health-related information. Established system must obtain standards to enable systems to exchange information reliably and securely. It also requires critical mass of health IT adoption within the delivery system to create and share health-related information electronically.

IV. ELECTRONIC DOCUMENTATION: BENEFITS AND BARRIERS

A. Benefits of Electronic Medical Records

EMRs and health information exchange can help clinicians provide higher quality and safer care for their patients. By adopting EMR in a meaningful way, clinicians can:

- **Know more about their patients.** Information in EMRs can be used to coordinate and improve the quality of patient care.
- **Make better clinical decisions.** With more comprehensive information readily and securely available, clinicians will have the information they need about treatments and conditions—even best practices for patient populations—when making treatment decisions.
- **Save money.** EHRs require an initial investment of time and money. But clinicians who have implemented them have reported reductions in the amount of time spent locating paper files, transcribing and spending time on the phone with labs or pharmacies; more accurate coding; and reductions in reporting burden.[6,7]

There are many benefits to utilizing an EMR. The most critical reason is the availability and improved access to clinical information. By having one point of entry for patient information in an organization, clinicians have access to all patient information as necessary, including patient demographics and accurate and complete payment sources. Having complete and reliable patient information immediately available improves communication with the patient concerning their care, and allows for better case management, team communication, and decision making. By improving the quality and readability of documentation, there is also great potential for improved reimbursement. An EMR also provides the ability to streamline business processes by reducing redundant front office activities and eliminating use of forms and paper in general. Hard copy medical records take up large amounts of space and have the potential of being misfiled or lost. The storage of discharged EMRs is simpler, cheaper, and easier to retrieve, and can be backed up or saved in duplicate on networks or disks.

EMRs have the ability to provide a practical delivery mechanism for clinical practice guidelines, which assist with clinical decision making. It also allows for a clinician to evaluate and assess valuable sources of data providing new information about quality outcomes and practice styles. EMRs have the ability to track and report consistent, positive, and effective outcomes by entering coded data that facilitate advanced computer-based decision support. This will aid in identifying inconsistencies in utilization of care that compromise quality, and will also assist in standardizing care and minimizing quality disparities. The ability to easily identify and report outcomes serves to empower research feedback loops that can help turn American healthcare into a self-improving system, leading to a significant potential to lower overall healthcare costs. The coordination of care that results from effective use of an interoperable EMR improves the availability, timeliness, and accuracy of data. Sharing of patient information among authorized professionals improves, as well as continuity of care and timeliness of diagnosis and treatment.

An EMR will not only assist with clinical aspect of the practice setting, but it will also provide an enormous benefit to the clerical aspect of a practice. An integrated or end-to-end EMR system has several positive impacts that are detailed in the following section.

Scheduling Component.
Assists in decreasing patient and administrative staff time spent in managing appointments, while providing important practice management reports reflecting data related to patient visits (i.e., new patients, returning patients, cancellations, no shows, referral sources, and patterns).

Documentation and Billing Component.
Patient demographic data, both administrative and clinical in nature, collected prior to or at the start of care and merged with the clinical documentation completed by the clinician or other appropriate staff, provides for more accurate billing of services, and fewer opportunities for clinical errors as a result of improved legibility, accuracy, and accessibility of treatment and progress notes. This can reduce the possibilities for insurance denials or misinterpretations of data and may help decrease provider cost per visit and improve revenues. Electronic data will also improve interdepartmental and interprovider communication and increase the ability to have remote access to patient information. In addition, effective EMRs will increase full integration and documentation

of clinical information, increase timeliness of patient tracking and follow-up, reduce the time frame of administrative filing, finding, and pulling records, and will eliminate lost or damaged paper records.

Data Management Component. Electronic documentation has demonstrated increases in operational efficiency, clinical productivity, and office workflow. Improving workflow has been identified to be a primary motivation for implementing EMR systems.[8] Productivity is a key success factor in any business, including physical therapy, and clinicians who may be required to see a specific number of patients/clients per day and complete all necessary documentation within the framework of their working day will find that, after successful transition, EMRs will assist in tracking key indicators that can facilitate identification of trends that would require a call to action to facilitate the effective management of the clinical practice.

A fully implemented EMR may increase revenue due to allowing for a more complete charge capture of services that are efficiently and correctly documented. EMRs assist in decreasing under-coding or up-coding of services, thus avoiding audit paybacks, and will reduce billing errors and turnaround time, as well as staff time spent on data entry. EMRs facilitate claims submission and third-party payment, and importantly, effective systems will assist providers in meeting the compliance requirements of CMS and other third-party payers, thereby reducing the risk of reimbursement denial and duplication of services. Revenue can be enhanced further with an EMR that has the ability to monitor the payment patterns of the payers. This becomes critical since some third-party payment rates are better than others, and if a facility knows which physicians are referring patients with better insurance payment rates, that facility could improve their net profits without having an effect on productivity by focusing their marketing on those physicians. If a facility knows which insurance companies do not reimburse well for treatment, marketing of those physicians who refer those patients could be reduced.

B. Barriers to Adoption of Electronic Medical Records

Given the benefits to implementation and use of an EMR, there are also significant barriers that should be considered and addressed in order to be best prepared for this opportunity. Understanding these barriers, and potential solutions to them, will greatly assist physical therapists in the successful transition from paper documentation to an EMR. Implementation of an EMR has been demonstrated to follow the 80/20 rule, where 80% of work of implementation is spent on issues of change management and 20% is spent on technical issues related to the technology itself. The various barriers to EMR implementation can be categorized into four main types: financial barriers, technological barriers, attitudinal and behavioral barriers, and organizational change barriers.[8] Each area of a potential barrier also presents with potential solutions for addressing these barriers that should assist the physical therapist in easing the transition process.

Financial Barriers. Typically, the most significant barriers to the adoption of an EMR are the high initial "up-front" costs related to purchase of hardware and software, installation, interfacing with existing programs, administrative and clinical training, and having adequate and appropriate space to house necessary hardware, such as servers. After the initial cost, there are also ongoing costs associated with technical support, hardware updates, and ongoing maintenance. There is also often an underdeveloped business case made to support transition, meaning there may be an uncertain return on investment (ROI) and slow financial benefits to the outlay of initial costs. Finally, high initial time costs are also of concern, meaning the time spent with EMR installation, training, and motivating and cheerleading staff can be a drain on staff resources that could otherwise be focused on patient care and other revenue-generating activities.

One of the potential solutions to the financial burden may include considering a modular system that allows for obtaining an EMR system incrementally with smaller up-front investment. This "building" of a full-scale EMR system over time may work if there is no intention to purchase an integrated product. A company/practice may also use a phased implementation approach, purchasing or renting more complex EMR components in a planned manner for a later implementation process or adding hardware (laptop computers, workstations, etc.) as the number of users or utilization of the software increases. If initial financial outlay is a concern, it is advisable to strongly consider an "application service provider" (ASP), which is defined completely later in this chapter. The ASP model reduces specific costs associated with EMR, specifically software upgrades, server, and other hardware costs, to decrease the initial costs in the areas of hardware and maintenance. It is important to recognize that ROI cost is not instant, since cost savings are realized in the medium to long term, and are also associated with elimination of paper chart, encounter forms, integration of referrals, decrease in data entry and transcription, and improvement in claim capture. EMRs also have the potential to increase the "bottom-line" annual financial return of investment through increasing billing revenue with more complete capture of services provided. An EMR should facilitate a decrease in coding and billing errors and improve the turnaround time of a claims eventual payment.

Another impact of successful adoption should be reduced staff time performing data entry, decreased patient and administrative staff time making appointments and filing activities related to paper charts, and a decrease in staff turnover due to efficiency gains with an EMR that are not present with handwritten processes. Research also shows that EMRs have the potential to save provider time in the long run by enhancing clinical processes and workflow practice efficiency; improving the clinicians' ability to make sound clinical decisions in a timely manner; decreasing provider documentation and dictation time by using templates with documentation prompts; increasing timeliness of patient tracking and follow-up; increasing full integration and documentation of clinical records; and improving the legibility, accuracy, and accessibility of documentation leading to reduced denials on medical review. Clear data exist that demonstrate net financial benefits from successful implementation of EMRs, with some studies citing between $20,000 and $86,400 per physician/healthcare provider over a 5-year period, and others recovering up to 11.9% of net patient service revenue attributed to excessive administrative complexity costs, which are typically eliminated after successful EMR adoption.[6–8]

Technological Barriers.
Technological barriers include inadequate technical support, inadequate data exchange and fragmentation, inadequate Internet connectivity, issues of customization, security and privacy issues, usability issues, and the current lack of interoperability standards incorporated into EMR programs. Regarding technical support, often there is considerable time spent obtaining support from various software, hardware, networking, backup, and service vendors and limited clinician knowledge of technical troubleshooting. Insufficient equipment or equipment inadequacy may cause a problem due to limited access to workstations, older hardware, lack of adequate backup, and storage limitations. Internet connectivity that is inadequate or inconsistent can slow and/or decrease the efficiency of the system. The lack of ability to customize EMR systems to fit specific office needs, including diagnosis-specific forms and documentation shortcuts, can also present barriers. Concerns for privacy, confidentiality, and security of EMR and Internet-based communication can also pose barriers to the implementation and use of an EMR. A system may have inadequate data exchange, data fragmentation, or lack interoperability. EMR systems require standards to be met in areas related to content, information capture and representation, quality assurance, and clinical decision support. Any deficit in these standards produces a risk for a technological barrier. "Usability," or the ease with which healthcare providers can employ the EMR technology in order to achieve the goal related to this transition, is one of the major factors hindering widespread adoption of EMRs.[7] Usability has a strong, often direct, relationship with clinical productivity, error rate, user fatigue, and user satisfaction—critical factors for EMR adoption. Clinicians lose productivity during the training days, and potentially for months afterward, as they adapt to the new tools and workflow.

In order to limit some of the technological barriers, it is important to arrange for comprehensive technical and process support. Technical support is a critical component of successful EMR implementation, and comprehensive technical support from vendors needs to be included in contract negotiations (see *Training and Support*). This is often overlooked or eliminated from contracts by the provider due to cost concerns; however, doing so is generally short sighted. Major EMR advocacy groups such as the Healthcare Information and Management Systems Society (HIMSS) (www.himss.org), professional organizations, vendors, and major healthcare organizations are developing IT systems that adequately communicate and exchange healthcare data. Data-producing organizations are increasingly using data standards such as HL7 (Health Level Seven), a standard for exchanging information between medical applications that defines a format for the transmission of health-related information. In regards to customization concerns, when purchasing or renting an EMR system, make sure your contract has adequate terms for the provision of complimentary changes and adequate support to customize the EMR system to meet the needs, including the management of data, of your particular practice (see *Customization Ability*).

Privacy, confidentiality, and security concerns are mitigated by the fact that all data exchanged between EMR servers must be encrypted to protect confidentiality, and must comply with the privacy and security requirements promulgated within the Health Insurance Portability and Accountably Act (HIPAA). It is critical that vendors implement administrative, physical, and technical safeguards to maintain data confidentiality, integrity, and availability. Typically, vendors are well aware of these requirements, and these safeguards are built into systems. Providers should verify this compliance with any EMR vendor with whom they are considering contracting. However, often providers, in an attempt to develop shortcuts in practice, may not use these protection systems, and therefore, even though the EMR offers these protections, confidentiality and privacy can be breached easily. One such shortcut is not logging out of the program after each use so that anyone can access the data from the same computer, or providers that use the same log in information for each provider or employee (often the login of the practice owner or department manager). Both of these situations should be avoided!

Attitudinal and Behavioral Barriers.
Resistance to change is cited repeatedly in the literature as the primary barrier to successful implementation of an EMR. This and other attitudinal and behavioral barriers of office staff and clinicians generally focus on the concern about how IT systems will change the delivery of care and relationships between and among providers and patients. Staff may have an aversion to clinical applications of technology and a belief that use of EMRs will decrease clinical productivity and effect financial reimbursement. Attaining technical competency can develop into a barrier if providers are uncomfortable with computers or use of technology in necessary communications. Also, electronically inputting information may initially take practitioners more time than writing or dictating, especially if current handwritten notes are substandard.

The lack of clear leadership in transitioning to an EMR is also a major behavioral barrier. The lack of leadership may cause staff to build a resistance to change and even have an underlying fear of job loss. Some clinicians, due to a lack of understanding of the technology, may see the clinical decision support tools provided in more sophisticated EMR solutions as a "cook book" approach to treatment, causing a perception that the healthcare provider will lose individuality or choice. There are also varying ranges of acceptance, technological access, and computer literacy among patients and healthcare consumers, who may also have concerns about access, content, and dissemination of private information.

The initial disruption of a facility or practice's administrative and clinical services workflow associated with the introduction of new IT systems, and how to align these systems into this workflow, often is met with significant resistance, as there is clearly an initial disruption in some financial, clinical, and organizational processes in moving to a paperless system. Finally, the lack of financial incentives available to physical therapists for implementation of EMR systems from the government may cause therapists to avoid "biting the bullet" and planning now for such a transition.

The appropriate use and implementation of an EMR system can overcome these attitudinal and behavioral barriers and create solutions for moving forward with efficiency and effectiveness. An effective EMR system can increase provider–patient communication abilities, and improve patient satisfaction and patient self-care abilities according to several studies.[8] Examples of such communications that could save time and enhance provider effectiveness includes the use of e-mail messaging rather than phone calls, allowing for a better identification of patient needs. Interoffice electronic communication can increase communication and coordination between healthcare providers and support staff. Coordination of care is impacted by improving the availability, timeliness, and accuracy of messages among healthcare providers, the sharing of patient information among authorized professionals, and the continuity of care and timeliness of diagnosis and treatment.

Additionally, concerns about technical competency are in decline, further reducing attitudinal barriers. Provider and consumer attitudes toward the use of EMRs have progressed in a positive direction dramatically over the years, keeping pace with legislative initiatives and advances in the area. Studies from almost a decade ago clearly demonstrated an increased use of computers/Internet by physicians and other healthcare providers. In 2001, a study reported 75% of MDs used computers and 70% used Internet.[9] In 2002, an AMA study of practice managers and administrators reported almost 100% used computers, 85% had networked computers, 74% used Internet for administrative and clinical functions, and 79% used the Web to access medical research data.[10] Yet despite these numbers, a 2008 study published in the *New England Journal of Medicine (NEJM)* found that only 4% of physicians reported having an extensive, fully functional electronic records system, and 13% reported having a basic system.[1] So although it has been almost a decade during which comfort with IT has been demonstrated by healthcare providers, these various groups of healthcare providers have been slow to adopt meaningful use of HIT for electronic documentation.

Additional studies have demonstrated increased consumer comfort with information technology over the past decade. Consumers are increasingly using the Internet to obtain health information and communicate with their healthcare providers. By 2003, a survey through the American Health Information Management Association (AHIMA) identified that 22% of Americans aged 65 and older used the Internet.[11] There has been an increase in e-communication between clinicians and their patients, and more than half of e-mail users want to communicate electronically with their healthcare providers. Almost a decade ago, an AMA survey stated more than 30% of physicians are interested in e-communication with the patients and believe that electronic communication leads to improved continuity of care.[12] It is highly likely that studies conducted today would find these numbers to be quite a bit greater.

It is important to identify an "EMR champion" or a practice should not attempt to implement a transition at all. One of the best predictors of success in the transition to use of an EMR is leadership by a designated individual in the user community.[13] EMR implementation requires the commitment of an individual who effectively creates and communicates a shared vision, empowers staff to act on the vision, plans short-term "wins," and embraces an IT culture for continuous quality improvement. Simply put, it is essential to identify a person to be the EMR advocate in the practice or facility, and it is important to know that it is often not the practice owner who best meets this responsibility!

Finally, although physical therapists are not included in the list of the ARRA-identified eligible providers (EPs) able to receive incentive payments for implementation of an EMR, not having those funds available does not absolve the therapist, and all other providers excluded from compensation for this process, from having to meet the requirements of EMR adoption by the 2014 government-imposed timeline. The lack of financial incentives makes it all the more critical for physical therapists to perform due diligence in identifying the best EMR system for them.

Organizational Change Barriers. The final barriers to adopting an EMR are those related to organizational change. The concern that technology may interfere with the therapist–patient communication and relationship is often cited as a primary barrier. Migration away from paper to a paperless system can be difficult if the process is not appropriately planned. Workflow redesign can be difficult, particularly in gaining consensus in regards to the various aspects of the workflow in the facility or practice. Customization and standardization can be challenging and take time in order to be effective. Resource allocations and responsibilities are likely to change, and process issues are exposed, which can cause hard feelings among staff. There will also be, without a doubt, temporary reductions in productivity due to training in new tools, and an uncertainty about the types of training and skills needed to adopt IT systems for healthcare quality.

In attempting to mitigate these barriers, it is important to understand that the use of therapist–patient e-mail communications may optimize face-to-face interactions, and has the potential to increase patient satisfaction and patient self-care and compliance. It is important to avoid parallel paper and electronic data entry, as doing so will likely cause frustration as well as increase the time commitment necessary to effectively transition to a paperless system. To facilitate the transition away from paper, administrative staff can enter information in advance from paper to paperless systems, and scan recent reports and transfer past information from paper charts into the new EMR system. If the technology choice does not include adopting an integrated solution, it is important to set up efficient data exchange systems between your practices scheduling, documentation, and billing software. Efficiencies are maximized when information is entered only once electronically and passed automatically through to the necessary interfaces and processed seamlessly. Organizational change barriers are minimized when there is a well-planned work process redesign to eliminate paper-based clinical processes, and because EMR implementation in a provider's office changes how the practice does almost everything, staff needs adequate training in order to maximize success. These areas will be discussed more fully in the section *Strategic Recommendations for Successful Implementation*.

V. PHYSICAL THERAPIST PRACTICE AND THE EMR: PITFALLS AND KEY POINTS TO CONSIDER

Physical therapists should be aware of the various pitfalls that exist in the current EMR marketplace. The pitfalls described in this section represent some of the most common issues that may inhibit successful implementation of an EMR within a physical therapy clinic/facility and, if understood and addressed in context of the setting, can be avoided:

- **System selected/implemented without understanding documentation requirements.** Documentation is the bane of most therapists' existence, and unfortunately, it is a skill that most therapists have not taken adequate time to develop. In looking for an EMR, therapists tend to search for programs that will allow them to complete a note in a matter of seconds or minutes, and to be sure, there are some programs that allow this to occur. However, choosing a system before understanding the documentation requirements that are consistent with the standards of practice, state licensing laws, third-party requirements, and other regulations could result in significant time and money spent on a system that might be fast, but that will not assist the therapist in providing effective, efficient, and compliant documentation consistent with medical necessity or regulatory requirements. Staying current on the documentation requirements for physical therapist practice will ensure that any EMR selected is consistent with those requirements. Shortcuts are nice, but if a therapist ends up having to pay back all of the third-party payment received because the product of their electronic documentation does not pass muster, then the therapist has not done themselves or their patients any good!

- **System developed without adequate clinician input.** Many EMR systems are developed without the knowledgeable input of clinicians who understand best practice and who can provide the necessary information, requirements, and regulatory nuance to the programmers who drive the content into the EMR system. Be sure to look for an EMR program that has not only had the involvement of physical therapists, but be sure those therapists have appropriate credentials and expertise in the rules, regulations, standards, and clinical guidelines governing the practice of physical therapy.

- **Limited practice management options built into system.** Providers have to decide if they will invest in an integrated (or end-to-end) system, which includes scheduling, documentation, billing, and practice management, or focus only on a documentation system, in hopes of integrating with the scheduling or billing software already in use (see the section *Determining the Right EMR: Criteria for Consideration*). The greatest efficiencies are gained with a system that allows for robust practice management capabilities, providing data that will assist in growing and maintaining a healthy business, provide outcomes, and allow for efficient and effective practice management over the entire process of the patient/client interface.

- **Equating an electronic documentation system (i.e., word processing-based system) to a true electronic medical/health record.** If providers do not understand the true benefits of an EMR, they are likely to equate a simple word processing system or a depository of data with the power of an EMR. While word processing systems will assist in creating legible documents, and may allow the flexibility of designing or customizing a template to meet specific needs, they typically do not integrate evidence-based practice or assist in improving quality of care by incorporating clinical decision support systems. It is worth the investment in time to understand the development of a system and its ability to incorporate the elements of a true EMR system.

- **Software is not compliant with current rules/regulations.** Providers often believe that an EMR system inherently incorporates third-party rules and regulations into its programming, and that using these systems will protect the therapist from deficiencies and paybacks in the event of an audit. The rules and regulations governing therapy services are complex, and remaining compliant with them takes a considerable effort. Many EMR systems profess to incorporate compliance rules related to documentation, coding, and billing, but the provider needs to ensure that due diligence is performed on these systems to identify and understand the process in which this occurs. Client–server-based systems can have difficulty maintaining compliance due to the significant lag time in providing updated versions of software, while ASP products should be able to maintain such compliance much more easily (see the section *Determining the Right EMR: Criteria for Consideration*).

- **Software that was originally designed for different market.** Many EMR products being marketed to physical therapy professionals have actually been designed for the physician or other healthcare provider marketplace, and either therapists customize these EMR products to meet their individual needs or the vendor may retrofit its product for the therapy marketplace. These approaches make compliance with professional standards and rules/regulations pertaining to physical therapy services difficult and often create significant barriers to successful EMR adoption.

- **Lack of due diligence in evaluating systems/vendors.** Making the decision to purchase an EMR based on word-of-mouth recommendations, the amount of users, or aggressive sales techniques without performing adequate due diligence will likely lead to a difficult transition and, possibly, even a mismatch between expectations and what is delivered as an outcome of using the program. Take the time to have staff use the program with real patients in order to make the most appropriate decisions. A large majority of vendors recognize that allowing a practice/facility/therapist to try the system before committing to purchasing or leasing the system can only assist in the successful outcome. Finally, be sure to check references of those who have been using the software!

- **Lack of inclusion of key staff in decision-making process.** Obtaining "buy-in" from your key staff is critical in contributing to a successful transition to an EMR. Your staff will be the ones using the system and learning how to incorporate it into their daily routine. Make sure to include them in your marketplace assessment, if not for each product you review, at least for the two to three that you identify as your top choices. Bringing your staff into the process early on, so that they are part of the decision making process, has been shown to be important in a successful transition.[14]

- **Having tunnel vision during process.** There are many choices that will need to be made in selecting the right EMR, and often choices are made based on biases before even beginning to explore the potential options available. For example, some clinicians feel strongly that they want to use a client/server system so that they maintain their data on a local hard drive, and will not even entertain the idea of an ASP model for fear of not having access to their data when and where they want it. Yet, ASP systems can actually offer more security than a typical server-based system, in that backup and redundancy systems are in place to ensure secure access to your data from any Internet-compatible computer, and they generally can meet many other needs that client–server systems cannot. The key is to recognize any biases that may exist, and do your best to set them aside as you perform your analysis of various products.

- **Focusing only on immediate needs.** It is all too common for clinicians to focus on their most immediate need in adopting a system. Usually, this means trying to gain efficiencies so that you can spend less time on documentation and related activities and more time treating patients. While this is certainly an important reason for adopting an EMR, focusing only on this aspect, without also ensuring that professional standards, compliance, audit protection, evidence-based practice guidelines, and clinical decision support systems are also integrated, will likely result in short-term feelings of success. That is until your coding, documentation, medical necessity, or outcomes are questioned by third-party payers, review organizations, or licensing board!

- **Lack of adequate system training before, during, and after implementation.** Lack of adequate training is one of the biggest obstacles to successful implementation of an EMR. See the section *Training and Support*, and ensure that adequate resources are dedicated to this critical area.

- **Lack of anticipation of reduced productivity during initial implementation.** An understandable (and valid) concern regarding EMR adoption is related to decreased practitioner productivity during implementation and its impact on day-to-day operations. It is typical for productivity to decrease during the early stages of implementation, and it is critical to anticipate and plan for this reduction. One study identified that a manager in a large paper-based practice said he expected "2–3 weeks of disastrous inefficiency followed by 4–6 months of relative inefficiency."[2] While implementation of an EMR system typically does not result in this reality, not anticipating and planning for a reduction in productivity can result in a less than successful attempt at EMR adoption. Modifying therapist schedules, phasing in implementation, and appropriate scheduling of implementation processes in less busy times will all help to mitigate these productivity losses, and allow for an easier transition and achievement of a more productive clinic. The desired result is less time spent on administrative tasks and more on the clinical management of patients.

- **Lack of an understanding of the true purpose and value of an EMR.** If you have gotten this far, you should be recognizing that the value of an effective EMR system is far greater than simply the use of electronic documentation. By understanding and embracing this paradigm change as a health professional in the U.S. healthcare system, along with the evolution of evidence-based care, providers will recognize that a transition to an effective EMR system will change almost everything about a practice. While this process can be stressful, the outcome of taking this step will be demonstrated in the use of efficient EMR that will not only improve documentation skills, capture clinical services with correct coding, and enhance revenue, but will result in an improved quality of care, enhanced outcomes, and greater patient satisfaction.

VI. COMPUTERS AT THE POINT OF CARE: INTRODUCING HEALTH INFORMATION TECHNOLOGY INTO THE THERAPIST/PATIENT RELATIONSHIP

The gains in operational efficiency and use of clinical decision support to impact patient/client management and outcomes are best recognized when an EMR is used while the therapist is actually interacting with the patient, or at the "point of care".

20

While detrimental effects on provider–patient rapport are often cited as a barrier to implementation of a point-of-care (PoC) EMR system in a busy practice, studies have demonstrated that patients did not indicate a sense of loss of rapport with their healthcare providers when an EMR was used during their outpatient visit, and in fact, in-room computing appeared to have positive effects on provider–patient interactions and care experience.[15–17]

Communication skills and information processing are the cornerstones of achieving quality in healthcare. Computers play a pivotal role in information management for many industries, in that their ability to store, correlate, and retrieve enormous quantities of information quickly and accurately makes them ideally suited to manage voluminous amounts of information.[16] However, computers potentially alter the traditional manner that therapists, physicians, and other healthcare providers use to communicate with patients. Treatment room computers can add complexity to the organization and flow of the visit by increasing the amount of clinical information available or introducing additional physical tasks, which have the potential to shift the clinician's attention and involvement away from the patient to the keyboard and monitor. Effective use of computers in the outpatient treatment room is often dependent upon clinicians' baseline skills that are carried forward and are amplified, positively or negatively, in their effects on clinician–patient communications.[17] For those with greater visit organization skills, the presence of a computer provides a new tool to help organize relevant clinical data as well as visit tasks. For those with poorer organization skills, the presence of computers can multiply the sense of disorganization of the visit and can extend its length. Studies have demonstrated that clinicians who integrated data-gathering (interview) and data-recording (written chart entry) activities into their conversations with patients prior to implementation of an EMR were able to seamlessly integrate the computer into their visits, both initially and at 6 months following implementation of an EMR.[17]

Clinicians' comfort with, and ability to navigate on, a computer, influences whether its use during a visit facilitates or impedes communication. Typing abilities and organization of information efficiently affects overall communication with the patient. The ability to use an EMR to effectively recall and share data/information on patient status or progress (often using visually appealing graphs or charts) will typically enhance clinician–patient communication. Effective use of computers should appear seamless and natural.

Some factors and barriers to communication include nonverbal behavior, computer navigation, mastery of skills, and spatial organization. The visual and cognitive attention required for a clinician to enter and retrieve data while maintaining the flow of the visit can be complex. There are three key ways by which clinicians can maintain communication with patients during computer use. The first is verbally, by maintaining conversation when looking at computer screen or typing. The second is visually, by making eye contact with the patient intermittently during computer use. The literature demonstrates that maintaining or reestablishing eye contact at least every 15 seconds or when talking to a patient provides the necessary connection with the patient.[17] The third key way is postural, where the clinician positions his/her head or torso toward the patient rather than having their back to the patient during computer use. Studies show that clinicians who are able to use frequent eye contact and proper bodily orientation and vocalization are able to stay connected to their patients as they use a computer.[17]

Physical configuration of the computer, the monitor, treatment table, and clinician's chair can make communication more or less challenging. Computer location should easily permit the clinician to alternate attention between the computer and the monitor while simultaneously entering information, and positioning the monitor in such a way to allow sharing of the information on the monitor with patients will enhance communication and understanding by the patient.[15,17]

Longitudinal studies have been published on the impact of treatment room computing on physician–patient interactions. One such study reviewed overall visit satisfaction, satisfaction with the physician's level of familiarity, and communication about medical issues and degree of comprehension with decisions made during visit all increased with PoC EMR use.[18] The study showed significant increase in the level of overall patient satisfaction during the visit after introduction of the computer into the treatment room in the 7th month after introduction as compared to baseline. Moreover, there was no significant drop in overall satisfaction immediately after computer introduction.

The use of computers resulted in the patient's perceptions that physicians were more familiar with them as persons and with their medical history.[15] There was an increased satisfaction with a level of communication about their medical care, including the explanation of diagnosis and treatment, the patient's participation in the decision-making process, and focus on prevention of illness and promoting good health. Further, patient satisfaction is not significantly different after introduction of the computer in the areas of the personal manner of interaction with the physician, the perception of physician's concern for their emotional and physical well-being, and how carefully their physician listened to them. Studies reveal that a majority of patients in family medicine clinics believe that computer use has a positive effect on the overall quality of care at the visit.[16] All areas of review demonstrated that patient satisfaction improved significantly over baseline levels by 7 months after implementation of an EMR. Few studies have found that introducing computers into treatment rooms had an adverse effect on physician–patient communications. However, it is important to understand that there are differences between the effects of providers learning to use computers and EMRs in treatment rooms while they are also trying to engage with patients, versus the experienced computer user who is able to more easily integrate the familiar use of computers into treatment rooms during outpatient visits.

Incorporating PoC documentation requires an understanding of the differences in hardware requirements necessary for efficient and effective practice. Applying an EMR at PoC requires a computer be taken into the treatment area with the patient. As a result, the most effective and efficient alternatives for electronic documentation that can facilitate PoC documentation include laptops, personal digital assistants (PDAs), netbooks, iPads, and the like. Some laptops and other devices have touch screen and electronic signature capture capabilities that can improve the speed of documentation and overall productivity. The technology available for PoC EMR use will only continue to improve as healthcare professionals become more and more comfortable with incorporating technology into the therapist/patient relationship.

Workstations, although still in widespread use, may make transition to an efficient and effective PoC paradigm more difficult. A workstation is usually a desktop computer that may have a printer attached. Based on the number of users, a kiosk can be set up in a central location where clinicians can document information as time allows. Because the computer is in a central location, clinicians typically have to document their clinical findings, interventions, and other notes on paper while they are with the patient, and then enter the information into the computer or wait for access to the kiosk. If a paper record is created before electronic entry, it actually increases documentation time and decreases efficiency.

Although workstations do not provide for the most efficient use of clinician's time and may limit productivity, some clinics/facilities may feel more comfortable by "dipping their toe in the water," so to speak, and not investing in hardware for each clinician. Some have installed individual workstations at predetermined "desk" areas. Although this may provide each therapist a station, the lack of portability of the hardware may result in these being located away from the treatment area, which decreases the efficiency because the therapist must be at the station to document.

VII. PREPARING FOR THE TRANSITION TO AN EMR: STRATEGIC RECOMMENDATIONS FOR SUCCESSFUL IMPLEMENTATION

An effective implementation of an EMR changes almost every aspect of a physical therapist's practice. It is therefore critical to recognize that a successful EMR implementation process starts long before the physical deployment of the application on-site. The implementation plan needs to be thought out well before selecting a vendor.

Each year, EMR systems are deployed in many healthcare provider practices throughout the country, typically with clear clinical and financial objectives. However, some of these systems are later uninstalled by practices after they have found them to be too costly in terms of lost time, productivity, and revenue. So how does a practice become one of the success stories instead of one of the casualties? The answer does not necessarily lie in choosing the right EMR system, although that is certainly important. Instead, the answer lies in making sure the practice has the kind of culture that is compatible with an EMR initiative—and in laying the groundwork for a successful implementation long before the EMR system is up and running.[19]

Although the shift to an EMR system may be mandated, its primary success or failure will depend upon the readiness of the practice's employees to embrace change, because as process changes go, this will likely be one of the biggest they have ever encountered! Planning strategically to go through this process will provide the best potential for successful transition to an EMR. The following 10 steps provide a basic framework for moving from a paper to a paperless system:

1. Identify an EMR "champion."
One of the best predictors of success in an EMR implementation is clinician leadership. EMR implementation requires the commitment of a therapist leader, a sort of "EMR champion," who creates and communicates a shared vision, empowers staff to act on the vision, plans short-term wins, and embraces an IT culture for quality improvement.[13] Identification of this "champion" is one of the most important decisions that will effect the success of the implementation process, and he or she should typically be a clinician who has the respect of the rest of the staff and, if it is not the owner of the practice or manager of the rehabilitation department, has a direct line of communication to that person.

2. Perform a workflow analysis.
There is almost always an initial disruption of office workflow associated with the introduction of new IT systems, and knowing how to align these systems into the practitioner workflow is critical for a successful implementation. In addition, there is also an initial disruption in some financial, clinical, and organizational processes in moving to a paperless system as well.

It is important for a practice to conduct a thorough assessment of its current workflow prior to initiating an EMR transition. Not only does this provide the practice with an excellent baseline for assessing its EMR needs, but it also will help to identify and reduce or eliminate any potential bottlenecks that could impede the EMR progress once it is installed or adopted. Just as important, the practice can begin to establish some reasonable expectations for the EMR system. For example, planning to initiate the use of an EMR on a Monday with an expectation that things will run smoothly at 100% productivity by that Friday is not realistic!

It is prudent to prepare to incorporate an EMR system in your daily office workflow by knowing your patient demographics, staff roles, practice environment, and office processes and work patterns. Begin to analyze the workflow of your office by reviewing current workflow from intake to discharge, taking special care to perform a forensic review of your current processes related to coding, billing, and documentation. This process includes a review of the current roles and functions related to administrative operations as well, identifying who is currently doing what tasks. The greatest efficiency and effectiveness will be gained by matching the required tasks to the talent of specific staff, providing the training necessary to maximize success, and involving your staff in this redesign process. This initial process will allow you to identify areas of deficiency and develop a plan to correct those deficiencies. It is generally best to diagram the workflow process by using flow maps and flowcharts to make it easier to identify waste, bottlenecks, and inefficiencies. Once these have been identified, use small tests of change to find solutions to patient flow problems. This will then allow you to promote implementation of an EMR into an efficient process, rather than incorporating historical inefficiencies into your new workflow.

3. Determine what data are desired as an output from your EMR system.
The workflow analysis should help you to understand the relationship between data collection and information that is produced and utilized. In order to do this, it is

important to determine the purpose of data collections and information sharing—such as diagnosis classification, outcomes identification, justification for skilled care, marketing, and adherence to third-party requirements. A clinician must determine what information is important to their practice from a clinical and administrative perspective. It is necessary to determine the target audiences (such as other therapists, physicians, case managers, and third-party payers) and their likely use of information, since each of these stakeholders will want or require different things from the output of your EMR.

Determining the data to be collected in your EMR system and the method of input of that data starts by understanding compliance requirements. Therapists will often complain that documenting in an EMR system takes much longer than when handwriting their documentation, without the understanding that their current documentation skills may not be sufficient, or that their current documentation does not meet professional standards or regulatory requirements. One of the biggest benefits of adopting an EMR system should be the assistance it provides in adhering to compliance requirements, so it is important to recognize current areas of deficiency and use the transition to an EMR to assist in improving compliance literacy. It will also be necessary to determine the most effective interface to efficiently input data into the system for your staff, and establish what application hardware (workstations, laptops, or handhelds) will be used for documentation.

Vendors will often identify the myriad of reports available in their systems as a reason to consider their product, when in truth there are a handful of reports that will provide you the most valuable data for the successful management of your practice. Be careful not to find yourself buried under piles of data that do not help you to manage your practice at a high level, sometimes referred to as "analysis paralysis." Ensure your EMR system can seamlessly translate your practice's key data elements into meaningful and usable information that will assist you in efficiently understanding the profile of your practice.

4. Include clinical input into development and decision-making process.
Implementing an EMR will likely challenge your current paradigm, and therefore, it is important to assess the impact of the pending adoption of an EMR system on the organization itself. This is often best initiated by including the perspectives of therapists who will be using the system in the end. Including key staff in the marketplace analysis and in the review of any system that may potentially be adopted will go a long way in helping staff "buy-in" into EMR implementation. However, it is important to remember that gaining consensus from everyone on the final product to adopt may take time, and agreement on any customization and standardization may be a difficult process. This is time well spent as long as the expectations for an outcome from this process are clear to all involved. Discussing timelines for decision making regarding choices related to EMR choices may assist in this process.

5. Understand the concepts of documentation, medical necessity, and regulatory requirements prior to the decision-making process.
Becoming aware of and staying current in professional standards, third-party payment policy, regulatory requirements, and coding and documentation guidelines and requirements are critical, but often-overlooked components of patient/client management. Understanding these aspects of practice will likely help avoid system choices that may not provide the necessary data capture to provide essential alerts related to compliance in these areas. An EMR that takes these areas into consideration should ensure the efficient clinical decision support the clinician requires to meet medical necessity requirements as defined by various third-party payers, allowing for a greater focus on patient care with less frustration, or a faulty sense of security related to compliance issues. Unfortunately, there are too many EMR products that do not accurately incorporate appropriate compliance requirements into the coding and documentation software. As a result, the therapist who is unaware of these requirements, or has not taken the time to remain current in this critical area, may end up submitting false claims to third-party payers.

Although a thorough discussion of what constitutes a false claim and the potential penalties associated with this is beyond the scope of this chapter, awareness of compliance requirements allows a critical analysis of potential systems prior to purchase commitment. It is strongly recommended that a practice undergo a documentation and coding audit both pre- and post-implementation to establish baseline adherence to professional requirements and ensure a successful transition and implementation to a complaint paperless system.

6. Determine desired system characteristics.

There are many different ways and types of documenting, both on paper and in an EMR. On paper, blank sheets may be used to document the various components of the record. Templates, "fill-in-the-blank" forms for specific types of evaluations and treatments, and assorted flow sheets and checklists are also used. EMR systems also offer very similar characteristics and formats. There are template-driven systems that allow a clinician to fill in the blanks, and there are knowledge-based driven systems that allow a clinician to document in any way they deem necessary. Knowledge-based systems that integrate clinical decision support will provide a huge advantage in incorporating evidence-based practice, compliance standards, and outcomes ability into a practice, and while data entry may be a bit more structured, the benefits usually far outweigh any downside. And as with paper or manual entry, once an EMR format is adopted, there should be consistency in the utilization and content capture among therapists and within a practice or facility.

7. Test system performance and usability.

Clinicians can easily become frustrated with a poorly performing system. An EMR must meet or exceed user expectations. It is best to plan your implementation in advance and test the product carefully (preferably before making that final purchase!) to ensure adequate software and hardware system performance. It is also important to select a system that will support future growth and functionality. Rules and regulations are always changing, and it is important to ensure that these changes can be incorporated into an EMR system timely and completely. And remember, usability is a key factor in a successful implementation, so spend some time testing the system to make sure it is intuitive, makes sense to the clinicians and administrative personnel who will be using it, and matches the flow of patient examination. One of the best ways to do this is by participating in any opportunity for beta testing of a new or developing program. Doing so not only provides the ability to "test-drive" the system, but participating in a beta opportunity is an excellent way to contribute to the development of a system and incorporate individual practice processes into a system that may be selected for adoption.

8. Don't "work around" standards.

It is crucial not to "work around" standards that are incorporated into EMR systems. Coded observations and quantitative results are necessary for incorporation of automatic clinical guidelines, driving clinical decision support systems, and other high-level functions. Ensuring data quality is paramount to achieving the full functionality of an EMR and for providing credible clinical outcomes. If users find themselves creating "work-arounds" to meet payer or other stakeholder requirements, the system is not working for you! Adoption of an EMR should also include an acknowledgement that these standards exist and are important, and result in a commitment to necessary data capture and adherence to future data standards.

9. Avoid duplicate processes.

It is critical to understand that regardless of the system identified, efficiencies and productivity increases will only be gained if providers avoid parallel paper and electronic data entry. For clinicians, utilizing a PoC process where data are entered directly into the system while the therapist is with the patient, as described previously, is the most efficient system. In addition, during any transition, having adminstrative staff enter information in advance from paper to paperless systems is helpful, so that demographic and health history information is entered in advance of the visit and key reports are scanned into EMR so that they are easily accessible to the clinician when needed. Ultimately, maximal efficiencies are gained when work processes are redesigned to eliminate paper-based clinical processes and move to an effective paperless system. By setting deadlines for specific paper processes to transition to electronic interfaces, staff can keep track of their own progress in avoiding inefficient duplication of efforts.

10. Don't skimp on training.

Training of staff is often minimized or underestimated. Training is critical to successful software implementation and use. If a facility does not know how to use a software application or what it is capable of doing, they will not receive the full benefits of it. This can lead to eventual dissatisfaction with the application. Levels of training can vary from having to travel for training, on-site training, Web-based training and tutorials, and manuals for self-paced education and training. But regardless, training should be multidimensional, including system navigation, training in new roles and workflow, and training methods to ensure data integrity. Therapists should take full advantage of training available as part of any EMR choice. The next section will provide greater insight into this most important aspect of EMR implementation.

VIII. Training and Support

The key to successful implementation and use of hardware or software is the type of training and support a facility receives as it transitions to an EMR. Software programs touted as being the most efficient and effective will quickly become ineffective if the end user does not know how to use the application. Typically, software companies usually provide some customer service and technical support for an agreed-upon period of time. Most vendors will offer higher levels or extended coverage for an additional cost, and these costs can be on a per-usage, monthly, or annual basis. The skill level of the end users will dictate the level of customer service and support a facility requires. Product and technical support and services should not be neglected or negotiated out of a contract to save money. Most importantly, all training should be reinforced by the facility itself by making sure they utilize a "train the trainer" method with their staff in order to ensure that in the event of staff turnover, remaining staff could train new staff or system training is procured.

The method of training should be carefully considered and planned to effectively and efficiently meet the needs of the clinic/facility. Traveling for training can be useful to eliminate distractions from everyday clinical functions, but can be costly for larger facilities and ongoing new employee training. On-site training is very useful because a trainer can see how a facility operates and provide suggestions of how their system can be best implemented into the facility's workflow. However, on-site training can be expensive and cost prohibitive if a facility must bring in a trainer every time it needs additional training or has a new employee. Self-paced manuals are typically included with the software but, for some providers, can also be the least effective method of training. The manuals will always be available as a refresher or for new employees but will not necessarily provide a facility with helpful hints of how an application can be best implemented in a facility.

Web-based technology has improved dramatically in the last few years, making training through the Internet both informative and extremely useful. There are several options for Web-based training, including self-paced tutorials, recorded Web training, and live Web-based training. Self-paced tutorials and videos are similar to viewing a slide or PowerPoint presentation, guiding you through the application. Recorded Web-based training often provides the user with more useful information, with helpful tips and tricks not always available in a self-paced tutorial. Live Web-based training is a real-time session with a trainer via the Web with the added ability to share computer screens, making training specific to the issues identified. This method provides the end user with live training without the expense and inconvenience of traveling.

As an added benefit, staff training on EMR implementation and office redesign has the potential to increase individual skills, confidence, and familiarity with IT systems. Preparation for actual EMR training can be broken down into three basic steps:[20]

1. **Identify current skill levels of staff.** Employee baseline skill levels and comfort with computers will vary depending upon the age and background of employees. Younger employees most likely have grown up using cell phones, texting, and

e-mailing, and are extremely comfortable with technology as a part of their daily routines; these are the people you probably need to worry about least! Other employees may come from a generation that is less "tech-savvy," making it imperative that their baseline computer skill level be determined before rolling out an EMR. Many EMR "failures" are really failures of planning on the part of practice owners and administration. No matter what training method or schedule you choose, make sure that those with less computer literacy have learned the basics of PC or Mac applications and Web browsing (for ASP users) before scheduling your training sessions.

2. **Bring everyone up to the necessary skill level.** Determine the core skills that will be needed with the new EMR system. These core skills will be based, in part, on whether an ASP-based system or a client–server one is selected. ASP systems are Web based, and more and more people are becoming comfortable with using the Internet. But there are certain basic skills that should not be taken for granted: turning a computer on and off, setting a default printer, following password protocols, and logging on and off properly are small things that can frustrate users if they are not comfortable with these and other basic actions.

3. **Design a training plan for the new EMR.** Whatever method you choose, a training plan will need to be developed based on the skills of particular staff. Start with the basics of the system and then use a building block approach, adding on common tasks that all employees need to use (such as scheduling), followed by increasingly complex functions depending on an employee's particular job tasks. Basic EMR training should incorporate basic terminology, workflow, security, usability, and communications. After a general orientation, it is best to identify some "super users" who will become very proficient with the system, and will help to train additional staff, particularly new staff who may come on after the initial implementation. These "super users" usually consist of clinicians who championed the new system, but could also include office managers, practice owners, or other key administrative staff. The "train the trainer" strategy has many benefits, including developing in-house "experts" who know the program well enough to problem-solve issues that may develop because of unique practice styles, culture, and workflows.

Although it is advisable to plan to minimize business interruption and monitor organizational progress while training, it is best to aim for training that is distraction free. With phones ringing and patients walking through the door, therapists and support staff can find themselves learning the system in 15-minute snatches—a formula for frustration. Careful planning will create longer blocks of uninterrupted learning. Ideally, shutting down the office completely allows for the most focus but may not be practical. If this is not an option, open the office late one morning or close early in the afternoon to dedicate the time necessary. If possible, schedule fewer patients than usual on training days or plan for training on light patient days. This will ensure that patient care is not negatively impacted. While it is usually prudent to accept the vendor's recommendation on training hours and schedule, it is not reasonable to try to learn everything all at once—this may just create "glazed-over" expressions and frustrations by trying to master new technology quickly.

It is important to instill the right culture through the right messaging as you embark on the training process. Getting therapists and other clinicians and staff mentally prepared for EMR training is another key to a successful launch.[21] Even in the most progressive offices, some therapists need a bit of a nudge (or a more forceful shove!) to embrace the new technology. This "encouragement" can typically occur by using a combination of selling the benefits of the new system and firmly announcing that the EMR train is leaving the station, whether they are on it or not! But be mindful, although encouragement and incentives often work better than threats, one resistant employee who may resent the added technology because they see it as a threat to their job security may, if allowed to spread this anxiety unchecked, derail the entire atmosphere and training process.

Finally, ongoing technical and professional support of an application after the initial training occurs is crucial to the overall success of the software implementation.

If the software application is not working correctly, it will have a significant negative impact on the efficiency and effectiveness of the staff and facility. Therapists need to understand how a particular vendor will provide ongoing training, both when new therapists need to learn the program and when enhancements to the software and new features have been incorporated. Levels of support can vary from continuous live support, to limited hours of support, to e-mail communication. Within these types of support, the level of expertise can vary significantly. Some companies will provide support strictly for technical difficulties associated with their software. Others will support the software and the hardware that their system runs on, while still others will have clinicians on staff who can assist a facility with more legal, ethical, and clinical decision-making issues. But the key here is simple: understand what support is available from the vendor, what the cost of that support is, and when that support is available to you. Negotiate any needed enhancements in this area prior to the purchase of the software. A live support line that is available 6 AM to 6 PM Eastern time won't do you much good if you have a problem at 4 PM Pacific time!

IX. EMR AND THIRD-PARTY PAYMENT: MINIMIZING RISK AND IMPROVING COMMUNICATION FOR PAYMENT OF PHYSICAL THERAPIST SERVICES

Documentation shapes the process of clinical reasoning and provides justification for payment of physical therapy services. Regulatory changes continually push even the best-prepared practitioner to work overtime to maintain the training, policies, and standards related to documentation and coding for clinical services. The issue of medical necessity has become a primary focus of payer and regulatory agency audits. Billing for services that are not adequately justified in medical records can become an issue of potential fraud or abuse, carrying a significant risk to the provider. The adoption of EMRs has been identified as one potential tool for reducing negative audit experiences as well as improving quality of care.

In the current healthcare reimbursement climate, it is common for insurance companies to request medical records for the purposes of determining whether payment for services already rendered will be provided or whether a refund for payments already made is required. Over the past few years, these incidents have become more frequent, driven in large part by third-party payers who recognize the lack of awareness and compliance by many therapy providers in the areas of documentation, coding, and billing practices.

The third-party focus on the payment for rehabilitation services is instructive, in that it provides an opportunity for therapists to examine their clinical programs to better demonstrate that what they do, and how they do it, is valuable and worthy of appropriate payment. Yet in many cases, physical therapy is perceived as unskilled or unnecessary and, therefore, is undervalued by the third party's reimbursement methodology. The physical therapist has the opportunity to change the third-party perception of physical therapy by doing a better job of reflecting the use of current evidence, demonstrating clinical reasoning in their approaches to patient care, and demonstrating successful outcomes of their clinical approaches through more accurate documentation, coding, and billing practices. An effective EMR can greatly assist in this process.

Audit flags are identifiers on claim forms or in documentation that alert auditors or reviewers to potential fraud, abuse, or over-utilization, and indicate that further investigation is necessary in order for the payer to justify payment of that particular claim. There are several common audit flags that providers should be aware of when evaluating potential EMR programs or self-auditing their own system. While some of these audit flags are not specific to electronic documentation and exist in handwritten documentation formats as well, EMR systems can increase the likelihood of some audit flags more than others (if for no other reason than the improved legibility of the record!). Awareness of these flags, and ensuring that the EMR you choose minimizes the risk of them, will greatly assist in reducing the potential of negative audits by third-party payers.

The following audit flags are seen commonly in many existing EMR systems:

- **Evaluation notes reduced to one page, without necessary information to justify medical necessity.** Too often, the desire to have reports printed to only one page to either save paper or provide physicians with summary reports because of fear that they don't want (or won't read) this clinical information causes therapists to minimize information they collect or that they enter into their EMR system. It is important to remember that there are a variety of stakeholders for whom therapy documentation is important: referral sources, third-party payers, colleagues, attorneys, etc. It is important to collect and report the data that will support medical necessity as well as minimize the risk in the event of any legal action. Many EMRs allow for various formats to be printed once the initial evaluation is complete and documented in the system. It is best to understand all the options available for reporting to third parties.

- **Canned and generalized "assessment" statements that do not give a proper representation of the patient's progress or justification of the need for therapy services.** The adoption of an EMR does provide significant efficiencies, one of which may be a menu of phrases that can be populated into various sections of documentation. Using these phrases repeatedly, without the ability to edit them or individualize them to the specific patient, may lead third-party payers to question the legitimacy or credibility of the documentation.

- **Generalized statements leading to standardized notes that go unchanged by clinicians from visit to visit.** Often, the review of documentation from EMR systems by third-party payers will identify notes that are essentially duplicated visit after visit, with only the date or some other small nuance modified. Although there may be great similarities between visits over a short period, typically, no two physical therapy visits will be identical, particularly if the patient is making progress toward established goals. Documentation should reflect the differences in provider interaction, progression of treatment, and patient response to treatment at each visit.

- **The signature area for the physician on the Medicare plan of care (POC) is printed on a separate page than the required POC elements.** Medicare requires that the physician or nonphysician provider (NPP) (per Medicare qualification requirements) certify a POC at least every 90 days. That POC must include, at a minimum, the patient's diagnosis, long-term treatment goals, and the frequency and duration of treatment. Often, a signature box prints out on a separate sheet of paper than these items, and in fact, often the signature box is the only item on the last page of the POC. In these circumstances, the Medicare contractor may have difficulty identifying if the required certification was referencing the required elements, and further, there is no guarantee that those elements can't be modified without the knowledge of the physician or NPP. Page numbers on the POC document are useful to indicate a signature is linked to information found on a previous page of the document.

- **Programs will often carry over previously measured objectives which are repeated each visit as if they are being obtained, but are actually just being repopulated from prior visits.** Documentation on each visit should pertain to data that are collected at each visit. Historical measures are appropriate to add to a visit if they are being compared to new data or referenced in regards to modifications in the POC. When these measures are simply included in a visit note and only reference historical data, this causes confusion and may be perceived as a lack of progress, since the values are not changing.

- **Minutes for each procedure identified in the EMR populate a unit charge for a CPT code regardless of the amount of time spent with the patient on that procedure.** One of the largest areas of audit is related to the accurate reporting of the time spent with a patient. The CPT codes that describe direct contact should be reported based on the time spent with the patient; however, the number of units of these codes submitted for payment on each visit cannot exceed the total time spent with the patient. Most programs populate units for any number of minutes identified (4, 8, 10, etc.) without aggregating the minutes, resulting in therapists submitting claims for payment that reflect more time spent than actually occurred. This type of billing could constitute a false claim and subject the provider to severe penalties.

- **Documentation of nonspecific subjective comments, functional status, or tests and measures on initial examination or follow-up visits.** Many EMR systems provide standardized measurements that reflect findings that are overly general and do not provide sufficient information from which to objectively measure progress throughout the rehabilitation program. One of the benefits of an EMR is the ability to collect specific data and use that data to measure objective progress throughout the episode of care. The absence of this level of specificity or objectivity will likely cause third-party payers to question the legitimacy of the care or medical necessity of the treatment provided.

- **Objective data populated in the medical record relates to impairments only, without relationship to objective measures identifying limitations in functional activity.** Although not specific to an EMR, therapists have historically focused their data collection on impairments, such as pain, strength, and range of motion. While limitations in these areas are important, limitations in impairments are only considered a basis for skilled therapy if they are impacting functional performance. An effective EMR will assist the physical therapist in establishing this relationship and minimizing audit risk in this area.

- **Goals that are nonspecific, not related to functional activity limitations, or not related to findings on examination.** An area of significant problem in therapy documentation is in goal development. Medical necessity and compliance adherence require therapy goals to be specific, objective, and functionally related. While not an audit flag specific to EMR, computerized documentation may cause these inadequacies to be more easily identified, thus increasing the likelihood of problems on audit. An effective EMR should provide the tools to enhance appropriate goal development using the data gathered and input during the examination process.

- **Focus of documented interventions is on activities the patient is performing, rather than the therapist interaction with the patient to justify the need for skilled care.** Historically, physical therapists have focused their documentation on lists of exercise and activities that the patient is performing, without providing any indication of how therapist involvement is necessary to meet the established goals. EMRs often provide significant detail on sets and repetitions of exercises, but offer no indication as to why the patient could not be performing those exercises at home or in a community health club. EMRs should assist the therapist in identifying their interactions with the patient to assist in justifying the need for skilled care.

- **The initial plan of care (POC) does not change, or is too general and does not provide specific detail necessary to drive interventions.** Compliance requirements and documentation standards require the parameters of specific interventions to be identified within the documentation. If these parameters are not identified in the initial POC, then they must be identified on each visit that they are provided. Further, when additions, deletions, or modifications to the established POC are made, the POC should be modified. EMRs often populate overly general elements in the POC (therapeutic exercise, manual therapy, etc.), or the POC is not modified in the documentation as it occurs.

- **Discharge notes do not summarize treatment, progress, or provide for recommendations for follow-up.** The absence of discharge summaries as a routine component of therapy documentation has been identified as a significant issue among third-party payers and review agencies. When they are documented, they often do not include the necessary components of a discharge note. EMRs, given their ability to collect, collate, and retrieve data, should provide significant value in complying with this aspect of professional responsibility. However, therapists must understand the required components of a discharge summary and ensure that the EMR system they adopt will trigger them to efficiently document this information.

While no EMR can assure that you will never be audited, an effective EMR, designed specifically with the rehabilitation professional in mind, can be a significant asset in ensuring compliance with third-party payment rules, practice act regulations, and standards of practice. This improved compliance can assist dramatically in reducing the risk of negative audit consequences and increasing the likelihood of enhanced revenue capture based on documented justification for billed services.

X. DETERMINING THE RIGHT EMR: CRITERIA FOR CONSIDERATION

When evaluating EMR systems, the application should fit into the workflow of the practice and assist in improving productivity. Any system that adds work to the practice's processes without adding efficiencies, or disrupts the workflow of the end users without significant benefits, will not be accepted, and will eventually have a negative impact on productivity levels. The EMR system should be intuitive to users, support them in documenting appropriate information, and assist with case management. If a system can provide these things, it will improve the clinician's efficiency and productivity, allowing them to spend more quality time with their patients. There are a multitude of criteria and features that physical therapists should review prior to purchasing and implementing a system.

There are three primary considerations in evaluating any software application:

- First, is it going to improve the workflow and functionality of the practice?
- Second, is the application going to improve productivity, case management, and reimbursement?
- Third, is the application going to improve compliance and practice management?

Once an application meets a facility's basic criteria, the next steps to evaluate are training and customer support. As was discussed in the previous section, training and support are key to user acceptance and obtaining maximum benefit from the system. After a system is implemented, there will be a learning curve before complete user acceptance and improved productivity. With practice and dedication to the system, the rewards of effective and efficient documentation, increased productivity, and increased revenues can be realized.

Key Features to Consider. There are many features provided in today's EMR systems, and the ability to identify key groups of these when evaluating the right EMR system for a particular clinic or facility is critical as a component of the due diligence necessary for successful implementation. The following is a noncomprehensive list of program features, grouped by category, which should assist the rehabilitation provider in this process, recognizing that there are many other sources of criteria analysis and feature recommendations that are available in the marketplace.

The first three features, ASP versus client–server, integrated systems versus best of breed, and the integration of clinical decision support systems are among the most important, and as a result are discussed in more detail.

A. Application Service Provider (ASP) versus Client–Server

With the growth in technology and the need for timely enhancements to EMR systems as well as the desire for providers to access medical records where and when it is convenient to them, the trend has been to shift from what is known as a client–server model to an ASP platform for EMR systems. This is one of the most significant decisions to be made in choosing an EMR.

In the client–server option, providers (or clients) host the EMR software on their internal computer responsible for running the software (called a server) and purchase the EMR licenses outright. This requires substantial capital as well as an internal IT staffing that can constantly stay on top of maintaining the server. Servers are typically out of date within 3–4 years, so this model is only for those clients that can afford to update and repair the internal network as needed. Also, software is a "fluid" product, and after purchasing, it is important to recognize that the vendor typically is continuing to modify and program new enhancements and features. With this model, it will be necessary to ensure not only that the vendor is making timely changes, particularly related to compliance and regulatory elements, but that a clinic is equipped to update and maintain a dedicated server with the new software on a regular basis.

In contrast, ASP is a remotely hosted software system accessed via an Internet Web browser, where the EMR application, the database (where all the patient data are stored), and server all reside in a central location outside the therapist's office and are maintained by the EMR vendor or other third party. The server is secure and HIPAA compliant, and clinicians and staff use a secure login to access the EMR, in the same way they would access a secure banking site. ASP allows clinicians to access the program and associated patient information at any time, from any place with Internet access.

Although ASP systems don't eliminate all hardware requirements (printers, scanners, and laptops or workstations are still necessary), they do allow for outsourcing the maintenance and repair of the critical server to outside IT professionals. This can be a significant time and money saver, and is one reason for the sharp increase in ASP system development over the past few years. EMR software updates (which can be challenging and time consuming for a client–server to keep up with) are done by the ASP vendor and included as part of the monthly service charge. The ASP vendor also is responsible for performing regular backups of patient data and providing redundant systems—crucial functions that can jeopardize a practice if done poorly (or not at all) by practices maintaining their own systems. And with an ASP system, the cost and hassle of replacing the server (typically the most expensive piece of hardware) every 3–4 years is eliminated.

From a cost perspective, in a client–server option, a practice purchases a perpetual license to the software. After the EMR is paid for (often in installment payments), the remaining financial obligation to the vendor is an annual support payment, which typically covers new updates and technical support. Annual support fees typically range from 18% to 20% of the retail cost of the software.[22]

In contrast, with an ASP option there is no upfront cost for the software. Users may pay a monthly fee for as long as the service is used, or other subscription-type payment models exist. Fees can range from $250 to $1000 per provider, per month, plus the cost of a reliable, high-bandwidth connection to the Internet. The ASP fee is typically inclusive, covering technical support, software upgrades, daily database backups, and any server maintenance. Training and implementation costs may or may not be included in the monthly fee for an ASP.

Often the ASP versus client–server decision primarily revolves around how much IT support, server maintenance, and data management a practice is willing to absorb. For practices that have the staff, ability, resources to maintain a server, perform the backups religiously, attend to the details of technical troubleshooting, and manage complex software upgrades, a client–server may be a good choice—and sometimes can be less expensive in the long run. But, if the tasks described above are daunting or terrifying, then ASP is a better choice for a practice. Experts will usually recommend the ASP model based on the ability to assess the past and see where large software companies (such as Microsoft) are heading, and because even if a provider has the wherewithal to handle the upgrades, maintenance, etc., it still does not prove to be financially advantageous to do so. In the long run, the ASP model has projected savings of up to 30% based on reduced labor costs related to maintenance and support and reduced ownership costs related to hardware expenses over client/server programs.[8]

B. Best-of-Breed versus Integrated (End-to-End) Systems

Most practices in the market for their first EMR already have computerized practice management (or billing) systems in place. In deciding on an EMR, they will need to make an important decision, which is whether or not to keep the existing practice management system and interface it with a new EMR (if possible), known as the "best-of-breed" approach, or purchase an integrated system that combines a new EMR with new practice management software, sometimes known as implementing an end-to-end solution.

With the best-of-breed approach, each software application is selected based on its inherent qualities. If the practice management and EMR systems selected come from different vendors and need to exchange data, it will be necessary to build an interface that allows this exchange. When combining EMR and practice management systems from different vendors, registration interfaces are the most common. This allows front desk staff to automatically send data for new patients entering a practice to the new EMR. Without a registration interface, staff must separately enter patient data into the practice management and EMR systems.

In contrast, integrated (or end-to-end) systems share the same database. This means that when front desk staff enters patient data into an integrated system, the information becomes instantly available to everyone in the office, using the scheduling, billing, or EMR portion of the system. With integrated systems, a single vendor provides the convenience of a single point of contact for support and technical concerns. In addition, the requirement to manage the technical aspects of building and maintaining an interface between the EMR and practice management systems is eliminated. Most importantly, there will be significant efficiency gains from the systems' shared applications. Because truly integrated systems share a common database, they allow sophisticated interactions between the EMR and practice management systems.[23] One such example of this is the development of clinical decision support systems, which function most effectively in a fully integrated EMR.

Another example is the integration of documentation with billing. In a fully integrated system, documentation during a visit populates the appropriate CPT codes, which are then sent electronically to the practice's billing department. This process will typically ensure that documentation supports the CPT codes billed to a third party. The billing staff then reviews the charges for proper coding and can quickly and efficiently post the claim. This type of seamless data exchange is difficult (and generally expensive) to achieve when interfacing between two separate systems.

Many tasks within therapy practices require different staff members to share data quickly and accurately. Integrated systems are built with this data sharing in mind; best-of-breed systems are not.

C. Clinical Decision Support Systems (CDSSs)

Computerized clinical decision support systems (CDSSs) are information systems (software) designed to improve clinical decision making about individual patients. In a CDSS, characteristics of individual patients are matched to a computerized knowledge base, and software algorithms generate patient-specific recommendations.[24] An EMR that integrates a CDSS provides a powerful tool to capture coded clinical information that can be linked to knowledge of evidence-based treatment to provide tailored recommendations *at the point of care*. So, by utilizing an EMR with an integrated CDSS while the therapist is actually examining or treating the patient, the clinician improves the ability to make sound clinical decisions in a timely manner and decrease documentation and dictation time by using evidence-based recommendations and other aspects of decision support. Appropriate systems *seamlessly* integrate into the current workflow of busy clinicians by suggesting actions at a time when a clinician is still in the process of clinical documentation. Such integrated clinical decision support should assist in closing the large and well-documented gap between best evidence and actual practice.

CDSSs are designed to facilitate clinical management. A provider can save time in the long run and improve the quality of care by enhancing clinical practices and workflow practice efficiency. Typical components suggested for inclusion in a CDSS related to rehabilitation care include the following:

- Actions and recommendations based on specific examinations/evaluation findings
- Clinical guidelines
- Electronic alerts
- Documentation prompts
- Reference materials
- Reports related to captured patient data

An additional critical element of CDSS is computerized *clinical reminders* or computer-generated suggestions about clinical care for individual patients that are informed by data stored in the EMR. These suggestions are based on programs that operationalize evidence-based practice as computable rules that are integrated into the clinical application. In addition to clinical reminders, more comprehensive CDSSs include administrative and compliance reminders as well.

Although there are barriers to implementation of CDSS, which include the failure of practitioners to use the CDSS, poor usability or integration into practitioner workflow, or practitioner nonacceptance of computer recommendations, compared with manual initiation, the automatic prompting of CDSS has been demonstrated to improve integration into practitioner workflow as well as provide better opportunities to correct inadvertent deficiencies in care.[24] Although some providers have voiced concern about increased practitioner dependence on CDSSs, with eroded capacity for independent decision making, others advocate strongly that the uses of CDSSs actually confirm the decision-making process while improving the efficiency and quality of care. CDSSs are considered so important to the future of quality healthcare that the ONCHIT included this criterion in the final rule establishing the initial set of standards, implementation specifications, and certification criteria for EHRs.

Additional features for consideration include the following:

D. Customization Ability

Many providers get caught up in the concept of "my workflow" versus the "EMR workflow." Some providers are looking for an EMR vendor to customize the system based on their current paper and clinical workflow, whether or not that workflow is efficient or based on evidence. EMRs have the ability to standardize the approach to physical therapy evaluation and intervention and reduce the unwarranted variation in physical therapist practice.

Unwarranted variation in practice has been identified as a root cause of excessive and inappropriate healthcare utilization, resulting in less-than-optimal quality and efficiency. This unwarranted variation is typically caused by the "unique approach" to the evaluation and treatment of patients that is maintained by individual healthcare providers. Often, it is a result of such things as working for an organization that dictates practice styles, following the teachings of the latest, greatest "guru," or simply the result of habit— "It's always been done it this way." Such variation may be further perpetuated by practice "philosophies" that physical therapists often tout as marketing or differentiating strategies for their practices or facilities.

Individual practitioner approaches, when not informed by the best current evidence, have become one of the root causes of what the third-party payer sees as excessive and potentially inappropriate utilization—the result of which may be demonstrated in less-than-optimal quality and efficiency of care. Physical therapy, as seen from the third-party perspective, is notorious for demonstrating unexplained variations in practice patterns. This is typically the result of efforts to put into place various clinical protocols or policies that may not be based in current best evidence, but instead use information gained in seminars or publications that are not consistently reflective of current evidence and out of context with other clinical programs and approaches. The physical therapist has the opportunity to change the third-party perception of physical therapy by doing a better job of reflecting the use of current evidence, demonstrating clinical reasoning in their approaches to patient care, and demonstrating successful outcomes of their clinical approaches through more accurate documentation, coding, and billing practices.

While it is important to ensure adequate provisions for customization, this customization should occur within the structure of a necessary standardization of approach, using best available evidence whenever possible. And while some customization is necessary, customization that eliminates necessary documentation requirements simply to reduce the time it takes to document or eliminate evidence-based clinical decision support can add to the unwarranted variation in physical therapist practice, resulting in decreased quality and effectiveness, increased cost, increasing audits, and demand for return of identified overpayments.

E. Compliance Adherence

Generally, compliance in the larger context means adherence to laws and regulations of the land, and when specifically applied to the medical world, a focus is on maintaining regulatory compliance in all activities of documentation, coding, and billing for professional services. A compliant process and environment is an absolute necessity when considering the manner in which regulatory organizations are closely monitoring all aspects of healthcare activities, including those related to patient quality of care, documentation of services to support charges, and other financial transactions between the provider and the beneficiary. How will a therapy practice ensure that what ends up in the chart accurately reflects the care that was provided to the patient, as well as the services that were billed? An effective EMR system should include the incorporation of compliance requirements and programming of payer/regulatory changes seamlessly and in a timely manner. Through utilizing an integrated EMR, the burden of assessing compliance is lessened dramatically. A well-designed system that incorporates these requirements and changes will greatly assist the clinical staff in performing their documentation, and it is this documentation that then automatically determines the services to be coded and billed, a process that is easily performed once reviewed by the responsible staff. Typically, ASP systems are significantly more timely and complete with compliance updates.

F. Focus on Functional Activities

Professional standards and third-party payer requirements focus on the attainment of measurable functional goals based on activities and impairments that are identified on the initial evaluation. When evaluating an EMR system for documentation abilities, a facility should look at its ability to: generate previous and current levels of function; identify measurable impairments and functional limitations; facilitate outcomes data collection; integrate the International Classification of Functioning, Disability, and Health (ICF); and develop and track measurable functional goals that identify the impact of noted impairments on activity performance.

G. Clinical Reporting Flexibility

We document for various reasons, and our documentation is read and utilized by many who are involved in the delivery and payment of our services. Physicians and third-party payers utilize documentation of therapy services for determining appropriateness of patients' responses and medical necessity, while state practice acts, compliance requirements, and medical/legal and risk management focus on specifics in documentation that could assist in malpractice or regulatory challenges. One report written in an ineffective and/or inefficient manner, while meeting the criteria for one set of eyes, will undoubtedly have another glaze over by the time they get to the third page of your initial evaluation report! The ability to generate multiple report formats as needed by the various entities that are the recipients of the documentation will simplify and reduce administrative work.

In choosing an EMR, look for a system that allows for documentation to be produced in a timely manner, is easy to review, and provides each intended recipient with the information they need (and want). Some applications generate template forms that may give a referral source the kind of information they need to make appropriate decisions concerning their patient's care, but may not include the information necessary to comply with your state practice act or third-party payment requirements. Other applications may provide too much information or be too "busy," making it difficult for the referral source to extract the information they are looking for. The ideal application would allow a clinician to document everything that is important and necessary to their clinical practice and patient/client management, and be able to report this information in a detailed evaluation or follow-up note that becomes part of the medical record, yet also provide a summary report that could be provided to the referral source with only the information they want and need. Providing the physician with the appropriate information to make him or her effective and productive may have a positive impact on the amount of referrals that physician sends, while still allowing the therapist to be compliant with necessary standards, rules, and regulations.

H. Tracking and Alert Systems

One of the greatest strengths of EMR systems, particularly those that integrate clinical decision support systems, is the ability to track various actions or statistics and notify the user based on predetermined parameters that are established by either the vendor or the end user. A few of the tracking and alert parameters to look for include the following:

Authorization and Resource Management. It is important that interventions and services that are medically necessary be reimbursed appropriately by either the third-party payer or the patient. Awareness of coverage limitations prior to treatment will allow clinicians to best manage patients within the limits of the patient's financial abilities. When evaluating EMR systems, a facility should seek features that assist with case management, tools to ensure optimal charge capture for documented services, and alerts to inform the clinicians before their patient's authorization expires. Having this information allows the therapist to make better clinical decisions and provide extended care for the patients who need it within the structure of the payment benefit. With such alerts, the clinician can educate the patient as to their coverage and take appropriate action to seek additional authorization, obtain payment for additional services directly from the patient, or discharge the patient.

One of the keys to managing a successful practice is the ability to manage the available resources related to payment for services. Payers manage their resources by limiting the number of covered visits or length of treatment under an insurance plan, the dollar amount paid per visit, or the duration of the benefit. If a patient is treated outside of the parameters established by the payer, the payer may refuse to pay for the treatment delivered. Having the ability to monitor the resource status of each patient will enable the clinician to develop an appropriate plan of care, manage the patient's care efficiently, maximize therapist productivity, and improve payment by informing patients prior to exceeding third-party payment limits and informing patients of their financial responsibility at the appropriate time.

Diagnosis, Intervention, and Functional Improvement. Medicare and many workers' compensation providers are requiring that clinicians have functional documentation to support continued care. Professional resources, including APTA's *Guide to Physical Therapist Practice*[25] and *Defensible Documentation*,[26] identify recommended examinations, tests and measures, and interventions, and proper documentation of these. There has been a greater demand for functional outcome-oriented documentation and the incorporation of evidence-based practice through research to justify therapy services. When a facility evaluates EMR systems, the system should be evaluated on its incorporation of these and other professional guidelines. The system should have the ability to generate the treating or physical therapist diagnosis in addition to the medical diagnosis, and track outcomes data related to interventions provided and functional status achieved at discharge. Being familiar with these resources, and others that are available, will assist in the review and decisions related to making an EMR choice.

Attendance and Utilization. It can be difficult to keep track of every active case in a facility. If a patient/client goes on vacation for a week, or cancels appointments as a result of illness, this patient entry can become lost and then therefore missing in the system. Certainly, lost or missing patients mean lost revenue in the short run, but there are trends like this that can also affect patient satisfaction or be reflected in more significant practice concerns. An effective EMR system should be able to track patients who have not been seen in a facility for an established period of time and alert the therapist when an active patient/client has not been seen in a set time, thus allowing the clinician to be able to take appropriate action in a timely fashion. By responding to these alerts, a clinician may be able to recapture lost visits, improve facility revenues, and better assist their patients in returning to a previous level of function. Besides attendance tracking, the ability to track utilization of services based on diagnosis code, insurance category, therapist, etc. will provide significant information to allow for practice growth through more efficient and effective management.

I. Dashboard Availability

Dashboards are one of the most intuitive and interactive ways to display data so that clinicians and managers can make intelligent, data-driven decisions about their practice on a daily basis. The best dashboards should allow for the flexibility to view both high-level reports as well as detailed listings, down to the patient account level. One of the benefits of having an EMR is the ability to report captured key data in an efficient manner to allow for efficient and effective practice management. There are several key areas that can be reported on dashboards within an EMR. For example, a patient dashboard will display a summary of all appropriate patient information stored in the EMR, and is updated in real time, without the need for manually updating the information. Data such as patient demographics, problems/diagnoses, notes, and other helpful information to make necessary clinical decisions are typical components of the patient dashboard. Financial dashboards will provide real-time data on dimensions of a practice, such as collection ratios, adjustment ratios, and extensive accounts receivable reporting. Practice management dashboards include such statistics as number of new patients, visits, and procedures, with the ability to identify each based on CPT code, diagnosis code, insurance type, and various other statistics.

These fundamental but evergreen calculations can provide quick and useful information when monitoring the health and stability of a practice or facility. Used as a management tool, these dashboard ratios and statistics paint a picture of fluctuations in payer patterns, practice billing operations, patient statistics, or other influencing factors that can help efficiently focus a practice's efforts in the overall management of clinical and administrative operations.

J. Financial/Revenue Report Availability

One area of responsibility for most office staff is the ability to report on the quantity of patients/clients treated, revenue generated, and money collected from co-pays (and durable medical equipment if the facility is a provider). By having this information readily available, a facility is able to quickly assess whether they are making or losing money. When choosing an EMR, a facility should be able to generate these reports quickly and easily, without having to do additional data entry.

K. Outcomes Reporting

Outcomes measurements, the ability to compare the results of an action or process over time, are part of the next wave of EMR applications. Certain outcomes, such as time from injury to release to partial or full employment, are easy to calculate and track if they are entered as dates. They can be recalled for specific procedures, clinicians, diagnoses, and payers. More advanced outcome measurements, such as improvement in the SF-36, DASH, or other scales can be integrated into existing EMRs. Maintaining outcomes in an integrated EMR will allow practices to monitor their outcomes, benchmark them against published standards, and participate in new pay-for-performance or value-based purchasing initiatives as they are created. When evaluating various EMR systems, remember that this is likely going to provide you an opportunity to track and report data that previously took hours, if not days, to identify, and embrace new methods to continue to provide better care.

L. Incorporation of Third-Party Payment Policy

Collecting payment for services provided is often a challenge. There are a plethora of reasons why a payer may deny or refuse to pay a claim, and moreover, payers also aim to ensure that there is documentation to support the bills submitted for payment. There are several different types of edits that can be applied to charges. The most common types of edit is known as the Correct Coding Initiative (CCI), and local medical review policies (LMRP) or local coverage decisions (LCD) often have crosswalks that identify diagnoses for which a particular CPT code will be considered for payment. There are also billing rules, such as cascading or multiple procedure reductions that may have an impact on how a facility submits a bill for payment. CCI edits are a Medicare Part B policy that evaluates claims when two or more CPT codes are submitted for payment, to see if one comprehensive code would be more appropriate (bundling). Medicare Part A and Part B local medical review policies are used to assist therapists in submitting correct claims for payment. In choosing an EMR, a facility should ensure the application takes any billing and coding edits into account to ensure efficient submission of claims and timely payment. Further, payers generally have contract-specific fee schedules, so any EMR you select should be able to support many different contractual fee schedules, as well as provide alerts if a particular insurance company does not cover a particular service or there is a need to submit charges with CPT codes that are different than would typically be associated with an intervention.

M. Legal Adherence and Risk Mitigation

In regards to the incorporation of HIPAA and other legal elements, there are many legal aspects in the day-to-day operations of a physical therapy business. When evaluating an EMR system for a facility, one should make sure that the application follows professional standards and Medicare guidelines for documentation, and is compliant with HIPAA regulations. There are also federal and state guidelines that need to be monitored. By implementing an EMR system that keeps current with the legal aspects of documentation, a facility can improve overall productivity and minimize risk of noncompliance.

In the past, making certain errors was a mistake, but in an environment that has ratcheted up the scrutiny, making certain errors may be considered fraud. Examples include overbilling and billing for treatment that was not actually rendered. It is a continual challenge to keep track of all the regulatory requirements, so an EMR system should assist with this. All data exchange must be encrypted to protect confidentiality, and it is essential to avoid access to patient data by unauthorized individuals in or associated with a practice. EMR systems typically implement safeguards to maintain data confidentiality, integrity, and availability. From an administrative perspective, these include access management and workforce security; from a physical perspective, such things as facility controls and workstation access; and from a technical focus, audit control, system integrity, and user authentication. When evaluating EMR systems, it is critical to ensure that the system will reduce exposure to fraud and risk, rather than making day-to-day activities more challenging to monitor and control.

N. Automation of Administrative Functions

An effective EMR system should have the ability to automate current administrative office functions such as appointment reminders, insurance eligibility, and patient follow-up. The inclusion of PoC documentation, coding, and billing alerts related to missing or incorrect information will greatly enhance administrative efficiency.

O. Adaptability to Future Changes

Even with the long history of EMR development that began almost 20 years ago, we are only in the early stages of EMR evolution, and the criteria for "meaningful use," standards for interoperability, and technical abilities of clinical decision support systems are still in their infancy. When shopping for a system, it is most important to consider those things that are not yet known in the industry or about your specific utilization of a system, and to consider the standards related to specific aspects of EMR that will likely be required in future. After all, the purchase of an EMR is a long-term investment in your practice and your profession.

XI. FINAL THOUGHTS

Most physical therapists recognize the importance, and value, of appropriate coding and documentation of clinical services, yet the process of learning and implementing all of the necessary information to adequately document the clinical care provided to patients, not to mention the time it can take to do so, can be overwhelming. However, if an appropriate and effective EMR system is implemented, the process of documentation can not only efficiently meet the clinical, legal, regulatory, and payment requirements that currently exist, but can also serve to enhance the patient encounter, facilitate improved functional outcomes, and increase a company's bottom line, while at the same time reducing the risk of punitive audits. To achieve these goals, it is critical for therapists to increase their "compliance IQ" as well as improve their "documentation hygiene," and then to embrace, after appropriate education and due diligence, the transition to an EMR. For in that transition, a computerized documentation system will not only assist physical therapists to meet new legislative requirements and become a significant administrative and compliance asset – it will also become a most valuable partner in the provision of efficient, effective, evidence-based physical therapy care.

REFERENCES

1. DesRoches CM, Campbell EG, Rao SR, Donelan K, Ferris TG, Jha A, et al. Electronic Health Records in Ambulatory Care—A National Survey of Physicians. *N Engl J Med* 2008;359(1):50–60. (http://www.contentnejmorg.zuom.info/cgi/reprint/359/1/50.pdf)

2. Zandieh SO, Yoon-Flannery K, Kuperman GJ, Langsam DJ, Hyman D, Kaushal R. Challenges to EHR Implementation in Electronic Versus Paper-based Office Practices. *J Gen Intern Med* 2008;23(6): 755–761.

3. Vreeman DJ, Taggard SL, Rhine MD, Worrell TW. Evidence for Electronic Health Record Systems in Physical Therapy. *Phys Ther* 2006;86(3): 434–446.

4. American Physical Therapy Association. Position Statement: *Support of Electronic Health Record in Physical Therapy* (HOD P06-08-18-12). June 2008. www.apta.org.

5. Department of HHS. *Defining Key Health Information Technology Terms*. April 28, 2008.

6. Blanchfield BB, Heffernan JL, Osgood B, Sheehan RR, Meyer GS. Saving Billions of Dollars—and Physicians' Time—by Streamlining Billing Practices. *Health Aff* 2010;29(6):1248–1254. (http://content.healthaffairs.org/cgi/content/abstract/hlthaff.2009.0075)

7. Wang SJ, Middleton B, Prosser LA, Bardon CG, Spurr CD, Carchidi PJ, et al. A Cost-Benefit Analysis of Electronic Medical Records in Primary Care. *Am J Med* 2003;114(5):397–403.

8. Miller RH, et al. *EHR Implementation: Barriers and Potential Solutions*. IMS HIT Initiative.

9. PR Newswire Association, Inc. *AMA Survey Finds Upsurge in Physician Usage and Regard for Internet*. 2001.

10. American Medical Association. Technology Use Increases at Physician Practices. Industry Watch, Health Management Technology, February, 2002.

11. Bodenheimer T, Grumbach K. Electronic Technology: A Spark to Revitalize Primary Care? *JAMA* 2003;290(2):259–264.

12. MM&M. *Use of Internet for Reaching Physicians Grows in Value*. June 20, 2002.

13. Miller RH, Sim I. Physicians' Use of Electronic Medical Records: Barriers and Solutions. *Health Aff* 2004;23(2):116–126.

14. Garret D, et al. *Electronic Health Records: Overcoming Challenges in Deployment and End-User Adoption*. Syntel, 2007. http://www.syntelinc.com/uploaded-Files/Syntel/Digital_Lounge/White_Papers/Syntel_EHR.pdf.

15. Hsu J, Huang J, Fung V, Robertson N, Jimison H, Frankel R. Health Information Technology and Physician-Patient Interactions: Impact of Computers on Communication during Outpatient Primary Care Visits. *J Am Med Inform Assoc* 2005;12(4): 474–480.

16. Garrison GM, Bernard ME, Rasmussen NH. 21st-Century Health Care: The Effect of Computer Use by Physicians on Patient Satisfaction at a Family Medicine Clinic. *Fam Med* 2002;34(5): 362–368.

17. Frankel R, Altschuler A, George S, Kinsman J, Jimison H, Robertson N. Effects of Exam-Room Computing on Clinician-Patient Communication. *J Gen Intern Med* 2005;20(8):677–682.

18. Gadd CS, Penrod LE. *Dichotomy Between Physicians' and Patients' Attitudes Regarding EMR Use During Outpatient Encounters*. Proceedings of the AIA Symposium, 2000, pp. 275–279. http://www.ncbi.nlm.nih.gov/pmc/articles/PMC2243826/

19. Koo CC. Getting Ready for EMR. *Health Management Technology*, August 2004. Nelson Publishing. http://www.providersedge.com/ehdocs/ehr_articles/Getting_Ready_for_an_EMR.pdf.

20. Polack P. Training Your Staff for EMR. *Medical Practice Trends*. October 29, 2008.

21. Lowes R. EMR Success: Training Is the Key. *Med Econ* 2004;81:TCP 11. http://www.providersedge.com/ehdocs/ehr_articles/EMR_Success-Training_is_the_Key.pdf.

22. Kane LR. Best EMRs for Small Practices. *Medscape Business Medicine*. May 21, 2009.

23. Kleaveland B. The Tech Doctor: Best-of-Breed or Integrated Systems? *Physicians Practice* 2007:17(9).

24. Garg AX, Adhikari NKJ, McDonald H, Rosas-Arellano MP, Devereaux PJ, Beyene J, et al. Effects of Computerized Clinical Decision Support Systems on Practitioner Performance and Patient Outcomes. *JAMA* 2005;293(10); 1223–1238.

25. American Physical Therapy Association. *Guide to Physical Therapist Practice*. http://guidetoptpractice.apta.org/.

26. American Physical Therapy Association. *APTA's Defensible Documentation for Patient/Client Management.* http://www.apta.org/AM/Template.cfm?Section=Documentation4&Template=/CM/HTMLDisplay.cfm&ContentID=70701.

27. Belden JR, Grayson R, Barnes J. *Defining and Testing EMR Usability: Principles and Proposed Methods of EMR Usability Evaluation and Rating.* HIMSS EHR Usability Task Force. June 2009. https://mospace.umsystem.edu/xmlui/bitstream/handle/10355/3719/DefiningTestingEMR.pdf?sequence=1.

ADDITIONAL REFERENCES

Blumen HE, Nemiccolo LD. The Convergence of Quality and Efficiency and the Role of Information Technology in Healthcare Reform. *Milliman Research Report.* June 1, 2009 pp. 1–12.

Center for Medicare and Medicaid Services (CMS) Proposes Definition of Meaningful Use of Certified Electronic Health Records (EHR) Technology. December 30, 2009. www.cms.hhs.gov.

Center for Medicare and Medicaid Services (CMS) Proposes Requirements for the Electronic Health (EHR) Medicare Incentive Program. December 30, 2009. www.cms.hhs.gov.

Dworkin LA, Krall M, Chin H, Robertson N, Harris J, Hughes. Experience Using Radio Frequency Laptops to Access the Electronic Medical Record in Exam Rooms. Proc AMIA Symp 1999:741–744. http://www.ncbi.nlm.nih.gov/articles/PMC2232612/pdf/procamiasymp00004-0778.pdf

Electronic Medical Records: Client/Server or ASP? May 14, 2007. www.emrexperts.com.

Halamka JD. Making the Most of Federal Health Information Technology Regulations. *Health Aff* (Millwood) 2010 Apr: 29(4):596–600.

Hogan SO, Kissam SM. Measuring Meaningful Use. *Health Aff* 2010;29(4):601–606. http://content.healthaffairs.org/cgi/content/abstract/29/4/601.

Oberg E. Electronic health Records: Can Technology Help Your Practice? *Integrative Med* December 2007/January 2008.

Reed G. Barriers to Successful EHR Implementation. May 1, 2007. www.EHRSCOPE.com.

Reinberg S. *Doctors Slow to Embrace Electronic Medical Records.* U.S. News & World Report. September 9, 2009.

Schnipper JL, Linder JA, Palchuk MB, et al. "Smart Forms" in an Electronic Medical Record. *J Am Med Inform Assoc* 2008;15(4):513–523.

Torda P, Han ES, Scholle SH. Easing the Adoption and Use of Electronic Health Records in Small Practices. *Health Aff* 2010;29(4):668–675. http://content.healthaffairs.org/cgi/content/abstract/29/4/668.

Walsh SH. The Clinician's perspective on Electronic Health Records and How They Can Affect Patient Care. *BMJ* 2004;328(7449):1184. http://www.bmj.com/content/328/7449/1184.extract.

www.FearonLevine.com

CHAPTER 11 REVIEW QUESTIONS

1. What constitutes fraud in the medical record?

2. Explain the history of EMR development leading up to the current mandate for transitioning to an EMR by 2014.

3. Explain the concept of "meaningful use" in regards to EMR adoption.

4. Explain the difference between an electronic medical record and electronic health record.

5. Compare and contrast ASP versus client/server EMR platforms.

6. Compare and contrast the benefits of point of care use of EMR versus workstations or documenting outside the patient visit.

7. What is the key to user acceptance and obtaining maximum system benefit? Defend your answer.

8. What are the three primary considerations when considering software?

9. What is the relationship between an EMR system and evidence-based practice?

12 Utilization Review and Utilization Management

I. INTRODUCTION

Documentation is the means of communicating information from the treating professional to all users of the medical record. It is the "what" therapists do and "how" it is performed. It is imperative to clearly and concisely communicate only the information that is relevant and necessary about care provided and the resulting condition of the patient or client.

As defined by the American Physical Therapy Association (APTA), "Utilization review (UR) is a system for reviewing the medical necessity, appropriateness and reasonableness of services proposed or provided to a patient or group of patients. This review is conducted on a prospective, concurrent and or retrospective basis to reduce the incidence of unnecessary and or inappropriate provision of services. UR is a process that has two primary purposes: to improve the quality of service (patient outcomes) and to ensure the efficient expenditure of money."[1] It also serves to:

- Ensure delivery of cost-effective high-quality physical therapy services
- Identify inappropriate or less effective and less efficient services with corrective action
- Assure of compliance with accreditation and licensing guidelines
- Ensure the continuum of care in a timely manner
- Assure that medically necessary care was delivered
- Facilitate avoidance of unnecessary care beyond goals, beyond point of progress
- Determine if delivery of service not indicated in plan
- Determine if service not rendered for problems identified
- Discover if no baseline level of care provision based on information provided
- Ensure referral(s) to other practitioners when out of the therapist's scope of "expertise" by training, experience, or otherwise
- Facilitate risk management (prevention of all types of loss)
- Identify the appropriate physical therapy personnel provided care for level of skill required or by virtue of third party payer requirements

Prospective review, a component of UR, may also be referred to as utilization management (UM). UM is based on the information derived from the review process both internal and external to the organization providing services, to ensure quality of service and effective and efficient delivery.

UR is considered a component of quality assurance and may be referred to as utilization review and quality assurance (URQA). In organizations or facilities with ongoing quality improvement or quality assurance programs and monitoring, URQA is often used.

Before 1965, UR was largely experimental and not performed by many providers. Medicare introduced a new era in accountability with a requirement for all hospitals participating in Medicare and Medicaid programs to forming UR committees and develop written UR plans. Initially the programs were not successful because the focus was on the fiscal portion of care, the interpretations were inconsistent, and coordination of benefits was often nonexistent. In 1972, professional standards review organizations (PSROs) primarily for physician services were initiated. PSROs employed nonphysicians and physicians to review the appropriateness and quality of medical services. Although nonphysicians performed the initial review and could affirm care, only a physician could deny services. Little was done with rehabilitation review however, the focus instead being on the medical aspects. Hospitals were required to subscribe to a concurrent review and care evaluation program. This process was the precursor to the eventual development of critical pathways in the 1980s and early 1990s associated with the growth of managed care.

PRSOs evolved into peer review organizations (PROs) in the early 1980s, concurrent with the advent of Medicare inpatient acute care diagnostic-related groups (DRGs), with a continued focus on medical services. Based on the Peer Review Improvement Act part of the Tax Equity and Fiscal Responsibility Act (1982), the PSRO program was replaced with the Utilization and Quality Control Peer Review Organization (PRO) program for utilization and quality monitoring. To increase consistency and effectiveness of quality review organizations, Congress established the PROs to monitor both quality and utilization.[2] The PROs emphasized retrospective reviews with standard pre-established review criteria based on professionally recognized treatment standards versus the concurrent review stressed by the PRSOs.

With the early growth of managed care organizations such as HMOs and PPOs, as well as hospital-based DRGs, there was an increased interest in productivity standards versus quality of care issues for physical therapy and other rehabilitation services. As a result, as organizations focused on therapist productivity versus quality of care, therapists practicing in the 1980s experienced some of the first denials for physical therapy services for Medicare beneficiaries. As costs to the Medicare program increased (cost shifting as a result of DRGs), Medicare UR was expanded to include skilled nursing facility physical therapy services, Part A for short-term skilled rehab, Part B for long-term residents, and outpatient services under Part B. This evolved from the Medicare initiative for improvement in efficiency, effectiveness, and medical necessity of care in the hospital inpatient arena. Application of UR by Medicare created added financial risk for physical therapists and organizations providing Part B services.

The practice of UR was and is not exclusive to Medicare. Coincident to the rise in Medicare denials for services, private payer sources looked to the Medicare system for cost containment measures. Application of UR practices facilitated examination of medical necessity, effectiveness, and efficiency of care with maximization of outcomes. In the 21st century, as costs for health care continue to grow exponentially, the rise in the interest of evidence-based practice is a result of the need for justification of care. By engaging in UR and UM practices, therapists should be able to justify care by clearly identifying medical necessity and documenting efficient and effective quality care. These practices can also provide outcome data to support efficacy of intervention and the concept of evidence-based practice.

II. INTERNAL UR/UM PRACTICES

Internal UR and UM practices are based on review of documentation by a UR designated professional. The therapist must know for whom they are writing, what information must be conveyed, and the purpose for which the information will be used. From a UR perspective, the purposes include reimbursement; effective and efficient utilization of internal resources, such as staff to monitor productivity; determination of staffing needs; consistency of content in the record; consistency and objectivity of goal setting; and effective and efficient selection of interventions and outcome data established by individual therapists. The way the information is recorded should be the same, regardless of the purpose of the review. This is a principle of health information management as described by the American Health Information Management Association (AHIMA).[3] An organization, as part of an ongoing quality management program, can review the content of the medical records for compliance. Concurrent and retrospective reviews can be utilized to ensure concurrent compliance, confirm content is legally admissible, revise guidelines for the future, develop clinical pathways, ensure effective and efficient care and outcomes, and provide educational input to staff for improvement in documentation process and content.

It is critical that the PT know the patient/client's insurance plan and what their benefits are. For example, if a plan is limited to 30 PT visits/year, it is 30 visits regardless of what the PT, physician, or patient believes is medically necessary or how episodes of illness or injury an individual may have in 1 year. Other insurers may allow for PT services for 60 days from the first visit. Therefore, visits and timing should be used appropriately. If pre-op visits are necessary, they should be scheduled sparingly. Ignorance of policy limitations will result in denial of any care rendered beyond the limit. Once a payer maximum is reached, private pay can be offered in most circumstances.

III. UTILIZATION REVIEW AND REIMBURSEMENT

From a reimbursement perspective, the documentation must present a clear picture of the episode of care. The elements in the record reviewed are the referral and or authorization (if required by the payer); the information included for the initial examination and evaluation, including the plan of care; all tests, measures and examinations performed and the objective data, documentation of continued care; and documentation of summation of episode of care (see Appendix E).[4]

Evidence of continued or continuing care includes documentation of intervention or services provided and current patient/client status, and documentation of reexamination. Colloquially, these entries are referred to as treatment notes, progress notes/reports, and periodic summaries (i.e., monthly, weekly, or as designated by policy). They can also be reflected in flow sheet format or variations in checklists and additional entry, although flow sheets and checklists may be the most likely component of a record to result in denial.

Documentation of summation of the episode of care occurs at the termination or discontinuation of therapy services for a specific episode. Termination or discontinuation may occur for a variety of reasons and must be clearly documented for UR purposes. Based on the APTA definitions,[1] termination of care occurs when a patient or client has met the established PT goals. However, discontinuation may result from a variety of reasons, such as lack of progress, illness, hospitalization, patient noncompliance (with very specific descriptions of what led to this conclusion), excessive absenteeism (with evidence that the patient was contacted and documented or that attempt to contact was documented) inappropriate patient behavior, physician decision, decision of third-party payer, or decision of a case manager. Noncompliance in this context is lack of patient compliance with instructions, thus impeding progress in an effective and efficient manner or potentially results in harm. Prolonged illness that prevents participation in scheduled therapy must result in discontinuation. However, recovery and renewed ability to participate can result in resumption of care, although if more than 1 or 2 weeks have passed and the physical status has changed, it may be considered a new episode of care or require a revised plan of care and communication with the physician (if not a self-referral).

The documentation should emphasize the disability and function versus impairment. The Nagi Disablement Model was the designated model in the last Guide to Physical Therapist Practice.[5] Although the APTA has now moved to the ICF Model (refer to Chapter 3), the components of the Nagi model for documentation purposes still work. The impairments are the pathological and physiological consequences of the disease or injury process. The functional limitations are the inability to perform a task in an efficient or competent manner as a result of the impairments. The relationship between the impairments and functional limitations should be clearly identifiable in the documentation as justification for care and appropriateness of intervention.

The review process takes each document included and examines it for relevancy to the whole picture of the patient's functional needs versus the current functional status. Because this is often based on the level or function of the patient prior to the "recent" functional change, it is imperative to clearly indicate the prior level of function in the initial examination and evaluation process. If an episode of care has ended, or the review is occurring at any point in time during the episode, the information contained in the initial report should be similar in structure and content to allow easy comparison of data. It is important to identify the reason for the referral, whether the examination concurs with the reason for referral (as indicated by the physician) and what the therapist's evaluation of the patient's potential for responding to therapeutic interventions will be. When considering the reason for referral, a clear indication should be made of the medical diagnosis versus the physical therapy diagnosis. Depending on the reason for care, they may be the same or different.

There are technical components that can be addressed with an overall review as described in detail in the APTA *Guidelines for Physical Therapy Documentation*, General Guidelines section (see Appendix E).[4]

IV. INITIAL EXAMINATION AND EVALUATION/CONSULTATION

The review of the examination and evaluation/consultation is performed to establish that the documentation provides clear, cohesive data that supports the evaluation conclusions. It is important to review each document/section as to its relevance to the patient/client management. This documentation should include a clear statement regarding the method of referral (self-referral in states and settings that allow for direct access or a referral from another practitioner). If the review is being performed by a third-party payer or by an internal representative, the meaning of all content must be evident.

V. INITIAL EPISODE OF PHYSICAL THERAPY CARE

The history is reviewed to determine the patient/client's medical diagnoses and factors that may affect the length of care or stay (LOS), frequency of intervention, or precautions necessary during the delivery of service, as well as evidence of informed consent. This will also allow the reviewer to determine if the appropriate risks and benefits were reviewed during the informed consent process. The care of the patient/client will be affected by the comorbidities documented and the demographic information obtained in the history. Information documented in the history, such as living environment, comorbidities, medications, caregiver, services (either concurrent or prior), and patient knowledge and expectations (goals), will need to be interpreted in the evaluation to determine the exact effect and relationship to the overall care and specifically to the treatment plan and goals established. The specific relationship of this information to the plan of care should be clearly documented and evident to the reviewer as he or she not make assumptions based on their experience or knowledge. The following sections illustrate the elements that should be clearly identified for sound documentation and review purposes.

Diagnosis/Date of Onset: The date of onset and medical and PT diagnoses are important both clinically and for reimbursement purposes. The diagnosis selected from the referral should reflect the medical condition that relates directly to the reason for the functional deficit(s). The diagnosis is the starting point for ensuring appropriate testing and examination and ultimately, appropriate interventions and goals. It is therefore important for the reviewer to see clear documentation of the differentiation between the primary diagnosis and the secondary diagnoses. Selection of the diagnosis is based on the factors surrounding the onset of symptoms/functional problem(s). As the onset may cross provider settings, it must reflect the circumstances surrounding the reason for physical therapy, as well as if the patient/client had previous physical therapy for the same condition. The reviewer may determine the diagnosis selected reflects a chronic condition or the onset of symptoms that may not reflect an acute condition. This would be a red flag to the reimbursement procedure and would require substantiation within the documentation to support the current provision of skilled service. The physical therapy diagnosis may be the same as the medical in some cases, but should also contain more functionally based diagnoses and those directly relating to physical therapy.

> **Author's Note:** If the condition is chronic, but there is an exacerbation, exacerbation with remission, a change in function, or need for new instruction or intervention this must be clearly indicated. In rarer cases, a patient's medical status may actually improve, justifying physical therapy as in a patient who arouses from a coma.

The UR process is important for ensuring that supportive documentation is in place because this drives the process for reimbursement purposes and internal decisions regarding appropriateness of services. The documentation must reflect why specific skilled intervention at this time is critical to the patient/client's functional status.

Secondary Diagnoses/Comorbidities: The review includes consideration of the secondary diagnoses/comorbidities as these can affect the selection of and response to therapy. Documentation should reflect the complexity of the medical conditions pertinent to the therapeutic process. Complexity of the medical condition is often omitted and can prevent the reviewer from accurately assessing the true needs of the patient/client.

■ Example 1

Initial referral and WB instructions: Medical: Fx R hip/ORIF, NWB × 6 weeks

PT Diagnosis: orthopedic gait abnormality, functional decline, weakness

Medical history: CAD s/p CABG × 3 years, HTN, DM Type 2

VI. MEDICATIONS

Documentation of the patient/client medication regime is important to the review process because it can affect the interventions performed during the patient/client care. UR should ensure that the medications and their complicating effects to the therapeutic process are clearly documented. Once identified the reviewer should look for the precautions and modifications to the treatment interventions that are related to the medications identified.

■ Example 2

Medications: atenolol, lasix, dalmane

Note: monitor pulse (observe for physical S&S of distress as atenolol-beta blocker, will keep pulse lower than otherwise expected), monitor for need to urinate (lasix), schedule mid to late morning (dalmane—for sleep)

VII. DEMOGRAPHIC INFORMATION

The relating of the demographic information such as age, gender, date of birth, primary and secondary languages, living environment, family/social support, and potential discharge plans/destinations can affect the rehabilitation potential. The reviewer should see those items that are relevant to the delivery of service and any additional services (referrals) that may be required to address the patient/client desired outcomes. A patient/client living alone in a home with stairs and the bathroom on the second floor, or a trailer has very different needs than a patient living in a one-bedroom apartment on the ground floor of an apartment building. These should be evident in the documentation of the history.

VIII. HISTORY OF PRIOR TREATMENT

A patient's history of prior treatment may include prior intervention for the same diagnosis by physicians, chiropractors, therapists, adjunctive treatments or alternative practitioners. This history can support the rehabilitation potential for return to prior level of function. It is important to relate what has benefited the patient/client in the past and/or current episode of care, especially in the prior therapy interventions for the exacerbations of the same diagnosis. However, if the interventions were primarily palliative without active patient/client involvement, although they may have helped, they may result in denial. The utilization of previously unsuccessful modalities and interventions would be hard to support. Utilizing interventions that have been successful are easily supported as the reasonable expectation would be substantiated by the prior response to the treatment. If no treatment has been given for this diagnosis or if it is a new problem, documentation of that can be beneficial as well. If the condition is recurring or episodic in nature, the reviewer may also look for instruction in techniques that may alter the potential for recurrence or exacerbation.

IX. DIAGNOSTIC TESTING AND EXAMINATION

Documentation of the performed diagnostic testing and examination assists in the determination of medical necessity and the rehabilitation potential of the patient/clients. All appropriate categories should be included with objective findings. Reducing data to numbers, in fraction format as possible, is universally understood. Reliable and valid tests and measures that can be administered at initial examination, periodically throughout care as indicated, and at the end of care, will facilitate justification of care. It should be noted that the Centers for Medicare & Medicaid Services (CMS) recommends specific tests and measures be included for Medicare B outpatients.

The APTA's Outpatient Physical Therapy Improvement in Movement Assessment Log (OPTIMAL) is an instrument that measures difficulty and self-confidence in performing 21 movements that a patient/client needs to accomplish in order to do various functional activities. In response to changes to the Medicare outpatient therapy cap exceptions process and documentation requirements for 2007, the Centers for Medicare & Medicaid Services (CMS) recommended OPTIMAL as a measurement instrument to document objective, measurable physical function of beneficiaries.[6]

Author's Note: Because the OPTIMAL is patient perception, additional objectives, tests and measures of function should be included.

X. COGNITION

Recording data on the cognitive ability of the patient is often a difficult task for the therapist. However, it is extremely important to the UR process and can, when well written, justify the necessity of the frequency and duration of the program determined by the therapist. Documentation of confusion or disorientation is often done in a vague manner and lacks sufficient information to determine the appropriate utilization of services. No reimbursement source would reimburse for services with a patient/client who is unable to follow the therapeutic program. Most therapists document orientation with a person, place, time scale, or statement of ability to follow a number of step directions. This can be augmented indicating the type of direction or instruction; verbal, tactile, or visual with the time needed to respond to the directions given. Appropriate utilization of services may need to be expanded due to the skill required to determine and present the appropriate stimulus to elicit the desired response. Local medical review policies and many payers have established guidelines that may limit coverage for certain diagnoses that affect cognition. These guidelines may require short interventions with more frequent assessments to clearly justify the appropriate utilization of services. In these cases providing documentation that the patient/client has appropriate cognition to participate in therapy and benefit is important to assure that the cognitive status will not interfere with the rehabilitation

XI. PATIENT/CLIENT GOALS

The patient/client goals should be written in objective and measurable language in order to determine, as the treatment progresses, that the therapist and patient/client are working toward the same outcomes. All goals must match problems identified in the initial exam (or reexams as indicated) utilizing the appropriate interventions to achieve reasonable goals. The therapist should include the patient and family and/or caregivers as appropriate in the discussion of anticipated goals to ensure the compliance with interventions and home instructions as family members or caregivers may need to be involved in the administration of these.

XII. PROFESSIONAL TERMINOLOGY

Although the language in the medical record must indicate the need for skilled care it must be universally understood. Choice of word combinations can influence reimbursement and determination of medical necessity. (See Tables 12-1 and 12-2 for a list of nondescriptive and descriptive phrases and common PT terms and their functional phrase alternative.) The concept of "training" should be empha-

TABLE 12-1 • Nondescriptive and Descriptive Phrases

Nondescriptive Phrases	Descriptive Phrase Alternative
1. Poor quad contraction	Per manual muscle test right quadriceps strength is poor.
2. Patient unable to balance unsupported in sitting	Patient exhibits sitting balance loss to the left and posteriorly when reaching for objects and requires contact guard assistance to correct.
3. Ambulation: Distance is improved from 30 feet to 200 feet × 3 in hallway	Neuromuscular electrical stimulation applied to facilitate strengthening exercises. Patient uses one crutch for safe gait due to knee buckling. Gait training with rolling walker and supervision of 1 for 200 feet × 3 (previously 30 feet with minimal/moderate assistance for balance). Base of support and stride length within normal limits without verbal cueing (previously moderate verbal cueing required).
4. Patient currently complains of a constant ache in the low back radiating into the right lateral leg, right anterior thigh, and right shin	Patient reports a 10, on a scale of 1 to 10, regarding pain in the low back radiating through the right lower extremity. Patient states difficulty falling asleep secondary to low back pain.
5. Initially, PROM R extremities WFL's, LLE: knee extension –30°; presently, ROM R extremities WFL's, LLE: –20° knee extension	Static stretch performed within patient tolerance to improve hip extension for rolling. Pain monitored. Passive range of motion right lower extremity is within functional limits. Left knee extension –20° (previously –30°).

SOURCE: Baeten, Moran, and Philippi.[7]

TABLE 12-2 • Common PT Terms and Functional Phrase Alternatives

Common PT Terms	Functional Phrase Alternative
Ambulated/Walked	Gait training
Confused	Attention span deficit
Debility/Deconditioning	Functional strength deficit
Declined	Functionally regressed
Did not appear to understand	Following ____ minutes of training demonstrated inconsistent …
Difficulty walking	Gait deviation
Endurance	Aerobic capacity, functional activity tolerance
Helped	Tactile facilitation
Improved	List comparative data such as:
	Presently ____ (Previously ____)
Observed/monitored	Evaluated/Analyzed
Pacing of activity	Instructed in energy conservation techniques
Patient unable to	Patient exhibits … (describe)
Performed lower extremity exercises	Performs individualized lower extremity exercise program emphasizing
Poor gait	Gait abnormality or gait disturbance
Practiced	Instructed
Reminders	Verbal instructions (avoid use of cues per CMS transmittal)
Some drainage	Indicate specific amount
Stable	Beginning to respond
Stays in bed	Confined to bed
Strengthening	Progressive resistive exercise
Walked	Ambulated or gait trained
	Note: as nurses use the term ambulation, PT should concentrate on using the term "gait training" which indicates skill
Water-pik™	High-pressure irrigation
Weakness	Strength deficit
Went to doctor	Transported to physician's office

SOURCE: Baeten, Moran, and Philippi.[7]

sized relative to functional activities such as gait training and transfer training, and the verbiage that is consistent with Current Procedural Terminology (CPT) codes should precede the entry content.

■ Example 3

Therapeutic Procedures: LLE: strengthening with manual resistance, PNF

Therapeutic Activities: transfer training bed to and from chair, sit to and from stand

The results of the tests and measures in any examination should identify the link between the information gathered in the history to specific tests and measures determining baselines for precautions and limitations and intervention. The reviewer should be able to discern the relationship between the selection/appropriateness of the tests and measures and the problems identified, including impairments and the resulting functional limitations and disabilities.

A. Cardiopulmonary

The examination should include documentation of the physiological and anatomical status of the cardiovascular/pulmonary system and vital signs. Including vascular signs are not consistently seen as important across provider venues, but can be significant in monitoring the response to interventions and therefore baselines performed at the time of the examination (especially when there are comorbidities such as cardiac or respiratory conditions listed in the history that may necessitate monitoring).

The interpretation of the relevance and significance should be documented and the limitations/precautions identified for the safe performance of functional activities.

This requires the skills of the therapist to determine the specific and individualized program that will safely progress the patient/client to their desired outcomes. The tests and measures expected in this area include aerobic capacity measured objectively during functional activities or standardized exercise protocols, cardiovascular and/or pulmonary signs and symptoms and the response to increased oxygen uptake in exercise or functional activity, oxygen saturation, ventilation/respiration, and physiological responses to positional changes (i.e., orthostatic hypotension). Borg's perceived exertion scale is a good example of a reliable and valid measure of a patient's perception of their exertion/work level. If the patient's primary referring diagnoses are cardiopulmonary, all measurements above would be expected by the reviewer.

XIII. INTEGUMENTARY

The presence of skin integrity issues can often lead to significant compensation of function. The utilization may be impacted based on the severity, size, and location of the change in wound or skin integrity. Many skin integrity issues also indicate a loss of sensation locally or regionally. The loss of superficial or deep sensation, proprioception, pain, or temperature sensation can significantly impact the patient/client's ability to perform functional activities in a safe and effective manner, necessitating teaching compensatory strategies. Therefore, where present or indicated, the reviewer should see assessments and teaching compensation in the plan of care, consistent with goals of learning.

XIV. MUSCULOSKELETAL RANGE OF MOTION AND MUSCLE PERFORMANCE

These categories of examination indicate the patient/client status of range of motion, flexibility, strength, muscle performance, joint integrity, presence or absence of atrophy, and symmetry of the body (height and weight and other anthropometric measurements may be included as well). Strength can be measured manually by manual muscle testing or instruments developed for the same purpose. Regardless of the numbering system the therapist uses, clear documentation must be made of the strength in numbers expressed as fractions versus verbiage, as in colloquial English, good is better than normal. Percentages should be avoided in some cases numeric systems may be misleading in patients with limited endurance, and descriptive verbiage may be preferable.

■ Example 4

Kendall System: expressed in terms of the fractions for baselines and goals of strength (MMT)

Normal	5/5
Good	4/5
Fair	3/5
Poor	2/5
Trace	1/5
None	0/5

■ Example 5

Range of Motion Scale from the American Academy of Orthopedic Surgeons:

Shoulder Flexion Active 180°/180°. Example: R shoulder flexion: 120°/180° actively
Knee Flexion R/L 135°/135°
Cervical Rotation R/L 80°/80°

XV. NEUROMUSCULAR

The reviewer will be expecting the measurement of tone, synergies, motor control, and the way in which the patient/client accomplishes gross coordinated movement such as balance, gait, transfers, transitions, and the coordination of these activities. The tests and measures expected to be seen in this area include use of assistive and adaptive devices, CNS integrity, cranial and peripheral nerve integrity, motor function including dexterity, coordination, agility, neuromotor development and sensory integration, pain, posture as related to position and gravity, and reflex integrity. The relationship to self-care and home management, work, community, and leisure integration or reintegration should appear in the problem summary.

The tests and measures should be carefully chosen to clearly and objectively establish the decline in function seen by the therapist and should be apparent to the reviewer to support the frequency and duration selected. The measurements should be documented in consistent terminology throughout the examination and should reflect standardized testing methods. Utilization is supported by the comparison of the results to the age-appropriate norms. Where available, disease specific objective tests and measures and well as reliable functional tests and measures should be used at initial exam and discharge. They can also be used as intervention strategies as indicated and to assess progress. This will help the UR reviewer determine effectiveness of care.

XVI. DOCUMENTATION OF THE CONTINUUM OF CARE

Colloquially called progress notes, daily notes, treatment notes, or progress notes/reports, continuation of care documents are reviewed to determine the continued need for skilled intervention. The documentation provides the comparative data to justify the skilled physical therapy services rendered and should reflect measurable, functional progress (progress notes/reports). The documents may have different formats, however, all need the same identification information and basic content, regardless of format and should be titled to assist any reader of reviewer in easy identification of a document. The documentation should contain all available information to relate the skill required.

Each visit or encounter should be documented and authenticated with the applicable signature and professional designation. This is typically the therapist signature with license held followed by the license number (e.g., *Patricia Smith, PT* # 12345 or *Susan Smith*, PTA # 12345.). Inclusion of the license number ensures that the reviewer can determine a licensed individual rendered skilled care and may avoid a technical denial. In the case of a student physical therapist, the signature should be the student's legal name followed by SPT or SPTA (e.g., *Samuel Smith*, SPT) and then authenticated by the supervising PT or PTA. It is recommended that the students also print their names for easy identification as signatures are frequently illegible.

Documentation of supervision for treatment provided by physical therapist assistants is essential to denote the services were provided under the direction of a physical therapist. This may be done in a variety of ways.

■ Example 6

12/15/10, 2:30PM e.g., Discussed with *PT-Debra Stern*, PT progression of gait from walker to a cane. E...PTA *Regina Y. Brown*, PTA

Patient/client self-report should be included only as relevant to the therapy rendered. The utilization could be affected by statements documented either positive or negative reports. If the statements documented are negative, prognosticating statements such as "I don't see anything happening" or "I'm not making progress" service will likely not be viewed as appropriate. The positive, prognosticating statements such as "I am able to bathe myself now" or "I can get my hand over my head now" would support continued services based on the plan established. However, if quotes are included such as "I played a round of golf this weekend" is included and the patient is being treated for acute bursitis of the shoulder, any treatment rendered after this statement is documented may be denied. The reviewer will look for indications that the patient is an integral part of the review of goals and progress and would expect to see this reflected in the subjective statements documented.

Identification of specific interventions in objective, codeable terms is also important. The documentation in this section is one that can create the greatest challenge for the therapist. There are two areas affected during the UR of this section. The first is the correlation of the modalities and procedures given to the billing submitted to the third-party payer. These documents must match. The modalities also must adhere to the guidelines of the third-party payer in terms of covered services and should be accompanied by the appropriate physician's order for them to be recognized as billable services. Changes in treatment strategies will be reviewed for compliance to the required physician approvals necessary to comply with the procedures for each payer source. The reviewer also looks to see if the treatment strategies are relevant and effective for the problems identified and if the strategies are causing the expected progress as outlined in the goals. A lack of progress, should it be evident, would prompt the reviewer to look for alternative treatment strategies or goal revision to be implemented in a timely manner. The expectation of the UR is that the modalities rendered correspond to the services billed, that they are within the coverage guidelines established by the third-party payer, and that they are effective for the problems identified in the plan of care. All components must match.

Changes in patient/client status as they relate to the plan of care (adverse reactions to the interventions, and factors that affect the frequency or intensity of the interventions and progression toward goals) are usually documented as part of the assessment section. Content should reflect the thought process of the therapist and should relate the objective information documented with the patient/clients response and how that impacts the progression toward the stated goals. The assessment of the interventions given and the effect they have on the patients' progress relative to function are the only justification allowing UR to support continued treatment. This provides support for third-party payers to continue to reimburse for the services rendered. Documentation can support changes in modalities/procedures, frequency/intensity, and continuance/discontinuance.

Communication and consultation with other health care providers and family/significant other/patient is also reviewed for the development of patient-oriented goals and the coordination of interventions to meet those goals. It is important to see that all health care professionals are working in concert to achieve the goals established and that there is no duplication of services between the providers, especially if the same CPT code is used on the same day by different services such as PT and OT. Note: see Chapter 5 on coding.

XVII. DOCUMENTATION OF REEXAMINATION

Reexamination, also called recertification by some providers and Medicare, is necessary to support continued interventions beyond the original period certified (allowed) by the third-party payer. This documentation may also require physician approval to be accepted by some third-party payers.

To effectively advocate for the patient/client, the reexamination by the physical therapist should assess the effectiveness of the plan given, state the changes to be implemented and the expected outcomes based on the changes made if indicated. The documentation should also reflect the positive prognosticating factors supporting the revised plan of care including all interventions and outcomes to be carried over from the initial examination/evaluation. Revisions to the plan may be necessary to change modalities or procedures based on patient/client progress, adverse or more rapid response to modalities originally planned, or new medical problems occurring during the delivery of service. Patient/clients with multiple comorbid presentation may require modifications to their plan as their comorbidities may alter the response to treatment and, although every effort should be made to account for this at the time of the evaluation, there may be extenuating circumstances that affect the response. It is through the reexamination that physical therapists can advocate for the unique needs of the patient/client to achieve the desired outcomes that may fall outside the established parameters of the third-party payer standard guidelines. If a specified number of visits was preauthorized, and additional visits are indicated, from a UR perspective, it is better for the PT to make the request than a nonprofessional as the PT can communicate as professional to professional and respond to questions.

XVIII. DOCUMENTATION OF SUMMATION OF EPISODE OF CARE

Termination of care falls into two general categories: (1) the patient/client met the goals and expected outcomes or (2) the care was discontinued as a result of a change in the patient/client desire, medical condition, financial resources, or ability to benefit from intervention as based on the therapist's determination. Regardless of the reason for discontinuation of care the documentation should include a summary of the care from start to finish. Among the items that should be listed are the length of episode, number of visits, the current physical/functional status compared to initial findings, the degree of goals achieved or not achieved, complications during the provision of service, and the discharge/discontinuance plan, including any written or verbal directions related to the patient/client's continued care such as home programs, referrals, follow-up physical therapy, family/caregiver training, and equipment provided.

This report should provide the justification for the skilled intervention from the last progress report. It must also justify the overall progress made from the beginning of care and why this progress could only be made through the interventions provided. The therapist should also indicate the expectations for the carryover into the home, work, or play environment and the potential for retaining the achieved functional improvements. The reviewer's ability to determine reasonableness of the plan of care is dependent on the therapist clearly and briefly documenting what happened during the course of treatment.

XIX. UTILIZATION MANAGEMENT

UM is the establishment of policies that minimize the occurrence of denial of payment. This starts from the moment a patient/client walks into the facility. It is important to have policies that will establish important demographic and identifying information with what information is to be verified and who will perform that part of the information gathering.

Proactive UM should include need for and presence of a correct referral or authorization (unless self-referral in direct access states). The policy should address all applicable guidelines, including state and federal, for your setting, with compliance to the strictest regulation. CMS Medicare no longer requires a physician prescription to bill for services, but requires that a patient be under the care of a physician and that the physician sign the plan of care. The referral process whether physician, NPP or self is important as it is from this point the patient/client enters your practice. If the physician/NPP referral should have an order for physical therapy evaluation, a medical diagnosis that relates to the reason for the problem, and any specific information the practitioner needs to relate to you regarding the patient/client treatment.

> **Author's Note:** If the medical diagnosis indicated by the physician is not appropriate, the PT should contact the physician or referring health care practitioner and request a telephone order to change it. For example:
>
> Dx: s/p THR x 6 years. At 6 years post, this is an inappropriate diagnosis.

The referral may specify a body part and the treatment of any other part without physician approval would precipitate a denial. It is therefore necessary for the therapist to carefully review the referral and assess the problems to ascertain if further discussion with the physician is necessary. States with direct access allow the provision of therapy services without a physician referral or prescription. However, billing third-party payers may require a physician referral to receive payment for PT services.

Ensuring payment also requires the determination of the primary payer and verifying that insurance is active and the extent of the coverage the patient/client is entitled to. Patient/clients often are lost in the legal language of the insurance policy and may need direction to determine the extent of coverage. This can become a tangled process and result in significant delay if not outright denial, if done after the treatment has begun. With the changing networks and insurances, it is necessary to know what contracts are current and which types of policies are accepted at a facility. Insurance companies have multiple products and each may require its own contract to become a provider. A therapist could have a valid contract with a company's Preferred Provider program and not with the HMO program. It is important to look at or copy the patient/client's insurance card both front and back. Calling to verify insurance or having direct data access can benefit both the patient/client, and the provider and most insurance cards have customer service and verification phone numbers on the back of the card. The verification process can allow you to determine if there are copayments or out-of-pocket expenses that need to be met and if there are limits on the number of visits per year. A facility that is not a designated carrier/provider may be able to receive payment but would need to assist the patient/client in verifying the insurance allows for out-of-network benefits prior to the start of care. Although the cost may be higher than in network, the patient/client may elect to utilize this option. Some insurance companies require preauthorizations. This means the PT must request permission to evaluate and treat the patient.

The determination of the primary insurance is dependent on the reason for referral. One of the common mistakes made by a therapist is to verify the health insurance only to complete the history taking in the examination and determine the major complaint is due to an auto accident. If the patient was in an accident, there may be other insurance that should be billed first (i.e., personal injury protection [PIP], automobile insurance, or homeowners). Payment from these would take precedence over the individuals' health insurance until the policy is exhausted or it is determined no litigation is pending. Knowing the correct insurance to bill can avoid delayed payment or no payment at all. With insurance verified, provider number in hand, and examination/evaluation completed, you are ready to submit the billing. However, preauthorization does not guarantee reimbursement. The documentation must support the therapy rendered.

XX. EXTERNAL REVIEW

This phase of the review process is performed after the claim is submitted for reimbursement to the insurance company. It is done for two purposes: to assist in the improvement in quality and service delivery and to ensure the efficient expenditure of monies. To make this determination, external review organizations employ a variety of nonlicensed and licensed staff. It is important to know who reviews your documentation as the claim is processed and what degree or experience they have.

> **Author's Note:** If all efforts are made to ensure appropriate documentation content, justification for skilled services and elimination of technical errors, regardless of who the reviewer is, the record should withstand any review.

Utilization review organizations (UROs) no longer typically use nurses for the review/screening process. URO is now performed primarily by physical therapists and occupational therapists for rehabilitation services. If the claim is questionable, a physician may review for approval or denial. There are still UROs employing nurses for denial-level decisions or employing high school graduates without medical experience to review services. The federal Government Accountability Office (GAO) reported that 67% of UROs allow nurses to shorten the length of stay for patients, 62% allow nurses to convert inpatient to outpatient services, and 28% allow nurses to shift care to another provider. The experience of the nurses is varied and can range from new graduates to nurses with years of experience in the rehabilitation setting. Knowledge of who reviews the documentation you submit may help you determine the expectations. While a relationship with the reviewer is positive, many facilities deal with multiple UROs and can only rely on general expectations. The expectations of any reviewer are to read a clear, legible document that relates the therapist's efforts to resolve the patient's problems in a timely and efficient manner. The documentation should answer, not create, questions. The focus of the review is on effective use of the dollars spent. UROs that employ nonprofessionals to perform the reviews usually give a short (3-week) training about interpretation of medical reports and claims administration. The documentation for this review needs to clearly identify what the problem with the record/care is, and will request how the therapist is planning to address the problem with care or the record, and how long it will take to resolve or remedy the problems.

Decisions are made based on the available documentation and how professionally the documentation is presented. Presentation includes the legibility, organization, and meaningfulness of the documentation submitted. Documentation sufficient for a favorable decision includes a clear statement identifying the patient's/client's problem in functional terms, a reasonable treatment plan based on medical necessity, significant functionally oriented progress with measurable changes based on professional and community standards, and evidence of clinical decision-making. This is also known as reasonable and necessary care. For Medicare, there are four conditions identified for reasonable and necessary care:

1. The treatment is in accordance with accepted standard of practice, with specific and effective modalities for the patient's/client's condition.

2. The documentation denotes the complexity and sophistication of the condition of the patient such that the services of a physical therapist are required to safely perform the program. For instance, therapeutic exercise for a patient with cardiac history may require the skills of a therapist to monitor the level and intensity of the exercise program while maintaining cardiac precautions.

3. A reasonable expectation that the condition will improve significantly in a generally predictable and reasonable amount of time is based on the physician's assessment after appropriate consultation with a physical therapist. If this is not the case, it is necessary to establish a safe and effective home exercise program required in a specific disease state. This would be evident if the documentation shows the patient is meeting the goals established on the plan of care.

4. The amount, frequency, and duration are reasonable for the condition and functional deficits documented. The frequency and duration should be established as individualized as the modalities used. A reviewer may see a pattern of frequency and duration that identifies the provider for a more intensive review.

Patients/clients who have policies requiring preauthorization may require advocacy through critically documented communication with the payer to receive "reasonable and necessary" treatment from the treating therapist documentation of specific skilled interventions and measurable gains are necessary in each progress report and the payer may deny any visit not justified by the specific report. Requests for continuation of care would need to include the skills required to complete the rehabilitation and the specific number of visits required to accomplish the established goals. The expectation of the intermediary/carrier is that the patient/client take responsibility for their rehabilitation and, once trained in the specific technique, continues the progression on their own.

Management of unfavorable claims requires organization and attention to detail. Most third-party payers use a denial system similar to the Medicare system. Therefore, a basic knowledge of this system is beneficial. Once a claim is submitted, an unfavorable decision may result from the technical or clinical aspect. Technical denials are typically returned to the provider also referred to as RTPs (returns to providers). RTPs are due to incorrect identification information, illegibility, incomplete information, claim overlap with another provider's claim for the same or similar services, the appropriate qualifier does not accompany the submission, or the intermediary/carrier does not have a record of the provider number or participation identification.

Returned claims can be avoided by taking some simple steps. The insurance verification policy of any organization should include copying the beneficiary's insurance card and verifying eligibility before starting treatment. Medicare has eligibility information online through the Direct Data Entry (DDE) system. This system allows a provider to gather information such as exact coverage, other claims currently being billed, and the status of claims. The review of claims to be submitted should also ensure that all handwritten documents are accurate for technical information, including identification numbers and completeness. Names can be a major source of technical denials. The name on the documentation should match the name on the insurance including the suffix (Jr., Sr., or III), and avoid the use of nicknames. Knowledge of the proper billing codes and value codes can also eliminate RTP. Claims may also be denied if the services provided were noncovered items. Knowing the coverage of the policy in your particular practice setting will help a provider avoid this type of denial. Additionally, it is always the therapist's responsibility to know the laws and guidelines that govern the setting in which they operate in any state or locality. These problems are easily avoided through a process of review and establishment of proper policies.

Claims can also be denied based on the intermediary/carrier determination that the service was not reasonable and necessary. This is a judgment-based decision made from the documentation submitted with the claim. The appeal of these denials serve the facility and the profession alike as long as the documentation supports that therapy was necessary for the patients condition and the patients goals were achieved in a reasonable and predictable time. The appeal is dependent on the documentation and additional supportive statements related to the efficacy of the services provided. The decision to appeal a claim must be made based on an objective review of the services delivered. Procedures should be performed only when the documentation justifies the skilled interventions and the duration of care.

The Medicare program is divided into Part A, or inpatient services and Part B, outpatient services. The role of the therapist in preparation of the appeal may vary depending on the type of appeal. It could range from collecting and reviewing the documentation to participation in the hearing process depending on the size, personnel, and policies of the facility. Part A claims management is usually coordinated by administrative personnel and the therapist may have very little to do with the appeal. Part B (outpatient) appeals are very paperwork intensive and time sensitive. However, if there is a policy outlining the specific responsibilities of each person, the time involved is worth the potential outcome. This process allows you to defend the decisions made during the course of care and can affect future denials. The appeal allows you to advocate for all future patient/clients with a similar condition and care. Medicare has three levels of appeal: Additional Development Required (ADR), Hearings, and Administrative Law Judge (ALJ).

A level one ADR process occurs when a submitted claim has an error in the technical data. These claims are not reviewed based on medical necessity. The denial may result from a diagnosis not matching the services billed, an incorrect billing period, onset date or date treatment commenced, information crossing lines in electronic claims, incorrect name, and so on. The claim can be corrected and resubmitted for payment, unless a payer has policies that preclude this. The documentation must be received in the intermediary's office no later than 45 days from the ADR date. Each record should be submitted with a copy of the ADR attached. Records sent with multiple beneficiaries or multiple ADRs attached will cause delays that may result in automatic denials for lack of meeting the time deadlines. Organization and clarity is a must at this stage in the denials process.

Level two denials occur when the technical information does not support the physical therapy intervention. Examples of this are the claim exceeded the usual and expected number of treatments (with approximately 30 days used as a reference) the medical diagnosis selected did not clearly indicate the need for physical therapy or did not support the need for the PT services rendered, or the facility has been selected for a focused review and the intermediary has chosen to review all or a percentage of claims submitted. A new provider may be on a percentage review in this category to demonstrate to the intermediary their knowledge of the regulations and ability to provide care under the guidelines.

Since January 1, 2002, the percentage of claims reviewed at this level can only change after the intermediary/carrier has performed three educational seminars with the provider. These can be provided either in person or by teleconference. If the review at this level results in a denial the provider and the beneficiary receive a notice of claim determination, which gives the dates of service that were denied and a specific reason for the denial. The therapist or provider should review the documentation and determine if there is sufficient reason to appeal the claim. The benefits are not only the recovery of payment but also include education of the patient and intermediaries reviewer, validation of the treatment chosen, and the providers increased understanding of specific intermediary policy. The decision to appeal is based on three factors: if the documentation speaks to the reason for the denial; if the provider understands the payers regulations well enough to clearly explain why the treatment given fits in the guidelines stated; and lack of clear connection of all the factors for the reviewer, such as multiple comorbidities and key symptoms related to the diagnosis. If the facility decides to appeal the claim, a letter of support may accompany the request and can include information supporting the rationale for the interventions and duration. It may not include any new or conflicting information than what was originally submitted. A checklist for the completion of an appeal letter is helpful to target the specific reason for the request. Employing resources such as the State Insurance Commission, Department of Labor, Workers' Compensation Board, Professional organizations, physicians, family members, and the patient can provide support for an appeal. A well-educated therapist and client/patient can be the key ingredients to a successful request. Using the resources and substantiating the rationale for treatment can result in a successful claim review. If the claim is denied at this level, the provider may request a fair hearing.

Fair hearings are typically conducted by telephone. However, an in-person hearing or on-the-record hearings may be requested. The provider must notify the intermediary in writing as to the type of hearing requested and the intermediary/carrier will then provide written notice of the date and location of the hearing. The notification usually includes the name of the officer hearing the cases and the claims to be discussed/reviewed. There has been concern as to the qualifications of the fair hearing officers because there is not a clear credential requirement for this position.

On-the-record hearings are conducted based on documentation and written materials submitted to the fair hearing officer. There is no verbal communication between provider and payer in this type of hearing and this is usually the least likely option. More commonly chosen options are the telephone hearing or an in-person hearing. These require considerable organization and preparation as both review specific treatments relating them to the supportive research and intermediary regulations to justify the skills of a therapist as the only discipline able to effectively provide the treatment. The phone hearing should involve the treating therapist unless not available. If the therapist is not available, then the individual designated must be familiar with the guidelines for reasonable and necessary care and have sufficient knowledge of the claim to defend it. In-person hearings allow for the presentation of expert witnesses, research articles, history of payment for similar conditions, and any other pertinent information necessary to successfully defend the delivery of service. A list of the items and witnesses to be presented as well as the résumés of each witness should be provided to the hearing officer in advance of the hearing.

Determinations can only be based on the evidence offered at the hearing and the information from the previous appeal levels. Recourse beyond this level is conducted before an administrative judge and requires legal assistance and expert witnesses are not optional. To proceed beyond the fair hearing should be carefully considered as the cost may outweigh the benefit.

ALJ hearings are the last level of appeal and are considered when the hearing is unsuccessful. Larger providers who have sufficient claims and wish to set precedence in order to avoid future similar claims being denied usually select this appeal level.

If the decision of denial is overturned at any appeal level payment of the claim is made. If the decision to deny is upheld through the last attempted appeal level payment is withheld.

In summary, the therapist and all involved in the documenting and billing of services should read and understand the regulations and guidelines for all payers before initiating care. The policies and guidelines will assist the therapist in determining the patient/client eligibility and the allowable treatment modalities for each payer. The examination/evaluation provides the objective and measurable baseline data, which establishes the need for the skills of a physical therapist to carry out the plan of care and safely restore the function of the patient/client. All documentation must use consistent measures and tests that meet standard requirements with established norms for the population being treated. The progress reports must reflect the functional changes occurring as a direct result of the interventions and the critical decision-making performed to alter the program as needed to achieve the goals established. This step is critical when the progress made is not as rapid as predicted by the therapist on the evaluation. If events that were not predictable at the time of the evaluation occur, the documentation could show reason to justify continued intervention. It is essential that documentation be complete, accurate, and legible for submission of a good claim. Having this allows for the therapist to appeal decisions made by the third-party payers and advocate for the patient and profession.

XXI. SUMMARY

A reviewer must decide retrospectively if the therapeutic intervention was medically necessary, if the skilled services were required and if so, if they were required for all sessions based on the patient's progress and goals. For a concurrent review, the questions are the aforementioned as well as if skilled services will be required beyond the point of review based on the information provided. Specific forms can be developed for this purpose (see Table 12-3).

There are significant educational opportunities and benefits to having an active internal UR/UM process. This process can range from internal chart audits performed utilizing a check sheet to audits by a designated UR department. The results of a strong UR program provide the basis for a strong UM process. Adherence to policies and procedures can result in quality-oriented programs resulting in significant patient outcomes in a cost-effective and efficient manner.

According to Stern and Page, the record or the documentation of services provided will be the primary basis for determination of reimbursement.[8] The term primary is used because the reviewer may, depending on the organization, have the opportunity to question the providers or the individuals who actually provided the care. There may be records to use as baseline for prospective decision-making. If the documentation reflects the medical necessity of skilled service or intervention, and if the interventions are relevant and appropriate for the PT problems indicated, reimbursement and or appropriate continued care can be justified.

TABLE 12-3 • Therapy Content Review Worksheet

Reviewer: _____   Date: _____

This is an: _____ Internal review   _____ External review

Record reviewed is for: ____ outpatient   ___ inpatient

Review is: ____ retrospective   ___ concurrent

Treatment venue

  Acute care hospital: ____ inpatient/acute   _____ inpatient/acute rehab

                                                     _____ hospital outpatient

  SNF: ____ inpatient   _____ out-patient

  Rehab Hospital: ____ inpatient   _____ outpatient

  _____ CORF   ____ PT in private practice

  _____ Home health   ____ Outpatient

                        ____ Outpatient physician's office

  _____ Other: _____

Referral status: _____ self-referral/direct access or _____ physician: If physician referred, status of prescription: ___ in record, written ___ in record, verbal only ___ARNP/PA ___Other _____

General information: please indicate if the item is present by writing y for yes. If missing or incorrect, please put n for no. If not applicable, please put NA.

_____ entries are in ink (single color) (hard copy records only)

_____ informed consent indicated

_____ blank spaces are not left in entries

_____ cosignature is used for student entries/or for those pending licensure

_____ each category of entry is labeled: i.e., PT Evaluation, PT notes, Discharge Summary

_____ pages are numbered as appropriate, i.e., if multipage evaluation, pages are numbered

_____ indicates release to communicate with family members, caregivers, others

_____ treatments rendered are included in the initial plan of care or interim plans

_____ reason(s) for treatment and referral are indicated

_____ all required components are included

_____ all required components are identified

_____ patient response to treatment is indicated for individual entries

_____ consistent attendance is indicated or follow-up is indicated for missed appointments

_____ treatment is modified based on changes in function or response to interventions

_____ outcomes/goals are expected in a reasonable time frame

_____ based on the content, care rendered was skilled

_____ based on the content, care was reasonable and necessary

_____ all entries match: billing dates, visit dates, plan, interventions, goals

_____ signatures are original or electronic

_____ entry errors are corrected appropriately

Identification:

_____ patient/client's full name (on all pages)   _____ date of birth, age are included

_____ other identification as relevant   _____ all entries are dated/timed

_____ signatures include license #   _____ signatures include professional
                                                           designation

TABLE 12-3 · (Continued)

Initial Examination/Evaluation with Plan of Care

Please check yes or no to indicate if the item is included or is not included

Yes	no	Content item	yes	no	Content item
___	___	Medical history of presenting problem	___	___	Objective measures of systems dysfunction/functional problems
___	___	Primary medical diagnoses	___	___	Problem summary/ Indication of clinical judgment
___	___	Comorbidities/concurrent problems			
___	___	Physical Therapy diagnosis or problem	___	___	Objective, measurable goals that relate to identified problems
___	___	Precautions/contraindications	___	___	Goals are time defined by dates and days or weeks as indicated (circle which)
___	___	Barriers	___	___	Combination of impairment and functionally based goals that are related
___	___	Demographic information: Psychosocial, social, and environmental concerns			
			___	___	Indication of patient/client/ caregiver participation in goal setting
___	___	Cognition: Ability to communicate/understand			
___	___	Indication of patient/ client's knowledge of problem or responsible party	___	___	Treatment plan: Interventions in CPT codeable verbiage that matches problems and goals
___	___	Other services patient/ client is receiving related to episode of PT care	___	___	Patient/client/caregiver educational learning goals are included
			___	___	Frequency
___	___	Prior level of function relative to presenting problem	___	___	Duration
			___	___	Prognosis: Rehabilitation potential
___	___	Indication of collaboration with other professionals as indicated	___	___	Authentication: PT signature and designation
			___	___	License number

Does the venue or payer require a Physician Plan of Care (POC)?	___ yes	___ no
Does venue or payer require a plan of care by a physician extender if not a physician? If yes, professional designation: _____		
If yes, is all the information included from the above (except objective systems data)?	___ yes	___ no
Is the POC signed by the physician?	___ yes	___ no
Is the POC dated?	___ yes	___ no
Is the POC signed on the appropriate date, prior to intervention or within 30 days (if Medicare)?	___ yes	___ no

TABLE 12-3 • Therapy Content Review Worksheet (Continued)

Continuation of Care: PT treatment notes, progress notes, progress reports

There is an entry for each encounter/visit:	____ yes	____ no	
Each entry is authenticated?	____ yes	____ no	
Professional designation is included for all?	____ yes	____ no	
License number is indicated for all?	____ yes	____ no	
Co-signature as appropriate?	____ yes	____ no	____ not applicable

PT Treatment Notes (if applicable, if not, indicate NA)

Please check yes or no to indicate if the item is included or is not included

Yes	no	NA	Content item	yes	no	NA	Content item
____	____	____	Each entry is dated	____	____	____	Interventions match POC/findings
____	____	____	Time of visit/units is indicated	____	____	____	Equipment issued is indicated
____	____	____	Patient/client self-report in quotes as indicated	____	____	____	Instructions given are indicated
____	____	____	Indication of body areas treated	____	____	____	Response to treatment
____	____	____	Indication of procedures/interventions rendered in CPT codeable verbiage				Reflects communication with others as applicable
				____	____	____	Indicates if anyone else was present during sessions
____	____	____	Parameters of interventions included				
Other							

TABLE 12-3 • (Continued)

Progress Notes/Reports
Please check yes or no to indicate if the item is included or is not included

Yes	no	NA	Content item	yes	no	NA	Content item
___	___	___	Each entry is dated	___	___	___	Interventions match POC
___	___	___	Time of visit is indicated if single progress note for single day	___	___	___	Equipment issued is indicated
___	___	___	If entry is for a single or combination of visit days, dates are indicated and frequency of notes is appropriate for acuity	___	___	___	Reflects communication with others as indicated, including caregivers
				___	___	___	Instructions given are indicated
___	___	___	Indicates where treatment rendered/ who accompanied	___	___	___	Reflects communication with others as indicated, i.e., physicians, other team members, including phone calls, conversations, conferences
___	___	___	Patient/client self-report in quotes as indicated				
___	___	___	Indication of body areas treated	___	___	___	Reflects adjustments in plan
___	___	___	Indication of procedures/interventions rendered in CPT codeable parameters of interventions included	___	___	___	Indicates where treatment rendered
				___	___	___	Information matches previous entry information
___	___	___	Includes progress toward goals as established in initial examination/ evaluation or reexamination	___	___	___	Indicates how patient came to PT
___	___	___	Response to treatment is indicated				
___	___	___	Indicates change in status				

Other:

TABLE 12-3 • Therapy Content Review Worksheet (Continued)

Reexamination

Reexam is included as applicable to evaluate progress and modify or redirect? _____ Yes _____ no _____ NA

Please check yes or no to indicate if the item is included or is not included or NA for not applicable.

yes	no	NA	Content item	yes	no	NA	Content item
___	___	___	Entry is identified as reexam, recert or appropriate designation	___	___	___	Need for continued skilled intervention is included
___	___	___	Timely, every 30 days or as applicable for setting (60 days, then q 30 for CORFs)	___	___	___	Elements from progress notes/treatment notes included relative to system dysfunction, functional deficits
___	___	___	Updated functional status, progress toward initial or interim goals	___	___	___	Authentication: PT signature, professional designation
___	___	___	Goals modified to reflect changes: up or down				

Other:

Is a recertification signed by the physician required?	____Yes	____ no
If required, is it in the record?	____Yes	____ no
If in the record, is it signed and dated?	____Yes	____ no
Does it contain progress toward goals, interventions provided, and any goal and plan revisions as applicable?	____Yes	____ no

TABLE 12-3 • (Continued)

Summation of Episode of Care

A summation of care/discharge, summary is included? _____ yes _____ no

Please check yes or no to indicate if the item is included or is not included or NA for not applicable.

yes	no	NA	Content item	yes	no	NA	Content item
____	____	____	Entry is identified	____	____	____	Discharge instructions to patient/client/ caregivers
____	____	____	Summary of interventions				
____	____	____	Time frame of treatment: From:to	____	____	____	Indication of patient/ client/caretaker instruction
____	____	____	Reference to all problems, impairment and functional addressed in initial exam/eval	____	____	____	Instructions are signed off on and copy is in record
____	____	____	Goals/outcomes achieved relative to initial plan and revisions	____	____	____	Recommendations/plan regarding condition, communication post discharge including:
				____	____	____	Referrals for additional services
____	____	____	Indication of current functional status	____	____	____	Recommendations for follow-up PT
____	____	____	If goals not achieved, indication of reason	____	____	____	Equipment provided
____	____	____	Indication that referral source has been informed or communicated with	____	____	____	Recommendation for physician follow up
				____	____	____	Indication of where discharged to
				____	____	____	Indication of why being discharged
				____	____	____	Authentication: PT signature, professional designation

Other:

Signature of Reviewer: _____   Date: _____

Based on Stern Therapy Content Review Sheet Revised 2003, Stern.[8]

BlueCross BlueShield of Kansas City

An Independent Licensee of the
Blue Cross and Blue Shield Association

Member Grievance Form

Inquiry #_____

(For Internal Use Only)

In keeping with our commitment to provide our members with the very best service possible, Blue Cross and Blue Shield of Kansas City has established a formal procedure for receiving and responding to your concerns.

This form is for your use in filing a formal Grievance regarding any aspect of your Blue Cross and Blue Shield of Kansas City benefit plan, including care you receive from any physician, hospital, or other healthcare professional or organization as a member of this health plan. If you have further questions about this form or the Grievance Process, please call the Customer Service number printed on the front of your Identification card.

Please print or type the following information:

_____   _____
Member Name (Last, First, MI)   Complainant Name or Representative (Last, First, MI)

_____ (____)_____ (____)_____
Address   Daytime Phone   Evening Phone

_____   _____
City   State   Zip

_____   _____
Name of Employer or Group   Group Number (if applicable)   Member Identification Number

_____   _____
Provider Name (if appropriate)   Date of Service (if appropriate)

Explanation of Concern (Use separate sheet if necessary.)

_____

_____

_____

_____

_____

If you attempted to resolve the situation, please give details.

_____

_____

_____

_____

I certify that, to the best of my knowledge, the information provided above is complete and accurate.

_____   _____
Member/Complainant Signature   Date

Submit this form to Appeals Department, Blue Cross and Blue Shield of Kansas City, PO Box 417005, Kansas City, MO 64141-7005. We will acknowledge receipt of your Grievance within ten working days from the date we receive it.

80-62-43 03/08

Grievance Process

Definitions

♦ **Adverse Determination -** A determination that an admission, availability of care, continued stay, or other health-care service has been reviewed and, based upon the information provided, does not meet the requirements for Medical Necessity, appropriateness, healthcare setting, level of care or effectiveness, and payment for the requested service is therefore denied, reduced or terminated.

♦ **Inquiry** – A question or request for information or action. Usually can be resolved on initial contact with no follow-up action required.

♦ **Complaint** - An oral allegation of improper or inappropriate action, or an oral statement of dissatisfaction with covered services, post-service claims payment, or policies that do not fall within the definition of a Grievance.

♦ **Grievance** - A written complaint submitted by or on behalf of a member regarding:

a) The availability, delivery, or quality of healthcare services, including a complaint regarding an Adverse Determination made pursuant to utilization review;

b) Post-service claims payment, handling or reimbursement for healthcare services; or

c) Matters pertaining to the contractual relationship between a member and Blue Cross and Blue Shield of Kansas City

d) Grievances must be filed within 365 days of receipt of the denial.

♦ **Expedited Review** – a Complaint or Grievance that fits the description of a Grievance, but involved a situation where the time frame of the standard Grievance procedures:

a) Would seriously jeopardize the life or health of a member;

b) Would jeopardize the member's ability to regain maximum function; or

c) In the opinion of a physician with knowledge of the member's medical condition, would subject the member to severe pain that cannot be adequately managed without the requested care or treatment.

When you are dissatisfied with your dealings with Blue Cross and Blue Shield of Kansas City, you have the right to pursue your concern through the following mechanisms:

Procedures for Filing a Grievance

You are encouraged to discuss your concerns regarding your medical care with your physician or other healthcare provider. Your customer service representative (see the phone number on your Identification card) is also available to answer questions about claims and benefits.

However, if you are not fully satisfied with the response you receive, and wish to express your concern to a higher level, you may file a formal Grievance. To file a Grievance, you may complete this form, or you may write a letter outlining as many details as possible regarding the incident in question. Your completed form or letter can be faxed to 816-502-4912, Attn: Appeals Department, or mailed to the following address:

Appeals Department
Blue Cross and Blue Shield of KC
PO Box 417005
Kansas City, MO 64141-7005

We will acknowledge receipt of your Grievance within 10 working days and conduct a thorough review. We will respond to your Grievance within 20 working days. If we are not able to respond to your post-service Grievance within 20 working days we will notify you of the time frame extension but the entire time will not exceed 60 calendar days unless your plan requires a shorter time frame (pre-service Grievances will be handled within 20 working days).

Procedures for Filing a Second Level Grievance

If our response to your Grievance does not satisfy all your concerns, you may file a Second Level Grievance. We will acknowledge receipt of your communication within 10 working days, and review (with the assistance of a Grievance Advisory Panel) the results of our previous review, as well as any new information provided to us at the time of your latest request.

Our Grievance Advisory Panel consists of other enrollees and appropriate representatives of management that were not involved in the circumstances giving rise to the Grievance or in any subsequent investigation or determination of the Grievance.

If the Grievance involves an Adverse Determination, the panel will consist of a majority of persons that are appropriate

clinical peers in the same or similar specialty as would manage the case being reviewed who were not involved in the circumstances giving rise to the Grievance or in any subsequent investigation or determination of the Grievance.

The Panel will convene within 20 working days of the date of receipt of the Second Level Grievance, or we will notify you of the time extension. The entire time will not exceed 60 calendar days for post-service Grievances, unless your plan requires a shorter time frame (pre-service Grievances will be handled within 20 working days). You will be advised of the decision of the Grievance Advisory Panel within 5 working days of the Panel's determination.

Contact the State Department of Insurance

You may, at any time, contact the Kansas or Missouri Department of Insurance, whichever is appropriate. You may also have the right to an have your Grievance reviewed by an Independent Review Organization (IRO) at no cost to you.

Missouri Department of Insurance
PO Box 690
Jefferson City MO 65102-0690
Phone: 1-800-726-7390

Kansas Department of Insurance
420 SW 9th Street
Topeka, KS 66612-1678
Phone: 1-800-432-2484

Author's Note: APPEALS AND APPEAL TYPES

There are essentially four classifications of appeals: utilization management appeals, adverse determination appeals, coding and payments, and other. Some payers, such as BlueCross BlueShield, may have forms or formats that are required for appeals.

Appeal for additional visits: Components

Full name and address of practice/practitioner submitting claim with phone number, email

Date: date of appeal letter

To: name of person that signed the claim denial if identified on letter or title of person letter should be directed to, or reference to phone notification and name of representative if denial received by phone and the name of the payer

Re: name of client, claim number from denial notification client's insurance ID number and exactly what the appeal is for, e.g., Re: James Smith, Claim # 1234, Insurance ID # 23450 Group number: UW 212, Denial for PT visits February 19 – March 19, 2010; request for payment

Fr: The name of the physical therapist submitting the claim

Greeting: Business format with a colon:

Body: objective statement of services are being appealed, dates, clear objective description of client/patient problems focusing on function, summary of services rendered and functional outcomes, and description of services allowed under the policy.

The 12 physical therapy visits for Mr. Client rendered from February 19 to March 19, 2010 have been denied for reimbursement from ABC Insurance based on lack of medical necessity.

Mr. Client, 55 years old, suffers from Parkinson's disease. In January 2010, his condition exacerbated, resulting in incessant dyskinesia and three falls resulting in multiple soft tissue injuries, preventing him from working and resulting in painful and nonfunctional gait distances. He was referred by his physician to physical therapy for treatment of the injuries he suffered to his right hip and back, his onset of nonfunctional gait and balance dysfunction, coupled with fatigue and weakness in his lower extremities, hip and back.

As a result of the treatment rendered; therapeutic exercise; trunk and extremities, soft tissue mobilization, trunk, back, hip; neuromuscular reeducation, gait training and electrical stimulation (back and hip), Mr. Client has met all of his goals; safe, functional gait with a straight cane on indoor and outdoor surfaces, resolution of fall risk as evidenced by improvement on the timed up and go test from 20 seconds to 10 seconds, safe – pain free and independent transitional movement sit to and from stand and in and out of bed, muscle performance in functional ranges with the ability to tolerate moderate resistance across all major joints in the 4-/5 range, and 0/10 pain. He is independent in a home exercise program and has returned to work. His dyskinesia has lessened.

Based on a review of Mr. Client's health policy, he is covered for PT services up to 36 visits/year that are functionally oriented and result in measurable, significant change. These are the only PT services Mr. Client has received to date in 2010. The services Mr. Client received meet these criteria as described. We are, therefore, requesting reconsideration of the original claim for physical therapy services. Please see attached copy of claim form.

Very Truly Yours,

Debra Eric, PT, FL License 1234

Debra Eric, PT, FL License 1234

REFERENCES

1. American Physical Therapy Association (APTA). www.apta.org. Accessed April 9, 2011.

2. Peer Review Improvement Act of 1982 (Title I, Subtitle C of the Tax Equity and Fiscal Responsibility Act of 1982) (Public Law 97-248).

3. American Health Information Management Association (AHIMA). http://www.ahima.org/. Accessed April 8, 2011.

4. APTA Guidelines: Physical Therapy Documentation of Patient/Client Management. http://www.apta. org/AM/Template.cfm?Section=Policies_and_ Bylaws&TEMPLATE=/CM/ContentDisplay. cfm&CONTENTID=26134. Accessed April 8, 2011.

5. APTA. *Guide to Physical Therapist Practice*. Rev 2nd ed. Alexandria, VA, American Physical Therapy Association, 2003.

6. APTA's Outpatient Physical Therapy Improvement in Movement Assessment Log (OPTIMAL).http:// www.apta.org/AM/Template.cfm?Section=Resea rch&CONTENTID=36589&TEMPLATE=/CM/ ContentDisplay.cfm. Accessed April 10, 2011.

7. Baeten AM, Moran ML, Phillippi LM. *Documenting Physical Therapy: The Reviewer Perspective*. Woburn, MA, Butterworth-Heinemann, 215 pp., 1999.

8. Stern D, Page C. *The PAD: Practical Approach to Documentation. The Write Stuff*. Ft. Lauderdale, FL, 1994.

ADDITIONAL REFERENCES

Acquaviva J. *Effective documentation for Occupational Therapy*, 2nd ed. AOTA, 1998.

Centers for Medicare and Medicaid. http://www.cms. gov/manuals/downloads/clm104c29.pdf. Accessed April 10, 2011.

CHAPTER 12 REVIEW QUESTIONS

1. What is utilization review?

2. How does utilization review differ from utilization management?

3. Compare and contrast retrospective, concurrent, and prospective review processes.

4. What is the continuum of care in PT?

5. How does quality improvement or quality management relate to utilization review programs?

6. What does an external review organization base their decisions for payment on?

7. Define a technical error and give three examples. How can they be avoided?

8. Compare and contrast first- and second-level denials and their appropriate appeals.

9. Compare and contrast internal and external utilization review.

10. Explain the benefits of expressing examination findings in numeric terms.

11. How should a student physical therapist or student physical therapist assistant sign a medical record entry and how should a PT or PTA authenticate it?

12. Does –preauthorization of physical therapy services guarantee reimbursement? Provide rationale for your answer.

Appendices

A Abbreviations

Δ	change
↓	decrease
↑	increase
↔	to/from, in/out of
~	approximate
=	equals
<	less than
>	greater than
#	number
−	minus
+	plus
&	and
etc	etcetera
%	percentage
‖	parallel bars
@	each, at, before
'	foot
"	inch
°	degree
$\bar{p}$	after
$\bar{c}$	with
$\bar{s}$	without
♀	female
♂	male
¶	paragraph
A	artery
a	ante (L)
A	assistance, assessment
AA	atlantoaxial; adjusted age; active assist
AAA	abdominal aortic aneurysm
AAO X3	alert, awake, and oriented to date, person, place
ARRA	American Recovery Reinvestment Act
AAROM	active assisted range of motion
AARP	American Association of Retired Persons
Abd	abduction
ABG	arterial blood gases
AC	alternating current; acromioclavicular
a.c.	before a meal
ACA	anterior communicating artery; anterior cerebral artery
ACCE	academic coordinator of clinical education
ACL	anterior cruciate ligament
ACM	Arnold-Chiari malformation

ACSM	American College of Sports Medicine
AD	adduction, advanced directive, assistive device
ADA	American Dental Association, American Dietetics Association
ad lib	ad libitum (Latin), at pleasure
ADD	attention deficit disorder
ADHD	attention deficit hyperactivity disorder
ADL	activities of daily living
Adm	admitted
ADR	additional development required
AE(A)	above elbow amputation; preferred is transhumeral amputation
AF	atrial fibrillation, Arthritis Foundation
AFB	acid-fast bacillus
AFO	ankle foot orthosis
AFP	alpha-fetoprotein
AGA	appropriate for gestational age
AHA	American Heart Association, American Hospital Association
AHIMA	American Health Information Management Association
AI	aortic incompetence
AIDS	acquired immune deficiency syndrome
AIMS	Alberta infant motor scale
AK(A)	above knee amputation; preferred is transfemoral amputation
ALL	acute lymphocytic leukemia, anterior longitudinal ligament
ALJ	administrative law judge
ALS	amyotrophic lateral sclerosis; advanced life support
AM	morning
AMA	against medical advice; American Medical Association
amb.	ambulate, ambulation
AML	acute meylogenous leukemia, acute myelocytic leukemia
ANA	American Nursing Association
ANS	autonomic nervous system
ant.	anterior
AOTA	American Occupational Therapy Association
AP	anteroposterior, before dinner
APGAR	appearance, pulse, grimace, activity, respiration
APTA	American Physical Therapy Association
ARC	Association for Retarded Citizens
ARD	assessment reference dates
ARDS	adult respiratory distress syndrome
	acute respiratory distress syndrome
ARF	acute renal failure; acute respiratory failure
ARNP	Advanced Registered Nurse Practitioner
AROM	active range of motion
AS	aortic stenosis; ankylosing spondylitis
As & Bs	apnea and bradycardia
ASA	aspirin
ASAP	as soon as possible
ASD	atrial septal defect
ASHA	American Speech and Hearing Association
ASIS	anterior superior iliac spine
Asst, assist	assistance, assist
ATC	athletic trainer, certified
ATNR	asymmetric tonic neck reflex
AV	arteriovenous; atrioventricular; aortic valve
AVM	arteriovenous malformation
B	bilateral; both
BAER	brainstem auditory evoked response (hearing screening)
BBA	Balanced Budget Act
BBB	blood brain barrier; bundle-branch block

BCBS	Blue Cross and Blue Shield
BE	barium enema
BE(A)	below elbow amputation; preferred is transradial amputation
BIB	drink
BICU	burn intensive care unit
BID	bis in die (Latin); twice a day
Bil, bilat	bilateral
BIN	twice at night
BK(A)	below knee amputation; preferred is transtibial amputation
Bl	blood; bleeding
BM	bowel movement
BMI	body mass index
BMR	basal metabolic rate
BMT	bone marrow transplant
BOS	base of support
BP	blood pressure; bed pan
BPD	bronchopulmonary disease
BPH	benign prostatic hyperplasia or hypertrophy
bpm	beats per minute; breaths per minute
BPPV	benign paroxysmal positional vertigo
BR	bathroom
BRP	bathroom privileges
BS	breath sounds; blood sugar; bowel sounds
B/S	bedside
BSA	body surface area
BT	Blalock-Taussig (shunt)
BUN	blood urea nitrogen
Bw	body weight, birth weight
Bx	biopsy
$\bar{c}$	with, calorie
C	celsius/centigrade
C & S	culture and sensitivity
Ca	calcium, about
Cal	calories
CA	cancer; chronological age
CAA	care area assessment
CABG	coronary artery bypass graft
CAD	coronary artery disease
CARF	Commission on Accreditation of Rehabilitation Facilities
Cath	catheter
CBC	complete blood count
CC, C/C	chief complaint; carbon copy
Cc	cubic centimeter
CCCE	clinical coordinator of clinical education
CCI	Correct Coding Initiative
CCU	cardiac care unit, coronary care unit
CDC	Center for Disease Control and Prevention
CDMM	Clinical Decision Making Model
CEH	continuing education hour
CF	cystic fibrosis
CFS	chronic fatigue syndrome
CG, CGA	contact guard
CHAMPUS	Civilian Health and Medical Program-Uniformed Services
CHD	congenital heart disease
CHF	congestive heart failure
CI	clinical instructor, curie
CICU	coronary intensive care unit; cardiac intensive care unit
CK	creatine kinase

CLD	chronic liver disease, chronic lung disease
CLL	chronic lymphocytic leukemia
cm	centimeter
CMC	carpometacarpal (joint)
CME	continuing medical education
CML	chronic myelogenous leukemia
CMR	computerized medical record
CMS	Centers for Medicare & Medicaid Services (formerly Healthcare Finance Administration, HCFA)
CMV	cytomegalovirus
CNA	certified nursing assistant
CN	cranial nerve, tomorrow night
CN I	olfactory
CN II	optic
CN III	oculomotor
CN IV	trochlear
CN V	trigeminal
CN VI	abducens
CN VII	facial
CN VIII	vestibulocochlear
CN IX	glossopharyngeal
CN X	vagus
CN XI	accessory
CN XII	hypoglossal
c/o	complains of
CNS	central nervous system
CO	cardiac output; carbon monoxide, complains of
CO_2	carbon dioxide
Cont.	continued
COPD	chronic obstructive pulmonary disease/disorder
CORF	comprehensive outpatient rehabilitation facility
COTA	certified occupational therapist assistant
CP	cerebral palsy, chest pain, cold pack
CPAP	continuous positive airway pressure
CPI	clinical performance instrument
CPK	creatine phosphokinase
CPM	continuous passive motion
CPR	cardiopulmonary resuscitation, computerized-based patient record
CPT	current procedural terminology
CRPS	complex regional pain syndrome (formerly reflex sympathetic dystrophy)
CS	cesarean section, cervical spine
CSF	cerebrospinal fluid
CT	chest tube, computed axial tomography (CAT scan)
CV	cardiovascular, central venous
CVA	cerebrovascular accident
CVL	central venous line
CWI	crutch walking instructions
CXR	chest x-ray
D & C	dilation and curettage
DAFO	dynamic foot ankle orthosis
DC	direct current, doctor of chiropractic
D/C,DC,d/c	discharge, discontinue
DDD	degenerative disc disease
DDE	direct data entry
DDH	developmental dysplasia of hip
DDS	doctor of dental science

Dept.	department
DF	dorsiflexion
DHT	Dobhoff (feeding) tube
DIP	distal interphalangeal (joint)
DJD	degenerative joint disease
DLE	discoid lupus erythematosus; disseminated lupus erythematosus
DLT	double lung transplant
DM	diabetes mellitus
DMD	Duchenne muscular dystrophy, doctor of medical dentistry
DME	durable medical equipment
DNA	deoxyribonucleic acid
DNR	do not resuscitate
DO	disorder; doctor of osteopathy
DOA	dead on arrival; date of admission
DOB	date of birth
DOE	dyspnea on exertion
DOI	date of injury
DPT	diphtheria-pertussis-tetanus vaccine, doctor of physical therapy
DRGs	diagnostic related groups
DT	delirium tremens
DTR	deep tendon reflexes
DVT	deep vein thrombosis
Dx	diagnosis

EBP	evidence-based practice
EBV	Epstein Barr virus
ECF	extended care facility, extracellular fluid
ECG, EKG	electrocardiogram
ECMO	extracorporeal membrane oxygenation
ED	erectile dysfuncton
EEG	electroencephalogram
EENT	ears, eyes, nose, and throat
EF	ejection fraction
EFA	essential functional activities
EHR	electronic health record
EIA	exercise induced asthma
EID	easily identified depression
EIP	early intervention program
EKG	electrocardiogram
ELBW	extremely low birth weight
ELISA	enzyme-linked immunosorbent assay
ELS	Eaton-Lambert syndrome
EMG	electromyography
EMR	electronic medical record
EMS	emergency medical services
EMT	emergency medical technician
ENT	ears, nose, and throat
EOB	edge of bed
ER	emergency room; external rotation
ERT	estrogen replacement therapy
ES	electrical stimulation
ESR	erythrocyte sedimentation rate
ESRD	end stage renal disease
ETOH	alcohol (use/abuse)
ETT	endotracheal tube
Eval	evaluation
EX	exercise
EXT	extension, extensive

F	♀, fair, female
f/u	follow-up
FAQ	frequently asked questions
FAS	fetal alcohol syndrome
FBG	fasting blood glucose
FBS	fasting blood sugar
FES	functional electrical stimulation
FEV$_1$	forced expiratory volume in 1 second
FI	fiscal intermediary
FIM	Functional Independence Measure
FIN	Federal identification number
FL	functional limitation, Florida
Flex	flexion
FOB	father of baby
FOIA	Freedom of Information Act
FOR	functional outcome reporting
FOTO	Focus on Therapeutic Outcomes, Inc.
FSH	fascioscapulohumeral dystrophy
FSP	family service plan
Ft.	feet
FT	feeding tube; full term
FTT	failure to thrive
FUO	fever of unknown origin
Func	function, functional
FVC	forced vital capacity
FWB	full weight bearing
FWW	four wheeled walker, front wheeled rolling walker
Fx	fracture
G	good, guard
G tube	gastrostomy tube
G#P#A#	number of births, pregnancies, and abortions, gravida/para/abortus
GA	gestational age
GAO	Government Accountability office
GB	gallbladder
GBS	Guillain-Barré syndrome
GCS	Glasgow Coma Scale
GER	gastroesophageal reflux
GI	gastrointestinal
Gm	gram
GMFM	Gross Motor Function Measure
GPCI	geographic practice cost indices
Grava	gravida = number of births
GSW	gun shot wound
gt	gait, gait training
GU	genitourinary
GVHD	graft versus host disease
GYN	gynecology
H & P	history and physical
H	flu haemophilus influenza B, hydrogen, hour, hematocrit
h/o	history of
HA	headache
Hams, hs	hamstrings
Hb	hemoglobin
HBP	high blood pressure
HC	heelcords
HCFA	Health Care Financing Information (now CMS)
Hct	hematocrit
HCPCS	Healthcare Common Procedure Coding Systems

HCVD	hypertensive cardiovascular disease
HDL	high density lipoprotein
HEENT	head, ears, eyes, nose, and throat
HEP	home exercise program
Hg, Hgb	hemoglobin
HH	home health, hand held
HHA	home health aide, hand held assist, home health agency
HHS	Department of Health and Human Services
HIB	haemophilus influenza B (vaccine)
HICN	health insurance claim number
HIE	hypoxic-ischemic encephalopathy
HIM	health information management
HIPAA	Health Information and Portability Accountability Act
HIV	human immunodeficiency virus
HKAFO	hip knee ankle foot orthosis
HLA	human leukocyte antigen; homologous leukocytic antibodies
HLT	heart-lung transplant
HMD	hyaline membrane disease
HMO	Health Maintenance Organization
HNP	herniated nucleus pulposus
HO	heterotopic ossification; house officer
HOB	head of bed
HOH	hard of hearing
HP	hot pack
HPI	history of present illness
Hr.	hour
HR	heart rate
HRT	hormone replacement therapy
HS	at bedtime
HSV	herpes simplex virus
Ht	height
HT	heart transplant
HTN	Hypertension
HVGS	high volt galvanic stimulation
HX	history
I	independent
I & D	incision and drainage
I & O	input and output
IADL	independent/instrumental activities of daily living
IBS	irritable bowel syndrome
ICA	internal carotid artery
ICD	international classification of diseases
ICH	intracranial hemorrhage; intracerebral hemorrhage
ICP	intracranial pressure
ICU	intensive care unit
ID	infectious disease
IDDM	insulin dependent diabetes mellitus
IDEA	Individuals with Disabilities Education Act
IEP	individualized exercise program, individualized education plan
IF	interferential electrical stimulation
IFSP	Individual Family Support Plan
Ig	immunoglobulin
IM	intramuscular
Indep	independent
inf.	inferior
instr	instructions
Imp	impression
IPA	independent practice association

IPPB	intermittent positive pressure breathing
IPO	independent practice organization
IQ	intelligence quotient
IR	internal rotation
IRB	institutional review board
ITB	intrathecal baclofen, iliotibial band
IUD	intrauterine device
IUGR	intrauterine growth retardation
IV	intravenous
IVC	inferior vena cava
IVH	intraventricular hemorrhage
IVP	intravenous pyleogram
J tube	jejunostomy tube
JCAHO	Joint Commission on Accreditation of Healthcare Organizations
JP	Jackson-Pratt (drain)
JRA	juvenile rheumatoid arthritis
jt	Joint
KAFO	knee ankle foot orthosis
Kcal	kilocalories
Kg	kilogram
KUB	kidney, ureter, bladder; kidney and upper bladder
L	left, lower
L, l	liter
l/min	liters per minute
LAP	laparoscopy; laparotomy
LAQ	long arc quad
LBP	low back pain
LBQC	large based quad cane
LBW	low birth weight
LCL	lateral collateral ligament
LD	learning disability
LDL	low-density lipoprotein
LE	lower extremity
LFT	liver function tests
LG	limb girdle dystrophy
LGA	large for gestational age
Lim	limited
LLC	long leg cast
LLE	left lower extremity
LLL	left lower lobe
LLQ	left lower quadrant
LMN	lower motor neuron
LMRP	local medical review policies
LOB	loss of balance
LOC	loss of consciousness
LOS	length of stay
LP	lumbar puncture
LPN	licensed practical nurse
LS, L/S	lumbar spine
LT	lung transplant, light, left
LTCF	long-term care facility
LTD	limited
LTG	long-term goal
LTM	long-term memory
LUE	left upper extremity
LUL	left upper lobe

LUQ	left upper quadrant
M	male, ♂
MAC	medicare administrative contractor
MAO	monoamine oxidase
max	maximum; maximal
MCA	middle cerebral artery
MCL	medial collateral ligament
MCO	managed care organization
MCP	metacarpophalangeal (joint)
MD	muscular dystrophy, medical doctor
MDA	Muscular Dystrophy Association
MDS	medical data sheet, material data safety sheets, minimum data set
MED	minimal erythemal dose
MENS	microcurrent electrical stimulation
mets	metastasis
METs	metabolic equivalent of task
MFT	muscle function test
MFR	myofascial release
MH	moist heat
MHP	moist hot pack
MI	myocardial infarction
MICU	medical intensive care unit
min	minimal; minute
ml	milliliter
mm	millimeter
mm Hg	millimeters of mercury
MMPI	Minnesota Multiphasic Personality Inventory
MMR	measles, mumps, rubella (vaccine)
MMT	manual muscle test
mo	month; months old
mob.	mobilization, mobility
mod	moderate
MOI	mechanism of injury
MOM	milk of magnesia
MP	metacarpophalangeal joint (MCP), metatarsophalangeal joint (MTP)
mph	miles per hour
MRE	manual resistive exercise
MRI	magnetic resonance imaging
MS	multiple sclerosis; mitral stenosis
MSDS	material safety data sheet
MT	medical technologist; metatarsal
MTBI	minimal traumatic brain injury
MTP	metatarsophalangeal joint
MV	mitral valve
MVA	motor vehicle accident
MVP	mitral valve prolapse
MWD	microwave diathermy
N	normal; nausea
N & V	nausea and vomiting
N/A	not applicable, not assessed
NAD	no appreciable disease, nothing abnormal detected, no acute distress
NCQA	National Committee on Quality Assurance
NCV	nerve conduction velocity
NDT	neurodevelopmental technique or treatment
neb	nebulizer
NEC	necrotizing enterocolitis
Neg	negative (−)

NG	nasogastric
NGT	nasogastric tube
NICU	neonatal intensive care unit; neurological intensive care unit
NIDDM	non-insulin dependent diabetes mellitus
NIH	National Institute of Health
NIOSH	National Institute for Occupational Safety and Health
NKA	no known allergies
nl	normal
NMES	neuromuscular electrical stimulation
NPI	national provider identifier, nonprofit insitution
NPO	non per os (Latin); nothing by mouth
NPP	nonphysician practitioner
NSAID	non-steroidal anti-inflammatory drug
NSR	normal sinus rhythm
NWB	non-weight bearing
O	objective
O2, O_2	Oxygen
OA	osteoarthritis
OB	obstetrics
Obj	objective
OBRA	Omnibus Budget Reconciliation Act
OBS	organic brain syndrome
OD	overdose, doctor of optometry
OHTx	orthotopic heart transplant
OI	osteogenesis imperfecta
OIG	Office of the Inspector General
OLD	obstructive lung disease
OLT	orthotopic lung transplant
OM	otitis media
OMRA	Other Medicare Required Assessment
OOB	out-of-bed
OP	outpatient
OPV	oral polio vaccine
OR	operating room
ORIF	open reduction internal fixation
OSHA	Occupational Safety and Health Administration
OT	occupational therapy, occupational therapist
OTC	over-the-counter
OTR	occupational therapist, registered
Oz	ounce
$\bar{p}$	after
P	poor, plan
PA	pulmonary artery; posterior-anterior; physician's assistant
PAC	premature atrial contraction
Para.	number of pregnancies, paraplegic
Path	pathology
PCA	patient controlled analgesic; posterior cerebral artery; posterior communicating artery
pcl	posterior cruciate ligament
PCP	primary care physician
PD	Parkinson's disease; peritoneal dialysis
PDA	patent ductus arteriosus, personal data application
PDD	pervasive developmental delay
PE	pulmonary embolus; pulmonary edema
PEDI	Pediatric Evaluation of Disability Inventory
PEEP	positive end-expiratory pressure
PEG	percutaneous endoscopic gastrostomy

Per	by, through
PERRLA	pupils equal, round, react to light, accommodate
PET	positron emission tomography
PF	plantarflexion
P4P	pay for performance
Pharm D	doctor of pharmacy
PH	past history
PHI	protected health information, personal health information, personal history interview
PI	present illness
PICA	posterior inferior cerebellar artery; posterior inferior communicating artery
PICC	peripherally inserted central catheter
PICU	pediatric intensive care unit
PID	pelvic inflammatory disease
PIP	proximal interphalangeal (joint), personal injury protection
PKU	phenylketonuria
PLF/PLOF	prior level of function
PLL	posterior longitudinal ligament
PM	afternoon
PM & R	physical medicine and rehabilitation
PMH	past medical history
PMS	premenstrual syndrome
PNF	proprioceptive neuromuscular facilitation
PNI	peripheral nerve injury
PNS	peripheral nervous system
PO	per os (L); by mouth
POC	plan of care
POD	post-op day number
POMR	problem oriented medical record
Pos	positive (+)
POS	point of service plan
Poss	possible
post.	posterior
post-op	post operative
PPH	primary pulmonary hypertension
PPO	preferred provider organization
PPS	prospective payment system
PRE	progressive resistance exercises
Pre-op	pre-operative
Pron	pronation
PRN	as needed
PRO	peer review organization
PROM	passive range of motion; premature rupture of membranes
PSIS	posterior superior iliac spine
PSRO	professional standards review organization
Psych	psychology, psychiatric
Pt., pt	patient; point, pint
PT	physical therapy; physical therapist, prothrombin time
PTA	physical therapist assistant; prior to admission; post-traumatic amnesia
PTB	patellar tendon bearing (prosthesis)
PTIP	Physical therapist in independent practice
PTPP	Physical therapist in private practice (per CMS)
PVC	premature ventricular contraction
PVD	peripheral vascular disease
PVH	periventricular hemorrhage
PVL	periventricular leukomalacia
PWB	partial weight bearing

q	every
QA	Quality Assurance
QC	quad
qd	once daily
qh	every hour
QI	Quality improvement, quality indicator
qid	quater in die (Latin); four times a day
qiw	four times per week
qod	every other day
qt	quart
quad	quadriplegic
R	right
R/O, RO	rule out
RA	rheumatoid arthritis; right atrium, rehabilitation agency (certified)
RAC	recovery audit contractor
RAM	random access memory
RAD	reactive airway disease
RAI	resident assessment instrument
RAP	resident assessment protocol
RAS	reticular activating system
RBBB	right bundle branch block
RBC	red blood cell
RCA	right carotid artery
RD	registered dietician
RDS	respiratory distress syndrome
Re	regarding
Rehab	rehabilitation
REM	rapid eye movement
Reps	repetitions
RF	radio frequency, rectus femoris
RGO	reciprocating gait orthosis
RLE	right lower extremity
RLL	right lower lobe
RLQ	right lower quadrant
RML	right middle lobe
RN	registered nurse
ROM	range of motion, read only memory
ROP	retinopathy of prematurity
ROS	review of systems
RPE	rate of perceived exertion
RR	respiratory rate
RRR	regular rhythm and rate
RSD	reflex sympathetic dystrophy
RSV	respiratory syncytial virus
RT	respiratory therapy/therapist; recreational therapy; renal transplant
RTx	radiation therapy; renal transplant
RUE	right upper extremity
RUL	right upper lobe
RUQ	right upper quadrant
RUGs	resource utilization groups
RV	right ventricle
RVRBS	relative value resource based systems
RVU	relative value component/unit
RW	rolling walker
Rx	drug; treatment; therapy, prescription
$\bar{s}$	without
S	sine (Latin); subjective; supervision

S & S	signs and symptoms
S/P	status post
SA	Sinoatrial
SACH	solid ankle, cushion heel
SBA	stand-by assistance
SBQC	small based quad cane
SC	sternoclavicular
SCC	sickle cell crisis
SCD	sickle cell disease
SCFE	slipped capital femoral epiphysis
SCI	spinal cord injury
SCID	severe combined immunodeficiency disorder
SCIM	spinal cord independence measure
SCM	sternocleidomastoid
SD	seizure disorder; standard deviation
SDAT	senile dementia of the Alzheimer's type
SDR	selective dorsal rhizotomy
sec	second
sed	sedimentation
SED	suberythemal dose
SGA	small for gestational age
SI	sacroiliac; sensory integration
SICU	surgical intensive care unit
SIDS	sudden infant death syndrome
SLC	short leg cast
SLE	systemic lupus erythematosus
SLP	speech language pathology
SLR	straight leg raise
SMA	spinal muscular atrophy
SNF	skilled nursing facility
SOAP	subjective, objective, assessment, plan
SOB	short of breath
SOC	start of care date
SOMR	source oriented medical record
SPL	subjective pain level
SR	sinus rhythm
SSN	social security number
ST	speech therapy, speech therapist
Stat	immediately
Stats	statistics
STD	sexually transmitted disease
STG	short-term goal
STM	soft tissue massage, short term memory
Str	strength
STNR	symmetric tonic neck reflex
STSG	split thickness skin graft
sup	superior; supination, supervision
SV	stroke volume
SVC	superior vena cava
SVD	spontaneous vaginal delivery
SWD	shortwave diathermy
Sx	symptoms
Sz	seizure
T	trace
T & A	tonsillectomy and adenoidectomy
TA	tricuspid atresia
TAH	total abdominal hysterectomy
TAR	total ankle replacement

TB	tuberculosis
TBA	to be announced
TBI	traumatic brain injury
TBSA	total-body surface area
Tbsp	tablespoon
TCU	transitional care unit
TD	tardive dyskinesia
TEF	tracheoesophageal fistula
TENS	transcutaneous electrical nerve stimulation
TER	total elbow replacement
TES	threshold electrical stimulation
TGA	transposition of great arteries
THA	total hip arthroplasty
Ther ex	therapeutic exercise
THR	total hip replacement
TIA	transient ischemic attack
tid	three times a day
tin	three times a night
TIW	three times a week
TKA	total knee arthroplasty
TKE	terminal knee extension
TKR	total knee replacement
TLSO	thoracic lumbar spine orthosis
TMJ	temporomandibular joint
TO	telephone order
TOF	Tetralogy of Fallot
TOS	thoracic outlet syndrome
TPN	total parenteral nutrition
TPO	Time, Place, and Occasion
TPR	temperature, pulse, and respiration
Trng	training
TS, T/S	thoracic spine
TSA	total shoulder arthroplasty
Tsp	teaspoon
TTWB	toe-touch weight bearing
TUR	transurethral resection
Tx	treatment; traction; therapy; transplant
U	upper
UA	urinalysis
UE	upper extremity
UMN	upper motor neuron
UM	utilization management
UQ	upper quadrant
UR	utilization review
URA	utilization review organization
URI	upper respiratory infection
URQA	utilization review quality assurance
US	ultrasound
UTI	urinary tract infection
UV	ultraviolet
VA	Veterans administration, visual acuity
VAD	ventricular assistive device, vertebral axial decompression
VAS	visual analogue scale
VC	vital capacity
VD	venereal disease
vent	ventilator
VLBW	very low birth weight

VO	verbal order
Vol	volume
VPA	valproic acid
Vs	vital signs
VSD	ventricular septal defect
VT	ventricular tachycardia
W	walker
W/C, WC	wheelchair
W/O	without
WB	weight bearing
WBAT	weight bearing as tolerated
WBC	white blood cell, white blood count
WFL	within functional limits, within full limits
WHO	World Health Organization
WIC	women, infants, children
Wk	week
WNL	within normal limits
wp, wpl	whirlpool
wt	weight
$\overline{x}$	except, times
XRT	radiation therapy
Yd	yard
y.o.	years old
yr	year

Author's Note: All abbreviations should be used with caution. Abbreviations that may be "unique" to physical therapy may not be universally understood. Misinterpretation of abbreviations may lead to medical errors, putting patient's/clients at risk. Abbreviations that may represent different meanings are also risky, i.e., WFL. JCAHO does not recommend the use of abbreviations in documentation.

B CMS 700 Form and CS-1786 HIPPA Disclosure Form

DEPARTMENT OF HEALTH AND HUMAN SERVICES
CENTERS FOR MEDICARE & MEDICAID SERVICES

PLAN OF TREATMENT FOR OUTPATIENT REHABILITATION
(COMPLETE FOR INITIAL CLAIMS ONLY)

1. PATIENT'S LAST NAME	FIRST NAME	M.I.	2. PROVIDER NO.	3. HICN
4. PROVIDER NAME	5. MEDICAL RECORD NO. *(Optional)*		6. ONSET DATE	7. SOC. DATE
8. TYPE ☐ PT ☐ OT ☐ SLP ☐ CR ☐ RT ☐ PS ☐ SN ☐ SW	9. PRIMARY DIAGNOSIS *(Pertinent Medical D.X.)*		10. TREATMENT DIAGNOSIS	11. VISITS FROM SOC.

12. PLAN OF TREATMENT FUNCTIONAL GOALS	PLAN
GOALS *(Short Term)* OUTCOME *(Long Term)*	

13. SIGNATURE *(professional establishing POC including prof. designation)*	14. FREQ/DURATION *(e.g., 3/Wk. x 4 Wk.)*

I CERTIFY THE NEED FOR THESE SERVICES FURNISHED UNDER THIS PLAN OF TREATMENT AND WHILE UNDER MY CARE ☐ N/A

17. CERTIFICATION

15. PHYSICIAN SIGNATURE	16. DATE	FROM	THROUGH	N/A

18. ON FILE *(Print/type physician's name)*
☐

20. INITIAL ASSESSMENT *(History, medical complications, level of function at start of care. Reason for referral.)*	19. PRIOR HOSPITALIZATION
	FROM TO N/A

21. FUNCTIONAL LEVEL *(End of billing period)* PROGRESS REPORT   ☐ CONTINUE SERVICES **OR**   ☐ DC SERVICES

22. SERVICE DATES	
FROM	THROUGH

INSTRUCTIONS FOR COMPLETION OF FORM CMS-700

(Enter dates as 6 digits, month, day, year)

1. **Patient's Name** - Enter the patient's last name, first name, and middle initial as shown on the health insurance Medicare card.

2. **Provider Number** - Enter the number issued by Medicare to the billing provider *(i.e., 00–7000)*.

3. **HICN** - Enter the patient's health insurance number as shown on the health insurance Medicare card, certification award, utilization notice, temporary eligibility notice, or as reported by SSO.

4. **Provider Name** - Enter the name of the Medicare billing provider.

5. **Medical Record No.** - *(optional)* Enter the patient's medical/clinical record number used by the billing provider.

6. **Onset Date** - Enter the date of onset for the patient's primary medical diagnosis, if it is a new diagnosis, or the date of the most recent exacerbation of a previous diagnosis. If the exact date is not known enter 01 for the day *(i.e., 120191)*. The date matches occurrence code 11 on the UB-92.

7. **SOC** *(start of care)* **Date** - Enter the date services began at the billing provider (the date of the first Medicare billable visit which **remains the same on subsequent claims** until discharge or denial corresponds to occurrence code 35 for PT, 44 for OT, 45 for SLP, and 46 for CR on the UB-92).

8. **Type** - Check the type therapy billed; i.e., physical therapy (PT), occupational therapy (OT), speech-language pathology (SLP), cardiac rehabilitation (CR), respiratory therapy (RT), psychological services (PS), skilled nursing services (SN), or social services (SW).

9. **Primary Diagnosis** - Enter the pertinent written medical diagnosis resulting in the therapy disorder and relating to 50% or more of effort in the plan of treatment.

10. **Treatment Diagnosis** - Enter the written treatment diagnosis for which services are rendered. For example, for PT the primary medical diagnosis might be Degeneration of Cervical Intervertebral Disc while the PT treatment DX might be Frozen R Shoulder or, for SLP, while CVA might be the primary medical DX, the treatment DX might be Aphasia. If the same as the primary DX enter SAME.

11. **Visits from Start of Care** - Enter the **cumulative total** visits *(sessions)* completed since services were started at the billing provider for the diagnosis treated, through the last visit on this bill. *(Corresponds to UB-92 value code 50 for PT, 51 for OT, 52 for SLP, or 53 for cardiac rehab.)*

12. **Plan of Treatment/Functional Goals** - Enter brief current plan of treatment goals for the patient for this billing period. Enter the major short-term goals to reach overall long-term outcome. Enter the major plan of treatment to reach stated goals and outcome. Estimate time-frames to reach goals, when possible.

13. **Signature** - Enter the signature *(or name)* and the professional designation of the professional establishing the plan of treatment.

14. **Frequency/Duration** - Enter the current frequency and duration of your treatment; e.g., 3 times per week for 4 weeks is entered 3/Wk x 4Wk.

15. **Physician's Signature** - If the form CMS-700 is used for certification, the physician enters his/her signature. **If certification is required and the form is not being used for certification, check the ON FILE box in Item 18.** If the certification is not required for the type service rendered, check the N/A box.

16. **Date** - Enter the date of the physician's signature only if the form is used for certification.

17. **Certification** - Enter the inclusive dates of the certification, **even if the ON FILE box is checked in Item 18.** Check the N/A box if certification is not required.

18. **ON FILE** (Means certification signature and date) - Enter the **typed/printed name of the physician** who certified the plan of treatment that is on file at the billing provider. If certification is not required for the type of service checked in item 8, type/print the name of the physician who referred or ordered the service, **but do not check the ON FILE box.**

19. **Prior Hospitalization** - Enter the inclusive dates of recent hospitalization *(1st to DC day)* **pertinent** to the patient's current plan of treatment. Enter N/A if the hospital stay does not relate to the rehabilitation being rendered.

20. **Initial Assessment** - Enter only **current relevant history** from records or patient interview. Enter the major functional limitations stated, if possible, in objective measurable terms. Include only relevant surgical procedures, prior hospitalization and/or therapy for the same condition. Include only pertinent baseline tests and measurements from which to judge future progress or lack of progress.

21. **Functional Level** (end of billing period) - Enter the pertinent progress made and functional levels obtained at the end of the billing period compared to levels shown on initial assessment. Use objective terminology. Date progress when function can be consistently performed. When only a few visits have been made, enter a note indicating the training/treatment rendered and the patient's response if there is no change in function.

22. **Service Dates** - Enter the From and Through dates which represent this billing period *(should be monthly)*. Match the From and Through dates in field 6 on the UB-92. DO NOT use 00 in the date. Example: 01 08 91 for January 8, 1991.

CS-1786
Rev 5/2004

HIPAA Disclosure Authorization Form

Full Name _____

I hereby authorize _____ to use or disclose my
(Discloser)

protected health information related to _____
(Type of Information)

to _____ for the following purpose:
(Recipient)

_____

_____

I understand that I may inspect or copy the protected health information described by this authorization.
I understand that, at any time, this authorization may be revoked, when the office that receives this
authorization receives a written revocation, although that revocation will not be effective as to the disclosure
of records whose release I have previously authorized, or where other action has been taken in reliance on an
authorization I have signed. I understand that my health care and the payment for my health care will not be
affected if I refuse to sign this form.
I understand that information used or disclosed, pursuant to this authorization, could be subject to redisclosure
by the recipient and, if so, may not be subject to federal or state law protecting its confidentiality.

_____   _____
Date   Signature of Individual or Representative

_____
Authority or Relationship to Individual, if Representative

EXPIRATION DATE: This authorization will expire on _____

If no date or event is stated, the expiration date will be six years from the date of this authorization.

COPY PROVIDED: The subject of this authorization shall receive a copy of this authorization, when signed.

C CMS Forms 1450 and 1500 with Instructions

CMS 1450 Form

ST11843 1PLY UB-92

1	2		3 PATIENT CONTROL NO.	4 TYPE OF BILL

| 5 FED. TAX NO. | 6 STATEMENT COVERS PERIOD FROM THROUGH | 7 COV D. | 8 N-C D. | 9 C-I D. | 10 L-R D. | 11 |

12 PATIENT NAME

13 PATIENT ADDRESS

| 14 BIRTHDATE | 15 SEX | 16 MS | ADMISSION 17 DATE | 18 HR | 19 TYPE | 20 SRC | 21 D HR | 22 STAT | 23 MEDICAL RECORD NO. | CONDITION CODES 24 25 26 27 28 29 30 | 31 |

32 OCCURRENCE CODE DATE	33 OCCURRENCE CODE DATE	34 OCCURRENCE CODE DATE	35 OCCURRENCE CODE DATE	36 OCCURRENCE SPAN CODE FROM THROUGH	37 A B C
a					
b					

38

39 VALUE CODES CODE AMOUNT	40 VALUE CODES CODE AMOUNT	41 VALUE CODES CODE AMOUNT
a		
b		
c		
d		

42 REV. CD.	43 DESCRIPTION	44 HCPCS / RATES	45 SERV. DATE	46 SERV. UNITS	47 TOTAL CHARGES	48 NON-COVERED CHARGES	49
1							1
2							2
3							3
4							4
5							5
6							6
7							7
8							8
9							9
10							10
11							11
12							12
13							13
14							14
15							15
16							16
17							17
18							18
19							19
20							20
21							21
22							22
23							23

50 PAYER	51 PROVIDER NO.	52 REL INFO	53 ASG BEN	54 PRIOR PAYMENTS	55 EST. AMOUNT DUE	56
A						
B						
C						

| 57 | **DUE FROM PATIENT ▶** | | | |

58 INSURED'S NAME	59 P. REL	60 CERT. - SSN - HIC. - ID NO.	61 GROUP NAME	62 INSURANCE GROUP NO.
A					A
B					B
C					C

63 TREATMENT AUTHORIZATION CODES	64 ESC	65 EMPLOYER NAME	66 EMPLOYER LOCATION
A				A
B				B
C				C

| 67 PRIN. DIAG. CD. | 68 CODE | 69 CODE | 70 CODE | 71 CODE | 72 CODE | 73 CODE | 74 CODE | 75 CODE | 76 ADM. DIAG. CD. | 77 E-CODE | 78 |

79 P.C.	80 PRINCIPAL PROCEDURE CODE DATE	81 OTHER PROCEDURE CODE DATE	OTHER PROCEDURE CODE DATE	82 ATTENDING PHYS. ID
		A	B	
	OTHER PROCEDURE CODE DATE	OTHER PROCEDURE CODE DATE	OTHER PROCEDURE CODE DATE	83 OTHER PHYS. ID
	C	D	E	A
84 REMARKS				OTHER PHYS. ID
a				B
b				
c				
d				X

UB-92 HCFA-1450   OCR/ORIGINAL   I CERTIFY THE CERTIFICATIONS ON THE REVERSE APPLY TO THIS BILL AND ARE MADE A PART HEREOF.

CMS 1450 Form Instruction

UNIFORM BILL:

NOTICE: ANYONE WHO MISREPRESENTS OR FALSIFIES ESSENTIAL INFORMATION REQUESTED BY THIS FORM MAY UPON CONVICTION BE SUBJECT TO FINE AND IMPRISONMENT UNDER FEDERAL AND/OR STATE LAW.

Certifications relevant to the Bill and Information Shown on the Face Hereof: Signatures on the face hereof incorporate the following certifications or verifications where pertinent to this Bill:

1. If third party benefits are indicated as being assigned or in participation status, on the face thereof, appropriate assignments by the insured/beneficiary and signature of patient or parent or legal guardian covering authorization to release information are on file. Determinations as to the release of medical and financial information should be guided by the particular terms of the release forms that were executed by the patient or the patient's legal representative. The hospital agrees to save harmless, indemnify and defend any insurer who makes payment in reliance upon this certification, from and against any claim to the insurance proceeds when in fact no valid assignment of benefits to the hospital was made.

2. If patient occupied a private room or required private nursing for medical necessity, any required certifications are on file.

3. Physician's certifications and re-certifications, if required by contract or Federal regulations, are on file.

4. For Christian Science Sanitoriums, verifications and if necessary re-verifications of the patient's need for sanitorium services are on file.

5. Signature of patient or his/her representative on certifications, authorization to release information, and payment request, as required be Federal law and regulations (42 USC 1935f, 42 CFR 424.36, 10 USC 1071 thru 1086, 32 CFR 199) and, any other applicable contract regulations, is on file.

6. This claim, to the best of my knowledge, is correct and complete and is in conformance with the Civil Rights Act of 1964 as amended. Records adequately disclosing services will be maintained and necessary information will be furnished to such governmental agencies as required by applicable law.

7. For Medicare purposes:

   If the patient has indicated that other health insurance or a state medical assistance agency will pay part of his/her medical expenses and he/she wants information about his/her claim released to them upon their request, necessary authorization is on file. The patient's signature on the provider's request to bill Medicare authorizes any holder of medical and non-medical information, including employment status, and whether the person has employer group health insurance, liability, no-fault, workers' compensation, or other insurance which is responsible to pay for the services for which this Medicare claim is made.

8. For Medicaid purposes:

   This is to certify that the foregoing information is true, accurate, and complete.
   I understand that payment and satisfaction of this claim will be from Federal and State funds, and that any false claims, statements, or documents, or concealment of a material fact, may be prosecuted under applicable Federal or State Laws.

9. For CHAMPUS purposes:

   This is to certify that:

   (a) the information submitted as part of this claim is true, accurate and complete, and, the services shown on this form were medically indicated and necessary for the health of the patient;

   (b) the patient has represented that by a reported residential address outside a military treatment center catchment area he or she does not live within a catchment area of a U.S. military or U.S. Public Health Service medical facility, or if the patient resides within a catchment area of such a facility, a copy of a Non-Availability Statement (DD Form 1251) is on file, or the physician has certified to a medical emergency in any assistance where a copy of a Non-Availability Statement is not on file;

   (c) the patient or the patient's parent or guardian has responded directly to the provider's request to identify all health insurance coverages, and that all such coverages are identified on the face of the claim except those that are exclusively supplemental payments to CHAMPUS-determined benefits;

   (d) the amount billed to CHAMPUS has been billed after all such coverages have been billed and paid, excluding Medicaid, and the amount billed to CHAMPUS is that remaining claimed against CHAMPUS benefits;

   (e) the beneficiary's cost share has not been waived by consent or failure to exercise generally accepted billing and collection efforts; and,

   (f) any hospital-based physician under contract, the cost of whose services are allocated in the charges included in this bill, is not an employee or member of the Uniformed Services. For purposes of this certification, an employee of the Uniformed Services is an employee, appointed in civil service (refer to 5 USC 2105), including part-time or intermittent but excluding contract surgeons or other personnel employed by the Uniformed Services through personal service contracts. Similarly, member of the Uniformed Services does not apply to reserve members of the Uniformed Services not on active duty.

   (g) based on the Consolidated Omnibus Budget Reconciliation Act of 1986, all providers participating in Medicare must also participate in CHAMPUS for inpatient hospital services provided pursuant to admissions to hospitals occurring on or after January 1, 1987.

   (h) if CHAMPUS benefits are to be paid in a participating status, I agree to submit this claim to the appropriate CHAMPUS claims processor as a participating provider. I agree to accept the CHAMPUS-determined reasonable charge as the total charge for the medical services or supplies listed on the claim form. I will accept the CHAMPUS-determined reasonable charge even if it is less than the billed amount, and also agree to accept the amount paid by CHAMPUS, combined with the cost-share amount and deductible amount, if any, paid by or on behalf of the patient as full payment for the listed medical services or supplies. I will make no attempt to collect from the patient (or his or her parent or guardian) amounts over the CHAMPUS-determined reasonable charge. CHAMPUS will make any benefits payable directly to me, if I submit this claim as a participating provider.

ESTIMATED CONTRACT BENEFITS

CMS 1500 Form

PLEASE
DO NOT
STAPLE
IN THIS
AREA

CARRIER

HEALTH INSURANCE CLAIM FORM

PICA | | | | | | PICA

1. MEDICARE   MEDICAID   CHAMPUS   CHAMPVA   GROUP HEALTH PLAN   FECA BLK LUNG   OTHER   1a. INSURED'S I.D. NUMBER   (FOR PROGRAM IN ITEM 1)

(Medicare #)   (Medicaid #)   (Sponsor's SSN)   (VA File #)   (SSN or ID)   (SSN)   (ID)

2. PATIENT'S NAME (Last Name, First Name, Middle Initial)

3. PATIENT'S BIRTH DATE   MM   DD   YY   SEX   M   F

4. INSURED'S NAME (Last Name, First Name, Middle Initial)

5. PATIENT'S ADDRESS (No., Street)

6. PATIENT RELATIONSHIP TO INSURED   Self   Spouse   Child   Other

7. INSURED'S ADDRESS (No., Street)

CITY   STATE   8. PATIENT STATUS   Single   Married   Other

CITY   STATE

ZIP CODE   TELEPHONE (Include Area Code)   ( )

Employed   Full-Time Student   Part-Time Student

ZIP CODE   TELEPHONE (INCLUDE AREA CODE)   ( )

9. OTHER INSURED'S NAME (Last Name, First Name, Middle Initial)

10. IS PATIENT'S CONDITION RELATED TO:

11. INSURED'S POLICY GROUP OR FECA NUMBER

a. OTHER INSURED'S POLICY OR GROUP NUMBER

a. EMPLOYMENT? (CURRENT OR PREVIOUS)   YES   NO

a. INSURED'S DATE OF BIRTH   MM   DD   YY   SEX   M   F

b. OTHER INSURED'S DATE OF BIRTH   MM   DD   YY   SEX   M   F

b. AUTO ACCIDENT?   PLACE (State)   YES   NO

b. EMPLOYER'S NAME OR SCHOOL NAME

c. EMPLOYER'S NAME OR SCHOOL NAME

c. OTHER ACCIDENT?   YES   NO

c. INSURANCE PLAN NAME OR PROGRAM NAME

d. INSURANCE PLAN NAME OR PROGRAM NAME

10d. RESERVED FOR LOCAL USE

d. IS THERE ANOTHER HEALTH BENEFIT PLAN?   YES   NO   If yes, return to and complete item 9 a-d.

READ BACK OF FORM BEFORE COMPLETING & SIGNING THIS FORM.

12. PATIENT'S OR AUTHORIZED PERSON'S SIGNATURE I authorize the release of any medical or other information necessary to process this claim. I also request payment of government benefits either to myself or to the party who accepts assignment below.

SIGNED _____ DATE _____

13. INSURED'S OR AUTHORIZED PERSON'S SIGNATURE I authorize payment of medical benefits to the undersigned physician or supplier for services described below.

SIGNED _____

14. DATE OF CURRENT: MM   DD   YY   ILLNESS (First symptom) OR INJURY (Accident) OR PREGNANCY(LMP)

15. IF PATIENT HAS HAD SAME OR SIMILAR ILLNESS. GIVE FIRST DATE   MM   DD   YY

16. DATES PATIENT UNABLE TO WORK IN CURRENT OCCUPATION   MM   DD   YY   FROM   TO   MM   DD   YY

17. NAME OF REFERRING PHYSICIAN OR OTHER SOURCE

17a. I.D. NUMBER OF REFERRING PHYSICIAN

18. HOSPITALIZATION DATES RELATED TO CURRENT SERVICES   MM   DD   YY   FROM   TO   MM   DD   YY

19. RESERVED FOR LOCAL USE

20. OUTSIDE LAB?   YES   NO $ CHARGES

21. DIAGNOSIS OR NATURE OF ILLNESS OR INJURY. (RELATE ITEMS 1,2,3 OR 4 TO ITEM 24E BY LINE)

1. _____ 3. _____
2. _____ 4. _____

22. MEDICAID RESUBMISSION CODE   ORIGINAL REF. NO.

23. PRIOR AUTHORIZATION NUMBER

24. A			B	C	D		E	F	G	H	I	J	K
DATE(S) OF SERVICE From		To	Place of Service	Type of Service	PROCEDURES, SERVICES, OR SUPPLIES (Explain Unusual Circumstances)		DIAGNOSIS CODE	$ CHARGES	DAYS OR UNITS	EPSDT Family Plan	EMG	COB	RESERVED FOR LOCAL USE
MM	DD	YY	MM	DD	YY		CPT/HCPCS	MODIFIER						
1													
2													
3													
4													
5													
6													

25. FEDERAL TAX I.D. NUMBER   SSN EIN

26. PATIENT'S ACCOUNT NO.

27. ACCEPT ASSIGNMENT? (For govt. claims, see back)   YES   NO

28. TOTAL CHARGE $

29. AMOUNT PAID $

30. BALANCE DUE $

31. SIGNATURE OF PHYSICIAN OR SUPPLIER INCLUDING DEGREES OR CREDENTIALS (I certify that the statements on the reverse apply to this bill and are made a part thereof.)

SIGNED _____ DATE _____

32. NAME AND ADDRESS OF FACILITY WHERE SERVICES WERE RENDERED (If other than home or office)

33. PHYSICIAN'S, SUPPLIER'S BILLING NAME, ADDRESS, ZIP CODE & PHONE #

PIN#   GRP#

(APPROVED BY AMA COUNCIL ON MEDICAL SERVICE 8/88)

PLEASE PRINT OR TYPE

APPROVED OMB-0938-0008 FORM CMS-1500 (12-90), FORM RRB-1500,
APPROVED OMB-1215-0055 FORM OWCP-1500, APPROVED OMB-0720-0001 (CHAMPUS)

PATIENT AND INSURED INFORMATION

PHYSICIAN OR SUPPLIER INFORMATION

CMS 1500 Form Instruction

BECAUSE THIS FORM IS USED BY VARIOUS GOVERNMENT AND PRIVATE HEALTH PROGRAMS, SEE SEPARATE INSTRUCTIONS ISSUED BY APPLICABLE PROGRAMS.

NOTICE: Any person who knowingly files a statement of claim containing any misrepresentation or any false, incomplete or misleading information may be guilty of a criminal act punishable under law and may be subject to civil penalties.

REFERS TO GOVERNMENT PROGRAMS ONLY

MEDICARE AND CHAMPUS PAYMENTS: A patient's signature requests that payment be made and authorizes release of any information necessary to process the claim and certifies that the information provided in Blocks 1 through 12 is true, accurate and complete. In the case of a Medicare claim, the patient's signature authorizes any entity to release to Medicare medical and nonmedical information, including employment status, and whether the person has employer group health insurance, liability, no-fault, worker's compensation or other insurance which is responsible to pay for the services for which the Medicare claim is made. See 42 CFR 411.24(a). If item 9 is completed, the patient's signature authorizes release of the information to the health plan or agency shown. In Medicare assigned or CHAMPUS participation cases, the physician agrees to accept the charge determination of the Medicare carrier or CHAMPUS fiscal intermediary as the full charge, and the patient is responsible only for the deductible, coinsurance and noncovered services. Coinsurance and the deductible are based upon the charge determination of the Medicare carrier or CHAMPUS fiscal intermediary if this is less than the charge submitted. CHAMPUS is not a health insurance program but makes payment for health benefits provided through certain affiliations with the Uniformed Services. Information on the patient's sponsor should be provided in those items captioned in "Insured"; i.e., items 1a, 4, 6, 7, 9, and 11.

BLACK LUNG AND FECA CLAIMS

The provider agrees to accept the amount paid by the Government as payment in full. See Black Lung and FECA instructions regarding required procedure and diagnosis coding systems.

SIGNATURE OF PHYSICIAN OR SUPPLIER (MEDICARE, CHAMPUS, FECA AND BLACK LUNG)

I certify that the services shown on this form were medically indicated and necessary for the health of the patient and were personally furnished by me or were furnished incident to my professional service by my employee under my immediate personal supervision, except as otherwise expressly permitted by Medicare or CHAMPUS regulations.

For services to be considered as "incident" to a physician's professional service, 1) they must be rendered under the physician's immediate personal supervision by his/her employee, 2) they must be an integral, although incidental part of a covered physician's service, 3) they must be of kinds commonly furnished in physician's offices, and 4) the services of nonphysicians must be included on the physician's bills.

For CHAMPUS claims, I further certify that I (or any employee) who rendered services am not an active duty member of the Uniformed Services or a civilian employee of the United States Government or a contract employee of the United States Government, either civilian or military (refer to 5 USC 5536). For Black-Lung claims, I further certify that the services performed were for a Black Lung-related disorder.

No Part B Medicare benefits may be paid unless this form is received as required by existing law and regulations (42 CFR 424.32).

NOTICE: Any one who misrepresents or falsifies essential information to receive payment from Federal funds requested by this form may upon conviction be subject to fine and imprisonment under applicable Federal laws.

NOTICE TO PATIENT ABOUT THE COLLECTION AND USE OF MEDICARE, CHAMPUS, FECA, AND BLACK LUNG INFORMATION
(PRIVACY ACT STATEMENT)

We are authorized by CMS, CHAMPUS and OWCP to ask you for information needed in the administration of the Medicare, CHAMPUS, FECA, and Black Lung programs. Authority to collect information is in section 205(a), 1862, 1872 and 1874 of the Social Security Act as amended, 42 CFR 411.24(a) and 424.5(a) (6), and 44 USC 3101;41 CFR 101 et seq and 10 USC 1079 and 1086; 5 USC 8101 et seq; and 30 USC 901 et seq; 38 USC 613; E.O. 9397.

The information we obtain to complete claims under these programs is used to identify you and to determine your eligibility. It is also used to decide if the services and supplies you received are covered by these programs and to insure that proper payment is made.

The information may also be given to other providers of services, carriers, intermediaries, medical review boards, health plans, and other organizations or Federal agencies, for the effective administration of Federal provisions that require other third parties payers to pay primary to Federal program, and as otherwise necessary to administer these programs. For example, it may be necessary to disclose information about the benefits you have used to a hospital or doctor. Additional disclosures are made through routine uses for information contained in systems of records.

FOR MEDICARE CLAIMS: See the notice modifying system No. 09-70-0501, titled, 'Carrier Medicare Claims Record,' published in the Federal Register, Vol. 55 No. 177, page 37549, Wed. Sept. 12, 1990, or as updated and republished.

FOR OWCP CLAIMS: Department of Labor, Privacy Act of 1974, "Republication of Notice of Systems of Records," Federal Register Vol. 55 No. 40, Wed Feb. 28, 1990, See ESA-5, ESA-6, ESA-12, ESA-13, ESA-30, or as updated and republished.

FOR CHAMPUS CLAIMS: PRINCIPLE PURPOSE(S): To evaluate eligibility for medical care provided by civilian sources and to issue payment upon establishment of eligibility and determination that the services/supplies received are authorized by law.

ROUTINE USE(S): Information from claims and related documents may be given to the Dept. of Veterans Affairs, the Dept. of Health and Human Services and/or the Dept. of Transportation consistent with their statutory administrative responsibilities under CHAMPUS/CHAMPVA; to the Dept. of Justice for representation of the Secretary of Defense in civil actions; to the Internal Revenue Service, private collection agencies, and consumer reporting agencies in connection with recoupment claims; and to Congressional Offices in response to inquiries made at the request of the person to whom a record pertains. Appropriate disclosures may be made to other federal, state, local, foreign government agencies, private business entities, and individual providers of care, on matters relating to entitlement, claims adjudication, fraud, program abuse, utilization review, quality assurance, peer review, program integrity, third-party liability, coordination of benefits, and civil and criminal litigation related to the operation of CHAMPUS.

DISCLOSURES: Voluntary; however, failure to provide information will result in delay in payment or may result in denial of claim. With the one exception discussed below, there are no penalties under these programs for refusing to supply information. However, failure to furnish information regarding the medical services rendered or the amount charged would prevent payment of claims under these programs. Failure to furnish any other information, such as name or claim number, would delay payment of the claim. Failure to provide medical information under FECA could be deemed an obstruction.

It is mandatory that you tell us if you know that another party is responsible for paying for your treatment. Section 1128B of the Social Security Act and 31 USC 3801-3812 provide penalties for withholding this information.

You should be aware that P.L. 100-503, the "Computer Matching and Privacy Protection Act of 1988", permits the government to verify information by way of computer matches.

MEDICAID PAYMENTS (PROVIDER CERTIFICATION)

I hereby agree to keep such records as are necessary to disclose fully the extent of services provided to individuals under the State's Title XIX plan and to furnish information regarding any payments claimed for providing such services as the State Agency or Dept. of Health and Humans Services may request.

I further agree to accept, as payment in full, the amount paid by the Medicaid program for those claims submitted for payment under that program, with the exception of authorized deductible, coinsurance, co-payment or similar cost-sharing charge.

SIGNATURE OF PHYSICIAN (OR SUPPLIER): I certify that the services listed above were medically indicated and necessary to the health of this patient and were personally furnished by me or my employee under my personal direction.

NOTICE: This is to certify that the foregoing information is true, accurate and complete. I understand that payment and satisfaction of this claim will be from Federal and State funds, and that any false claims, statements, or documents, or concealment of a material fact, may be prosecuted under applicable Federal or State laws.

According to the Paperwork Reduction Act of 1995, no persons are required to respond to a collection of information unless it displays a valid OMB control number. The valid OMB control number for this information collection is 0938-0008. The time required to complete this information collection is estimated to average 10 minutes per response, including the time to review instructions, search existing data resources, gather the data needed, and complete and review the information collection. If you have any comments concerning the accuracy of the time estimate(s) or suggestions for improving this form, please write to: CMS, N2-14-26, 7500 Security Boulevard, Baltimore, Maryland 21244-1850.

D ICD-9 Code Terms

ICD-9 Codes That Support Medical Necessity (not an inclusive list) for billing purposes, the following diagnoses usually describe an acute event or a complex medical condition that is generally considered acceptable.

138	Late effects of acute poliomyelitis
274.0	Gouty arthropathy
332.0–332.1	Parkinson's disease
333.0	Other degenerative diseases of the basal ganglia
333.6	Idiopathic torsion dystonia
333.7	Symptomatic torsion dystonia
333.83	Spasmodic torticollis
333.84	Organic writers' cramp
333.91	Stiff-man syndrome
334.0–334.8	Spinocerebellar disease
335.0–335.8	Anterior horn cell disease
336.0–336.8	Other diseases of spinal cord
337.20–337.29	Reflex sympathetic dystrophy
340	Multiple sclerosis
341.1	Schilder's disease
341.8	Other demyelinating diseases of central nervous system
342.00–342.92	Hemiplegia and hemiparesis
343.0–343.8	Infantile cerebral palsy
344.00–344.89	Other paralytic syndromes
353.0–353.8	Nerve root and plexus disorders
354.0–354.8	Mononeuritis of upper limb and mononeuritis multiplex
355.0–355.79	Mononeuritis of lower limb
356.0–356.8	Hereditary and idiopathic peripheral neuropathy
357.0–357.8	Inflammatory and toxic neuropathy
358.0–358.8	Myoneural disorders
359.0–359.8	Muscular dystrophies and other myopathies
430	Subarachnoid hemorrhage
431	Intracerebral hemorrhage
432.0	Nontraumatic extradural hemorrhage
432.1	Subdural hemorrhage
436	Acute, but ill-defined, cerebrovascular disease
438.0–438.89	Late effects of cerebrovascular disease
440.23	Atherosclerosis of native arteries of extremities with ulceration
440.24	Atherosclerosis of native arteries of extremities with gangrene
454.0–454.2	Varicose veins of lower extremities
457.0	Postmastectomy lymphedema syndrome
457.1	Other lymphedema
681.00–681.11	Cellulitis and abscess of finger and toe

682.3–682.7	Other cellulitis and abscess
695.81–695.89	Other specified erythematous conditions
696.0	Psoriatic arthropathy
696.1	Other psoriasis
707.0–707.8	Chronic ulcer of skin
709.2	Scar conditions and fibrosis of skin
710.1	Systemic sclerosis
710.3	Dermatomyositis
710.4	Polymyositis
710.8	Other specified diffuse diseases of connective tissue
711.00–711.99	Arthropathy associated with infections
712.10–712.99	Crystal arthropathies
713.0–713.8	Arthropathy associated with other disorders classified elsewhere
714.0–714.9	Rheumatoid arthritis and other inflammatory polyarthropathies
715.00–715.98	Osteoarthrosis and allied disorders
716.00–716.99	Other and unspecified arthropathies
717.0–717.43	Internal derangement of knee
718.00–718.89	Other derangement of joint
719.00–719.89	Other disorders of joint
720.0–720.9	Ankylosing spondylitis and other inflammatory spondylopathies
721.0–721.91	Spondylosis and allied disorders
722.0–722.93	Intervertebral disc disorders
723.0–723.9	Other disorders of cervical region
724.0–724.8	Other disorders of back
725	Polymyalgia rheumatica
726.0–726.91	Peripheral enthesopathies and allied syndromes
727.00–727.89	Other disorders of synovium, tendon, and bursa
728.0–728.89	Disorders of muscle, ligament, and fascia
729.0–729.9	Other disorders of soft tissues
733.10–733.19	Pathologic fracture
754.1	Certain congenital musculoskeletal deformities of sternocleidomastoid muscle
755.30–755.39	Reduction deformities of lower limb
755.60–755.64	Other anomalies of lower limb, including pelvic girdle
781.0	Abnormal involuntary movements
781.2	Abnormality of gait
781.3	Lack of coordination
781.4	Transient paralysis of limb
781.8	Neurologic neglect syndrome
782.3	Edema
799.4	Cachexia
805.00–805.9	Fracture of vertebral column without mention of spinal cord injury
806.00–806.9	Fracture of vertebral column with spinal cord injury
807.00–807.4	Fracture of rib(s) and sternum
808.0–808.9	Fracture of pelvis
809.0–809.1	Ill-defined fractures of bones of trunk
810.00–810.13	Fracture of clavicle
811.00–811.19	Fracture of scapula
812.00–812.59	Fracture of humerus
813.00–813.93	Fracture of radius and ulna
814.00–814.19	Fracture of carpal bone(s)
815.00–815.19	Fracture of metacarpal bone(s)
816.00–816.13	Fracture of one or more phalanges of hand
817.0–817.1	Multiple fractures of hand bones
818.0–818.1	Ill-defined fractures of upper limb

820.00–820.9	Fracture of neck of femur
821.00–821.39	Fracture of other and unspecified parts of femur
822.0–822.1	Fracture of patella
823.00–823.92	Fracture of tibia and fibula
824.0–824.9	Fracture of ankle
825.0–825.39	Fracture of one or more tarsal and metatarsal bones
826.0–826.1	Fracture of one or more phalanges of foot
827.0–827.1	Other, multiple, and ill-defined fractures of lower limb
831.00–831.19	Dislocation of shoulder
832.00–832.19	Dislocation of elbow
833.00–833.19	Dislocation of wrist
834.00–834.12	Dislocation of finger
835.00–835.13	Dislocation of hip
836.0–836.69	Dislocation of knee
837.0–837.1	Dislocation of ankle
838.00–838.19	Dislocation of foot
840.0–840.9	Sprains and strains of shoulder and upper arm
841.0–841.9	Sprains and strains of elbow and forearm
842.00–842.19	Sprains and strains of wrist and hand
843.0–843.9	Sprains and strains of hip and thigh
844.0–844.9	Sprains and strains of knee and leg
845.00–845.19	Sprains and strains of ankle and foot
846.0–846.9	Sprains and strains of sacroiliac region
847.0–847.9	Sprains and strains of other and unspecified parts of back
880.00–880.29	Open wound of shoulder and upper arm
881.00–881.22	Open wound of elbow, forearm, and wrist
882.0–882.2	Open wound of hand except finger(s) alone
883.0–883.2	Open wound of finger(s)
884.0–884.2	Multiple and unspecified open wound of upper limb
885.0–885.1	Traumatic amputation of thumb (complete) (partial)
886.0–886.1	Traumatic amputation of other finger(s) (complete) (partial)
887.0–887.7	Traumatic amputation of arm and hand (complete) (partial)
890.0–890.2	Open wound of hip and thigh
891.0–891.2	Open wound of knee, leg (except thigh), and ankle
892.0–892.2	Open wound of foot except toe(s) alone
893.0–893.2	Open wound of toe(s)
896.0–896.3	Traumatic amputation of foot (complete) (partial)
897.0–897.7	Traumatic amputation of leg(s) (complete) (partial)
905.1–905.9	Late effects of musculoskeletal and connective tissue injuries
923.00–923.9	Contusion of upper limb
924.00–924.4	Contusion of lower limb
926.0–926.8	Crushing injury of trunk
927.00–927.8	Crushing injury of upper limb
928.00–928.8	Crushing injury of lower limb
929.0	Crushing injury of multiple sites, not elsewhere classified
942.20–942.59	Burn of trunk
943.20–943.59	Burn of upper limb, except wrist and hand
944.20–944.58	Burn of wrist(s) and hand(s)
945.20–945.59	Burn of lower limb(s)
946.2–946.5	Burns of multiple specified sites
948.00–948.99	Burns classified according to extent of body surface involved
951.4	Injury to facial nerve
952.00–952.9	Spinal cord injury without evidence of spinal bone injury

953.0–953.8	Injury to nerve roots and spinal plexus
955.0–955.9	Injury to peripheral nerve(s) of shoulder girdle and upper limb
956.0–956.9	Injury to peripheral nerve(s) of pelvic girdle and lower limb
997.61–997.62	Amputation stump complication
V43.61–V43.69	Organ or tissue replaced by joint
V43.7	Organ or tissue replaced by limb
V49.1–V49.77	Problems with limbs and other problems
V52.0	Fitting and adjustment of artificial arm (complete) (partial)
V52.1	Fitting and adjustment of artificial leg (complete) (partial)
V53.7	Fitting and adjustment of orthopedic devices
V54.0–V54.8	Other orthopedic aftercare

E

APTA Guidelines for Physical Therapy Documentation and Guidelines for Group Coding

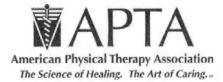

American Physical Therapy Association
The Science of Healing. The Art of Caring.™

GUIDELINES: PHYSICAL THERAPY DOCUMENTATION OF PATIENT/CLIENT MANAGEMENT

BOD G03-05-16-41 [Amended BOD 02-02-16-20; BOD 11-01-06-10; BOD 03-01-16-51; BOD 03-00-22-54; BOD 03-99-14-41; BOD 11-98-19-69; BOD 03-97-27-69; BOD 03-95-23-61; BOD 11-94-33-107; BOD 06-93-09-13; Initial BOD 03-93-21-55] [Guideline]

PREAMBLE

The American Physical Therapy Association (APTA) is committed to meeting the physical therapy needs of society, to meeting the needs and interests of its members, and to developing and improving the art and science of physical therapy, including practice, education, and research. To help meet these responsibilities, APTA's Board of Directors has approved the following guidelines for physical therapy documentation. It is recognized that these guidelines do not reflect all of the unique documentation requirements associated with the many specialty areas within the physical therapy profession. Applicable for both handwritten and electronic documentation systems, these guidelines are intended to be used as a foundation for the development of more specific documentation guidelines in clinical areas, while at the same time providing guidance for the physical therapy profession across all practice settings. Documentation may also need to address additional regulatory or payer requirements.

Finally, be aware that these guidelines are intended to address *documentation* of patient/client management, not to describe the provision of physical therapy services. Other APTA documents, including APTA Standards of Practice for Physical Therapy, Code of Ethics and Guide for Professional Conduct, and the Guide to Physical Therapist Practice, address provision of physical therapy services and patient/client management.

APTA POSITION ON DOCUMENTATION

Documentation Authority For Physical Therapy Services

Physical therapy examination, evaluation, diagnosis, prognosis, and plan of care (including interventions) shall be documented, dated, and authenticated by the physical therapist who performs the service. Interventions provided by the physical therapist or selected interventions provided by the physical therapist assistant under the direction and supervision of the physical therapist are documented, dated, and authenticated by the physical therapist or, when permissible by law, the physical therapist assistant.

Other notations or flow charts are considered a component of the documented record but do not meet the requirements of documentation in or of themselves.

Students in physical therapist or physical therapist assistant programs may document when the record is additionally authenticated by the physical therapist or, when permissible by law, documentation by physical therapist assistant students may be authenticated by a physical therapist assistant.

OPERATIONAL DEFINITIONS

Guidelines
APTA defines a "guideline" as a statement of advice.

Authentication

The process used to verify that an entry is complete, accurate, and final. Indications of authentication can include original written signatures and computer "signatures" on secured electronic record systems only.

The following describes the main documentation elements of patient/client management: (1) initial examination/evaluation, (2) visit/encounter, (3) reexamination, and (4) discharge or discontinuation summary.

Initial Examination/Evaluation

Documentation of the initial encounter is typically called the "initial examination," "initial evaluation," or "initial examination/evaluation." Completion of the initial examination/ evaluation is typically completed in one visit, but may occur over more than one visit. Documentation elements for the initial examination/evaluation include the following:

Examination: Includes data obtained from the history, systems review, and tests and measures.

Evaluation: Evaluation is a thought process that may not include formal documentation. It may include documentation of the assessment of the data collected in the examination and identification of problems pertinent to patient/client management.

Diagnosis: Indicates level of impairment, activity limitation, and participation restriction determined by the physical therapist. May be indicated by selecting one or more preferred practice patterns from the Guide to Physical Therapist Practice.

Prognosis: Provides documentation of the predicted level of improvement that might be attained through intervention and the amount of time required to reach that level. Prognosis is typically not a separate documentation element, but the components are included as part of the plan of care.

Plan of care: Typically stated in general terms, includes goals, interventions planned, proposed frequency and duration, and discharge plans.

Visit/Encounter

Documentation of a visit or encounter, often called a progress note or daily note, documents sequential implementation of the plan of care established by the physical therapist, including changes in patient/client status and variations and progressions of specific interventions used. Also may include specific plans for the next visit or visits.

Reexamination

Documentation of reexamination includes data from repeated or new examination elements and is provided to evaluate progress and to modify or redirect intervention.

Discharge or Discontinuation Summary

Documentation is required following conclusion of the current episode in the physical therapy intervention sequence, to summarize progression toward goals and discharge plans.

GENERAL GUIDELINES

- Documentation is required for every visit/encounter.
- All documentation must comply with the applicable jurisdictional/regulatory requirements.
- All handwritten entries shall be made in ink and will include original signatures. Electronic entries are made with appropriate security and confidentiality provisions.
- Charting errors should be corrected by drawing a single line through the error and initialing and dating the chart or through the appropriate mechanism for electronic

documentation that clearly indicates that a change was made without deletion of the original record.

- All documentation must include adequate identification of the patient/client and the physical therapist or physical therapist assistant:
  - o The patient's/client's full name and identification number, if applicable, must be included on all official documents.
  - o All entries must be dated and authenticated with the provider's full name and appropriate designation:
    - Documentation of examination, evaluation, diagnosis, prognosis, plan of care, and discharge summary must be authenticated by the physical therapist who provided the service.
    - Documentation of intervention in visit/encounter notes must be authenticated by the physical therapist or physical therapist assistant who provided the service.
    - Documentation by physical therapist or physical therapist assistant graduates or other physical therapists and physical therapist assistants pending receipt of an unrestricted license shall be authenticated by a licensed physical therapist, or, when permissible by law, documentation by physical therapist assistant graduates may be authenticated by a physical therapist assistant.
    - Documentation by students (SPT/SPTA) in physical therapist or physical therapist assistant programs must be additionally authenticated by the physical therapist or, when permissible by law, documentation by physical therapist assistant students may be authenticated by a physical therapist assistant.
- Documentation should include the referral mechanism by which physical therapy services are initiated. Examples include:
  - o Self-referral/direct access
  - o Request for consultation from another practitioner
- Documentation should include indication of no shows and cancellations.

INITIAL EXAMINATION/EVALUATION

<u>Examination (History, Systems Review, and Tests and Measures)</u>

History:
Documentation of history may include the following:
- General demographics
- Social history
- Employment/work (job/school/play)
- Growth and development
- Living environment
- General health status (self-report, family report, caregiver report)
- Social/health habits (past and current)
- Family history
- Medical/surgical history
- Current condition(s)/chief complaint(s)
- Functional status and activity level
- Medications
- Other clinical tests

Systems Review:
Documentation of systems review may include gathering data for the following systems:
- Cardiovascular/pulmonary

- ○ Blood pressure
- ○ Edema
- ○ Heart rate
- ○ Respiratory rate
- Integumentary
  - ○ Pliability (texture)
  - ○ Presence of scar formation
  - ○ Skin color
  - ○ Skin integrity
- Musculoskeletal
  - ○ Gross range of motion
  - ○ Gross strength
  - ○ Gross symmetry
  - ○ Height
  - ○ Weight
- Neuromuscular
  - ○ Gross coordinated movement (e.g., balance, locomotion, transfers,
    and transitions)
  - ○ Motor function (motor control, motor learning)

Documentation of systems review may also address communication ability, affect, cognition, language, and learning style:
- Ability to make needs known
- Consciousness
- Expected emotional/behavioral responses
- Learning preferences (e.g., *education needs, learning barriers*)
- Orientation (person, place, time)

Tests and Measures:
Documentation of tests and measures may include findings for the following categories:
- Aerobic capacity/endurance
  Examples of examination findings include:
  - ○ Aerobic capacity during functional activities
  - ○ Aerobic capacity during standardized exercise test protocols
  - ○ Cardiovascular signs and symptoms in response to increased oxygen demand with exercise or activity
  - ○ Pulmonary signs and symptoms in response to increased oxygen demand with exercise or activity

- Anthropometric characteristics
  Examples of examination findings include:
  - ○ Body composition
  - ○ Body dimensions
  - ○ Edema

- Arousal, attention, and cognition
  Examples of examination findings include:
  - ○ Arousal and attention
  - ○ Cognition
  - ○ Communication
  - ○ Consciousness
  - ○ Motivation

- o Orientation to time, person, place, and situation
- o Recall

- Assistive and adaptive devices
  Examples of examination findings include:
  - o Assistive or adaptive devices and equipment use during functional activities
  - o Components, alignment, fit, and ability to care for the assistive or adaptive devices and equipment
  - o Remediation of impairments, activity limitations, and participation restrictions with use of assistive or adaptive devices and equipment
  - o Safety during use of assistive or adaptive devices and equipment

- Circulation (arterial, venous, lymphatic)
  Examples of examination findings include:
  - o Cardiovascular signs
  - o Cardiovascular symptoms
  - o Physiological responses to position change

- Cranial and peripheral nerve integrity
  Examples of examination findings include:
  - o Electrophysiological integrity
  - o Motor distribution of the cranial nerves
  - o Motor distribution of the peripheral nerves
  - o Response to neural provocation
  - o Response to stimuli, including auditory, gustatory, olfactory, pharyngeal, vestibular, and visual
  - o Sensory distribution of the cranial nerves
  - o Sensory distribution of the peripheral nerves

- Environmental, home, and work (job/school/play) barriers
  Examples of examination findings include:
  - o Current and potential barriers
  - o Physical space and environment

- Ergonomics and body mechanics
  Examples of examination findings for *ergonomics* include:
  - o Dexterity and coordination during work
  - o Functional capacity and performance during work actions, tasks, or activities
  - o Safety in work environments
  - o Specific work conditions or activities
  - o Tools, devices, equipment, and work stations related to work actions, tasks, or activities
  Examples of examination findings for *body mechanics* include:
  - o Body mechanics during self-care, home management, work, community, or leisure actions, tasks, or activities

- Gait, locomotion, and balance
  Examples of examination findings include:
  - o Balance during functional activities with or without the use of assistive, adaptive, orthotic, protection, supportive, or prosthetic devices or equipment

- o Balance (dynamic and static) with or without the use of assistive, adaptive, orthotic, protective, supportive, or prosthetic devices or equipment
- o Gait and locomotion during functional activities with or without the use of assistive, adaptive, orthotic, protective, supportive, or prosthetic devices or equipment
- o Gait and locomotion with or without the use of assistive, adaptive, orthotic, protective, supportive, or prosthetic devices or equipment
- o Safety during gait, locomotion, and balance

- Integumentary integrity
  Examples of examination findings include:
  Associated skin:
  - o Activities, positioning, and postures that produce or relieve trauma to the skin
  - o Assistive, adaptive, orthotic, protective, supportive, or prosthetic devices and equipment that may produce or relieve trauma to the skin
  - o Skin characteristics

- Wound
  - o Activities, positioning, and postures that aggravate the wound or scar or that produce or relieve trauma
  - o Burn
  - o Signs of infection
  - o Wound characteristics
  - o Wound scar tissue characteristics

- Joint integrity and mobility
  Examples of examination findings include:
  - o Joint integrity and mobility
  - o Joint play movements
  - o Specific body parts

- Motor function
  Examples of examination findings include:
  - o Dexterity, coordination, and agility
  - o Electrophysiological integrity
  - o Hand function
  - o Initiation, modification, and control of movement patterns and voluntary postures

- Muscle performance
  Examples of examination findings include:
  - o Electrophysiological integrity
  - o Muscle strength, power, and endurance
  - o Muscle strength, power, and endurance during functional activities
  - o Muscle tension

- Neuromotor development and sensory integration
  Examples of examination findings include:
  - o Acquisition and evolution of motor skills
  - o Oral motor function, phonation, and speech production
  - o Sensorimotor integration

- Orthotic, protective, and supportive devices
  Examples of examination findings include:
  - Components, alignment, fit, and ability to care for the orthotic, protective, and supportive devices and equipment
  - Orthotic, protective, and supportive devices and equipment use during functional activities
  - Remediation of impairments, activity limitations, and participation restrictions with use of orthotic, protective, and supportive devices and equipment
  - Safety during use of orthotic, protective, and supportive devices and equipment

- Pain
  Examples of examination findings include:
  - Pain, soreness, and nocioception
  - Pain in specific body parts

- Posture
  Examples of examination findings include:
  - Postural alignment and position (dynamic)
  - Postural alignment and position (static)
  - Specific body parts

- Prosthetic requirements
  Examples of examination findings include:
  - Components, alignment, fit, and ability to care for prosthetic device
  - Prosthetic device use during functional activities
  - Remediation of impairments, activity limitations, and participation restrictions with use of the prosthetic device
  - Residual limb or adjacent segment
  - Safety during use of the prosthetic device

- Range of motion (including muscle length)
  Examples of examination findings include:
  - Functional ROM
  - Joint active and passive movement
  - Muscle length, soft tissue extensibility, and flexibility

- Reflex integrity
  Examples of examination findings include:
  - Deep reflexes
  - Electrophysiological integrity
  - Postural reflexes and reactions, including righting, equilibrium, and protective reactions
  - Primitive reflexes and reactions
  - Resistance to passive stretch
  - Superficial reflexes and reactions

- Self-care and home management (including activities of daily living and instrumental activities of daily living)
  Examples of examination findings include:
  - Ability to gain access to home environments

- - Ability to perform self-care and home management activities with or without assistive, adaptive, orthotic, protective, supportive, or prosthetic devices and equipment
    - Safety in self-care and home management activities and environments

  - Sensory integrity
    Examples of examination findings include:
    - Combined/cortical sensations
    - Deep sensations
    - Electrophysiological integrity

  - Ventilation and respiration
    Examples of examination findings include:
    - Pulmonary signs of respiration/gas exchange
    - Pulmonary signs of ventilatory function
    - Pulmonary symptoms

  - Work (job/school/play), community, and leisure integration or reintegration (including instrumental activities of daily living)
    Examples of examination findings include:
    - Ability to assume or resume work (job/school/plan), community, and leisure activities with or without assistive, adaptive, orthotic, protective, supportive, or prosthetic devices and equipment
    - Ability to gain access to work (job/school/play), community, and leisure environments
    - Safety in work (job/school/play), community, and leisure activities and environments

Evaluation
- Evaluation is a thought process that may not include formal documentation. However, the evaluation process may lead to documentation of impairments, activity limitations, and participation restrictions using formats such as:
  - A problem list
  - A statement of assessment of key factors (e.g., cognitive factors, co-morbidities, social support) influencing the patient/client status.

Diagnosis
- Documentation of a diagnosis determined by the physical therapist may include impairment, activity limitation, and participation restrictions.
  Examples include:
  - Impaired joint mobility, motor function, muscle performance, and range of motion associated with localized inflammation (4E)
  - Impaired motor function and sensory integrity associated with progressive disorders of the central nervous system (5E)
  - Impaired aerobic capacity/endurance associated with cardiovascular pump dysfunction or failure (6D)
  - Impaired integumentary integrity associated with partial-thickness skin involvement and scar formation (7C)

Prognosis
- Documentation of the prognosis is typically included in the plan of care. See below.

Plan of Care
- Documentation of the plan of care includes the following:

- Overall goals stated in measurable terms that indicate the predicted level of improvement in functioning
- A general statement of interventions to be used
- Proposed duration and frequency of service required to reach the goals
- Anticipated discharge plans

VISIT/ENCOUNTER

- Documentation of each visit/encounter shall include the following elements:
  - o Patient/client self-report (as appropriate)
  - o Identification of specific interventions provided, including frequency, intensity, and duration as appropriate. Examples include:
    - Knee extension, three sets, ten repetitions, 10# weight
    - Transfer training bed to chair with sliding board
    - Equipment provided
  - o Changes in patient/client impairment, activity limitation, and participation restriction status as they relate to the plan of care
  - o Response to interventions, including adverse reactions, if any
  - o Factors that modify frequency or intensity of intervention and progression goals, including patient/client adherence to patient/client-related instructions
  - o Communication/consultation with providers/patient/client/family/ significant other
  - o Documentation to plan for ongoing provision of services for the next visit(s), which is suggested to include, but not be limited to:
    - The interventions with objectives
    - Progression parameters
    - Precautions, if indicated

REEXAMINATION

- Documentation of reexamination shall include the following elements:
  - o Documentation of selected components of examination to update patient's/client's functioning, and/or disability status
  - o Interpretation of findings and, when indicated, revision of goals
  - o When indicated, revision of plan of care, as directly correlated with goals as documented

DISCHARGE/DISCONTINUATION SUMMARY

- Documentation of discharge or discontinuation shall include the following elements:
  - o Current physical/functional status
  - o Degree of goals achieved and reasons for goals not being achieved
  - o Discharge/discontinuation plan related to the patient/client's continuing care Examples include:
    - Home program
    - Referrals for additional services
    - Recommendations for follow-up physical therapy care
    - Family and caregiver training
    - Equipment provided

Relationship to Vision 2020: Professionalism
(Practice Department, ext 3176)

[Document updated: 12/14/2009]

Explanation of Reference Numbers:

BOD P00-00-00-00 stands for Board of Directors/month/year/page/vote in the Board of Directors Minutes; the "P" indicates that it is a position (see below). For example, BOD P11-97-06-18 means that this position can be found in the November 1997 Board of Directors minutes on Page 6 and that it was Vote 18.

P: Position | S: Standard | G: Guideline | Y: Policy | R: Procedure

American Physical Therapy Association

Retrieved from:
http://www.apta.org/AM/Template.cfm?Section=Home&TEMPLATE=/CM/ContentDisplay.
cfm&CONTENTID=22191

Recent Coding Issues and One-on-One and Group Patient Scenarios

Recent Coding Issues

CMS has established a correct coding initiative edit that prohibits billing for group therapy along with certain therapeutic procedure CPT codes (97110, 97112, 97116, 97140, 97530, 97532, 97533) in the same session unless a –59 modifier is used in certain settings. To be reimbursed for both services, the providers documentation must support that the group therapy and the therapeutic procedure were performed during separate time intervals.

Lastly, APTA does not interpret Transmittal 1753 as prohibiting payment for a supervised (unattended) modality and a one-on-one service being delivered to two patients in the same time interval. For example, Patient A is receiving unattended electrical stimulation at the same time as patient B is receiving therapeutic exercise…

These are intended to be examples of proper coding for billing purposes.

They are not intended to establish a standard for clinical practice.

1. MORE THAN ONE PATIENT IN THE CLINIC

Physical therapist sees patient A at 9:00 AM for 30 minutes of therapeutic exercise. At 9:15 AM patient B arrives and begins his visit with 15 minutes on the treadmill focusing on muscular recruitment and posture, assisted by a physical therapist assistant. At 9:30 the physical therapist sets up patient A to begin electrical stimulation (unattended). Following patient A's set up, the physical therapist begins working with patient B on gait training while patient A continues to receive electrical stimulation (unattended). At 9:55, the physical therapist briefly assesses Patient A following completion of the electrical stimulation and then patient A leaves the clinic. The physical therapist then completes Patient B's gait training and patient B leaves the clinic at 10:10 AM.

Coding:
Patient A: 97110 (therapeutic exercise) 2 units
97014 (electrical stimulation, unattended)
Patient B: 97116 (gait training) 2 units
97112 (neuromuscular reeducation) 1 unit

Rationale:
The physical therapist is one on one with Patient A from 9:00-9:30, and therefore two units of therapeutic exercise (97110) would be billed. Patient A's electrical stimulation (97014) is also billable as it is a supervised modality.

The time that Patient B spends with the physical therapist assistant from 9:15-9:30 is billable as one unit of neuromuscular reeducation (97112) as the physical therapist assistant is providing skilled therapy services under the supervision of the physical therapist. In addition, the time spent with the physical therapist from 9:30-10:10 is also billable as 2 more units of gait training (97116) because the physical therapist is one on one with Patient B. It is appropriate to bill 2 units of gait training rather than 3 units, because there were interruptions during the time frame.

2. MORE THAN ONE PATIENT, PT and PTA PROVIDERS

Patient A arrives at the physical therapists office at 8:30 a.m. and the physical therapist begins providing Patient A 30 minutes of therapeutic exercise. Patient B arrives for a 9:00 AM appointment and is seen by physical therapist briefly to assess need for modalities. The physical therapist determines that an ultrasound is appropriate to begin the treatment. The physical therapist examines the area to be treated, and directs the physical therapist assistant to position the patient and apply the ultrasound. The physical therapist then begins reviewing patient A's home exercise program. Patient A leaves the clinic at 9:15 AM. At 9:20, patient B's ultrasound is completed. The physical therapist assesses the patient following the application of ultrasound and begins a manual therapy technique to the area. At 9:45 AM patient B begins therapeutic exercises with a physical therapist assistant as instructed and directed by the physical therapist. At 10:00 AM Patient C arrives and the physical therapist begins treatment with 30 minutes of therapeutic exercises, ending with 15 minutes of ice to the area. At 10:15, patient B leaves after completing the therapeutic exercises.

Coding:
Patient A: 97110 (therapeutic exercise) 3 units
Patient B: 97035 (ultrasound)
97140 (manual therapy) 2 units
97110 (therapeutic exercise) 2 units
Patient C: 97110 (therapeutic exercise) 2 units

Rationale:
Patient A received three units of therapeutic exercise (97110). Patient A received two units of therapeutic exercise (97110) from 8:30-9:00. After patient B is set up for ultrasound (97035), the therapist continues with Patient A's home exercise program. This time is also billable as a direct one on one service (97110)

Patient B's ultrasound (97035) is a billable service because a physical therapist assistant (supervised by a physical therapist) is attending to Patient B. Patient B then receives manual therapy (97140) from 9:20-9:45, which amounts to two units. Patient B then receives therapeutic exercise (97110) from 9:45 to approximately 10:15, which amounts to two units.

Patient C receives 30 minutes of therapeutic exercise (97110), which amounts to two units. The time during which patient C is getting ice to the area for 15 minutes is not billable as hot/cold packs (97010) are bundled under the Medicare program.

3. GROUP AND ONE TO ONE PROCEDURES
Patients A, B, C and D are scheduled to see their physical therapist at 9:00 AM. They have all recently been fitted with lower limb prostheses. Patients A, B and C are below-knee amputees and patient D is an above-knee amputee. The physical therapist performs ADL training, including stump management techniques with these four patients for 60 minutes. During this 60 minute session, each of the four patients performs return demonstration of the techniques they are instructed in individually (for approximately 10-12 minutes each), with the therapist, one to one, to ensure compliance with the techniques in their home settings.

Coding:
Patient A: 97535 (self care/home management training)
97150 (group therapy)
Patient B: 97535 (self care/home management training)
97150 (group therapy)
Patient C: 97535 (self care/home management training)
97150 (group therapy)
Patient D: 97535 self care/home management training)
97150 (group therapy)

Rationale:
Patient A, B, C, and D would be considered as a group with a common, unifying element, therefore a group code (97150) would be billed for each patient. In addition, self care/home management training (CPT code 97535) would also be billed for each patient, because the physical therapist spends approximately 10-12 minutes of one-on-one time with each patient practicing the techniques individually. According to Program Memorandum, AB-00-39, the duration would be appropriate to bill one on one codes.

4. GROUP ONLY
Patients A, B, C and D are scheduled to see their physical therapist at 9:00 AM for aquatic therapy with therapeutic exercise. All four patients have arthritis. The physical therapist performs a total of 55 minutes of group exercise with these four individuals, allowing for a 5- minute rest after the first 20 minutes of continuous exercise. During the rest period the patients self-monitor their heart rates as they return to resting and compare their findings to previous sessions. The session ends with the therapist reminding patients to continue to perform their land-based home exercise programs.

Coding:
Patient A: 97150 (group therapy)
Patient B: 97150 (group therapy)
Patient C: 97150 (group therapy)
Patient D: 97150 (group therapy)

Rationale:
This is a group with a common unifying element (arthritis). The patients do not receive one-on-one treatment; therefore it is appropriate only to bill the group (97150).

5. GROUP COMBINED WITH MODALITIES AND ONE TO ONE

a. Patients A, B, C are scheduled for physical therapy at 9:00 AM. Patient A is being seen for a recent shoulder dislocation. Patients B and C are both recovering from rotator cuff surgery. After assessing each patient's shoulder, all three patients are provided skilled services simultaneously by the therapist while the therapist is in constant attendance. At 9:20, the physical therapist performs shoulder stabilization exercise techniques with patient A, while patient B and C continue with their strengthening exercises. Periodically the physical therapist will provide verbal cues to patients B and C to assure correct position and speed of their exercises. At 9:35, the physical therapist sets up Patient C on electrical stimulation (unattended) and shortly thereafter, patient A on ice. Following the set up of Patient C and A, the physical therapist performs manual techniques to Patient B's shoulder, while Patient A is receiving ice and Patient C is receiving electric stimulation to the shoulder. At 9:55 the physical therapist reviews Patient C's home exercise program, while Patients A and B perform the upper body ergometer for 10 minutes. Their visits all end at 10:05 AM.

Coding:
Patient A: 97150 (group therapy)
97110 (therapeutic exercise)
Patient B: 97150 (group therapy)
97140 (manual therapy)
Patient C: 97150 (group therapy)
97014 (electrical stimulation, unattended)
97110 (therapeutic exercise)

Rationale:
From 9:00-9:20, the patients are receiving group therapy services. The therapist is providing skilled services to all 3, while in constant attendance. Therefore, a group therapy code (97150) would be billed for each patient. From 9:20-9:35 a.m. the physical therapist provides one-on-one services to Patient A, and thus may be one unit of 97110 for Patient A. During that time frame, the physical therapist periodically looks up and makes comments to B and C; however, this time is not counted as billable for B and C, because the therapist is still attending to patient A with his hands during this brief encounter with patients B and C. From 9:40-9:55, patient B receives one-on-one manual therapy, which is therefore billable as 97140. Patient A is receiving ice during this time frame which is not a billable service under the Medicare program. Patient C is receiving unattended electrical stimulation (97014), which is billable as it does not have to be one-on-one. At 9:55, the physical therapist begins working with patient C on modifying and progressing a home exercise program which can be billed as 97110. The time that patient A and B spend performing the upper body ergometer is not billable, because the physical therapist is conducting the home program with patient C.

5b. Patients A, B, C are scheduled for physical therapy at 9:00 AM. Patient A is being seen for a recent shoulder dislocation. Patients B and C are both recovering from rotator cuff surgery. The physical therapist briefly assesses each patient's shoulder and begins shoulder stabilization exercise techniques with patient A, while patient B and C independently initiate their strengthening exercises. Periodically the physical therapist will provide verbal cues to patients B and C to assure correct position and speed of their exercises. At 9:35, the physical therapist performs manual techniques to Patient B's shoulder, while Patient A is receiving ice and Patient C is receiving electric stimulation to the shoulder. At 9:50 the physical therapist reviews Patient C's home exercise program, while Patients A and B perform the upper body ergometer for 10 minutes. Their visits all end at 10:00 AM.

Coding:
Patient A: 97110 (therapeutic exercise) 2 units
Patient B: 97140 (manual therapy)
Patient C: 97014 (electrical stimulation, unattended)
97110 (therapeutic exercise)

Rationale:
This scenario differs from 5a in that there is no group charge. The physical therapist would not bill group because there is not the initial 20 minutes with all three patients that occurred in scenario 5a.

Patient A receives shoulder stabilization exercise techniques from approximately 9:00-9:35, which would be considered two units of therapeutic exercise (97110). Periodically, the patient provides verbal cues to patients B and C. However, the time of patient B and C is not billed as either group or one-on-one, because the therapist is working one on one with Patient A. From 9:35-9:50, the therapist is performing manual techniques on Patient B's shoulder which is billable as one unit of manual therapy (97140). During this time frame, Patient A is receiving ice, which is not a billable service under the Medicare program, while Patient C is receiving unattended electrical stimulation (97014), which is billable, because it is not a one-on-one code. At 9:50, the physical therapist begins a one on one service with Patient C, review of the home exercise program that can be billed as therapeutic exercise (97110). However, the 10 minutes spent by A and B performing upper body ergometer is not billable as it is not supervised.

6. AGGREGATE TIME

Patient A arrives for their physical therapy appointment at 9:00 AM. The plan of care is currently focused on the patients need for balance training due to vestibular problems. The physical therapist performs 25 minutes of balance exercises with patient A. The patient rests for 5 minutes. Patient B has arrived for his appointment at 9:20. Patient B, who is being seen for complaints of back pain is seen by the physical therapist initially for 5 minutes of stretching to a tight hamstring. At 9:30 Patient B is instructed to continue stretching as the physical therapist returns to work with Patient A on techniques to improve coordination and balance when transitioning in and out of various postures. At 9:45 patient A and patient B are both on floor mats performing various exercises and stretches to improve movement and coordination. The Therapist provides alternating one to one interventions to both patients A and B for 15 minutes by moving between patients as they progress through their exercises. By 10 AM patient A had received a total of 48 minutes of one-on-one therapeutic interventions, Patient B had received a total of 12 minutes of one-on-one therapeutic interventions.

Coding:

Patient A: 97112 (neuromuscular reeducation) 3 units
Patient B: 97110 (therapeutic exercise) 1 unit

Rationale

From 9:00-9:25, patient A receives approximately 25 minutes of neuromuscular reeducation (97112) one on one. The therapist takes a break to see patient B and then moves back and spends more time with Patient A. Neither patient A nor patient B receives group. The one on one time spent alternating back and forth between A and B is incremental and aggregated. Thus, in the end patient A would be billed 3 units of neuromuscular reeducation (97112) and patient B would be billed one unit of therapeutic exercise (97110).

7a. SKILLED GROUP

Five patients are participating in an hour-long exercise program, with constant attendance from a physical therapist. At the beginning of this session, patients locate their exercise program that has been determined for them at a previous visit with their physical therapist. This written program is brought with them as they progress through the various exercise stations. During the period in which these patients are exercising simultaneously, the physical therapist provides clinical expertise and judgment, such as offering feedback, providing further individualized instruction, implementing modifications and progressions of the exercise program for each patient, or measuring each patient's response to treatment. The physical therapist is also there to attend to any patient who may experience difficulty while performing their exercises such as chest pain, dizziness, shortness of breath or other sudden emergencies.

Coding:

Patient A: 97150 (group therapy)
Patient B: 97150 (group therapy)
Patient C: 97150 (group therapy)
Patient D: 97150 (group therapy)
Patient E: 97150 (group therapy)

Rationale:

This is an example of a situation in which the therapist is overseeing more than one patient and is providing skilled services to them while in constant attendance. Group therapy (97150) could be billed for each patient in this circumstance.

7b. SUPERVISED EXERCISE

Eight patients are participating in an hour-long exercise program in a physical therapy clinic. At the beginning of this session, patients locate the exercise program that has been determined for them at a previous visit with their physical therapist. This written program is brought with them as they progress through the various exercise stations available in the gym. Each patient documents the exercise or activity that is completed with the specific parameters performed during that session. The physical therapist intermittently observes these eight individuals during their one-hour exercise period. The physical therapist is available to answer general questions an individual may have regarding the safe use of the equipment. The physical therapist is also there to attend to any patient who may experience difficulty while performing their exercises such as chest pain, dizziness, shortness of breath or other sudden emergencies.

For individual progression or changes to the patients exercise protocol, the patient is directed to the physical therapist that developed the plan for them initially, or the physical therapist that is currently responsible for their plan of care.

Coding:

Currently in CPT there is no code to appropriately describe the scenario as detailed above.

Rationale:

This care would not be considered skilled physical therapy and therefore is not a covered service under Medicare. Because it is a noncovered Medicare service, it would be possible for the therapist to collect out-of-pocket payment from the individuals.

8a. ONE-ON-ONE FOLLOWED BY GROUP INTERVENTION (PT & PTA)

Patient A arrives for a 9:00 AM appointment and is seen by the physical therapist for 15 minutes of manual therapy techniques followed by 15 minutes of PNF and manually resistive exercise for strengthening. At 9:15 AM, Patient B arrives and is seen by the physical therapist assistant for 15 minutes of manual stretching. At 9:30, Patient A is seen for 15 minutes of manual stretching by the PTA, while Patient B is seen by the physical therapist from 9:30 to 9:45 for manual therapy techniques. At 9:45, both patients A and B are working in the gym on strengthening exercises previously prescribed by the physical therapist, while the physical therapist assistant supervises both patients, providing verbal, visual and proprioceptive cueing to both patients for correct technique, speed and performance of exercises. Patient A leaves the clinic and 10:15 AM and Patient B leaves the clinic at 10:30 AM.

Coding:

Patient A: 97110 (therapeutic exercise) 2 units
97140 (manual therapy)
97150 (group therapy)
Patient B: 97110 (therapeutic exercise)
97140 (manual therapy)
97150 (group therapy)

Rationale:

Patient A received one on one manual therapyand therapeutic exercise from 9:00 –9:30. From 9:30-9:45, a physical therapist assistant provides one on one manual stretching, which is billable, because the physical therapist assistant may perform skilled one on one services under the supervision of the physical therapist. This amounts to two units of therapeutic exercise (97110) and one unit of manual therapy (97140).

From 9:15-9:30, Patient B receives manual stretching with the physical therapist assistant (under the supervision of the physical therapist), which is billable. During this time frame, patient B receives 15 minutes of manual stretching, which is counted as a therapeutic exercise (97110) because the physical therapist assistant may perform skilled one on one services. Patient B is then seen by the physical therapist one on one from 9:30-9:45, which may be billed as one unit of manual therapy (97140). Beginning at 9:45 the physical therapist assistant provides skilled services while in constant attendance with Patient A and Patient B simultaneously. Thus, it is appropriate to bill one until of group therapy (97150) for each patient for this time period.

8b. ONE-ON-ONE FOLLOWED BY GROUP INTERVENTION (PT & PT AIDE)

Patient A arrives for a 9:00 AM appointment and is seen by the physical therapist for 15 minutes of manual therapy techniques followed by 15 minutes of PNF and manually resistive exercise for strengthening. At 9:15 AM, Patient B arrives and performs a stretching program previously prescribed by the physical therapist for 15 minutes while an aide assists the patient on and off the floor mat. At 9:30, Patient A performs 15 minutes of stretching while an aide assists the patient on and off the floor, while Patient B is seen by the physical therapist from 9:30 to 9:45 for manual therapy techniques. At 9:45, both patients A and B begin working in the gym independently on strengthening exercises previously prescribed by the physical therapist, while an aide assists the patients with getting on and off equipment and checking off the completed exercises on an exercise flow sheet. Patient A leaves the clinic and 10:15 AM and Patient B leaves the clinic at 10:30 AM.

Coding:

Patient A: 97110 (therapeutic exercise)
97140 (manual therapy)
Patient B: 97140 (manual therapy)

Rationale:

Between 9:00 and 9:30 Patient A receives one unit of therapeutic exercise (97110) and one unit of manual therapy (97140).

The services patient B receives in the stretching program with the assistance of the aide would not be covered services as an aide cannot provide skilled services that would be covered by Medicare.

The time patient B spends one on one with the therapist from 9:30-9:45 would be billed as manual therapy (97140).

This scenario differs from 8a in that there is no group charge. The physical therapist would not bill the group because there is no physical therapist assistant (under the supervision of the physical therapist) providing services in this scenario as there is in 8a. An aide may not supervise group therapy. The time spent by A and B starting at 9:45 in the gym in not billable as the physical therapist is not in constant attendance. The supervision by the aide is not sufficient to permit billing.

1111 North Fairfax Street, Alexandria, VA 22314-1488
703/684-APTA (2782) * 800-999-2782 * 703/683-6748 (TDD)
703/684-7343 (fax)

F Goal Writing Exercise

Rewrite the following general goals into objective, measurable goals.

1. Decrease congestion

2. Improve standing posture

3. Independent with home exercises

4. Increase shoulder movements, all planes by 10 degrees

5. Decrease low back pain

6. Improve ambulation skills

7. Improve cervical rotation

8. Maximize functional ability

9. Decrease UE flexion synergy

10. Patient will be able to sit up

11. Improve motor planning

12. Reduce edema of the LUE

13. Increase endurance

14. Maintain spinal segment in place

15. Control balance

G Note Writing Exercise

1. Rewrite the following SOAP note in acceptable content format as a SOAP note.
2. Rewrite the following SOAP note in a narrative format with appropriate content and categorize the information.

NOTE # 1:
S: Fixed the lawnmower this weekend
O: Seen in dept. for cont with cybex protocol to BLE's 2 cycles r, 1 cycle L. Followed by balance beam, kicking ball, unilateral stance 15 sec. L unable to maintain L. Side <> side stepping. Side <> side gallop. Fast walking length of speech hall and back 196 in 45 sec 1st trial, 43 in 2nd, 36 in 3rd with encouragement. Kneeling–1/2 kneeling on mat 2 sets 10 reps. Amb 60′ with 8 hyperextensions 1st time, 4 2nd, 8 3rd.
A: Tol Rx well, fatigued with ex.
P: Continue

Note # 2:

S: Good spirits

O: Gait + advanced gait + balance techniques - instruction + practice.

A: Demonstrating good gait and balance with some proprioceptive L/E deficit + thus would advise to contact guard stand-by assistance for safety at present.

P: Continue as above

1. Write a chart entry for a patient that did not come to therapy today and did not call to cancel.

2. A patient is brought to PT but refuses to do anything and is disrupting others.

H Documentation Content Exercise

For the following intervention entries, please answer the following:

1. Is it written objectively with all appropriate objective information included?
2. Is the terminology correct for reimbursement and billing?
3. Is the intervention reproducible based on the information given?
4. If there is enough information to reproduce the treatment, defend your decision.
5. If there is not enough information to reproduce the treatment, what other information do you need?

1. Strengthening exercises to the LEs.

2. Massage to neck

3. Electrical stimulation to low back

4. Joint mobilization lumbar region

5. Gait training

6. Intermittent cervical traction in supine, head in neutral × 20 minutes, 25 pounds, 30 second hold, 15 second release

7. Stretching to R heelcords

8. Biofeedback for R UE

9. US to L calf

10. Back exercises

Documentation Content Examples

Appendix I

Physical Therapy Evaluation

Name: Grant Stern   **Date**: 10/26/11
DOB: 2/19/68   **SS#**: 213-36-8245
Referring Physician: C Brooks
Diagnosis: Medical: 820.9 fracture of neck of femur, unspecified, open L
PT treatment diagnosis: 781.2 gait abnormality (orthopedic)

Medical History: See attached General History for additional information.
43 y.o. male referred 10/25/11 with L femur fracture, s/p ORIF, hip pinning, 10/05/11 secondary to auto accident 10/04/11. Patient was a passenger. Hospitalized at BGMC 10/4 to 10/22/11. Other injuries included: multiple abrasions and lacerations extremities and face, which are in various stages of healing. No other medical problems prior to accident.
Meds: Percocet, PRN, Tylenol PRN for pain.
Social history: Married, lives in 2 story townhouse with stairs, bedrooms on second floor. 2 children, ages 3 and 5. Vocation: Middle school teacher in Broward County, but currently not working. Drives car with automatic transmission. Leisure: mountain biking, running.
Chief complaints: Unable to sleep, dependent on walker, unable to work, unable to enjoy leisure activities, unable to play with kids.
Precautions: 50% WB LLE
Barriers to learning: none
Home Barriers: stairs
Cognition:
     Intact, appropriate communication, accurate historian
Vital signs at rest: BP: 130 / 80   P: 84   RR: 16
Vitals following eval session: BP: 132 / 84   P: 86   RR: 18
Endurance:
     Becomes SOB with exertion. Requires 1 minute of rest for every 5 minutes of activity.
Pain:
     L hip: at rest 5/10, wakes him up at night 3 to 4x, when changes position
     With WB: 9/10   With movement: 8/10
Integument/Sensation:
     Surgical incision L lateral hip, staples out, incision closed, dark pink in appearance. Lacks sensation to light touch/pain along incision. Intact otherwise. Scabs on face and both lower extremities. No open areas noted.
     Mild edema in area of incision.
     Proprioception intact UEs & LEs.
DTRs:
     Normal

ADL: Per patient, I in toileting (elevated toilet seat) and showering. Uses shower chair at home with hand held shower head. I in self-feeding. Dresses in sitting using reacher and sock aid.

Mobility: Drove self to therapy, has compact type car.

    Bed mobility: I rolling L/R, scooting up and down, scooting L/R.

    Transfers: I: sit to supine, sit to stand, stand pivot using front wheel rolling walker (FWRW) and without, PWB 50% LLE. Able to transfer toward R and toward L, also I in all car transfers.

Gait: I with FWRW, 50% WB LLE on even surfaces and carpet. Demonstrates minimal WB on LLE with short stance, decreased stride and step length and step to pattern. Speed slow, at 40 meters per minute. Flexed posture with walker. Tendency to turn toward R, avoiding directional changes to L when possible. Initial contact with foot flat. Decreased hip flexion in swing phase. Distance limited to 50 to 75' (household).

    Unable to negotiate stairs in upright, and has been going up and down at home in sitting, bumping up and down on buttocks once per day.

Balance:

    Stable with FWRW

    Without walker: Single leg stance on R x 2 seconds with balance loss to left, able to I recover.

Strength:

UE s:	gross strength	5/5
RLE:	gross strength	5/5
LLE:	Hip flexion	2/5
	Abduction	2-/5
	Knee flexion	3-/5
	Extension	3-/5
	Ankle dorsiflexion	5/5
	Plantarflexion	4/5

Range of Motion:

    UE s: no deficits noted, intact

    RLE: no deficits noted, intact

		Active	Passive
LLE:	hip flexion	100°	120° with pain
	Abduction	10°	15°
	Adduction	to neutral	to neutral
	External rotation	10°	10°
	Internal rotation	10°	10°
	Knee flexion	80°	100°
	Extension	-5°	0°

Ankle dorsiflexion	8°	15°
Plantarflexion	40°	40°

Problem Summary:

Weakness LLE, ROM deficits LLE, Balance deficit in standing, Pain LLE, Gait walker dependent on even surfaces only, Abnormal gait pattern, Flexed posture in standing, endurance limitations, limited weight bearing

Gait limited to indoor surfaces primarily, household ambulator, unable to negotiate stairs in upright, unable to balance in upright for upright activities such as shaving, dresses in sit with assistive devices, fatigue secondary to inability to sleep through night, requires frequent rest during activity

Unable to work, unable to participate in play with children, unable to socialize or engage in leisure activities

Goals:

STGs: 11/08/11

Patient will be able to achieve gait with FWRW 200 feet on even and carpeted surfaces for safe standing in self-care.

Single leg stance on R x 20 seconds with balance loss to left, able to I recover.

MMT LLE: Hip flexion   3/5, Abduction   3/5

LTGs: 12/08/11

Patient will be able to achieve gait 200 feet with a straight cane on even surfaces, carpeted surfaces, and outdoors.

MMT LLE: Hip flexion	4/5, Abduction	4-/5
L Knee flexion	AROM 100°	PROM 130°

Return to work with straight cane

Requires 1 minute of rest for every 25 minutes of activity.

P: OP PT x 3 /week for 4 weeks to consist of gait training with FWRW and cane, crutches, progressive ther ex, neuromuscular re-ed, and cold pack LLE.

Signature: *Regina Brown*, PT 00723

SOAP Daily Note – Out-patient

Pt Name: Grant Stern   Date: 11/06/11
Time: 1:00 pm to 2:15 pm

Diagnosis: Medical: 820.9 fracture of neck of femur, unspecified, open L
PT treatment diagnosis: 781.2 gait abnormality (orthopedic)
Guide Section: 4H, 4I

S: Pt stated "Able to sleep through the night up to 6 hours now, as pain in my hip is no longer waking me up."
O: Precautions: PWB 50% LLE
22 minutes: 97116: Gait training: x3 trials each, contact guard with axillary crutches 4 point pattern; even surface x50 feet, grass, carpet, training stairs, 5 up/down; ascended/descended using crutches contact guard with verbal cues for crutch placement, and pattern. Tendency to for initial contact on left with whole foot, short stance on left without verbal cues.
15 minutes: 97110: Therapeutic procedure: in standing: Active: L hip abduction, adduction, flexion, procedure, circumduction x10 reps each, rest in between, holding handrail. Supine: Active L knee extension hamstring stretch x2, 30 sec hold, quad sets/glut sets bilaterally: x5 reps, 20 sec hold. Strength: L hip flexion 3+/5; abduction 3+/5.
18 minutes: 97112: Neuromuscular re-education: Balance training without crutches: single leg stance on R, eyes open minimal assist 10% (or limited assist 10%) for balance. Balance loss to the left, after 10 secs, 10 reps. Assist required to right self.
15 minutes: 97010: Cold pack L hip patient in R sidelying, pillow between knees for comfort following gait and exercise. Instructed to use axillary crutches at home instead of FWRW, on indoor surfaces only at present for safety and to continue with home exercises as previously instructed.

A: Progressed from front wheeled rolling walker to axillary crutches in order to increase mobility on uneven surfaces, including curbs and stairs. Skin on hip intact prior and following application of cold pack, mild hyperemia present. Patient is progressing toward his established goals of I on all surfaces with crutches, as well as increasing the strength of the L hip musculature.

P: Will continue with OP PT x 3/week for gait training, progressive ther ex, neuromuscular re-ed and cold pack. Plan to add resistance for ther ex next visit, 2#s.

Signature: *Lynn Robert*, PT 0001234

For billing purposes: Non-Medicare

Diagnosis: Medical: 820.9 fracture of neck of femur, unspecified, open L

PT treatment diagnosis: 781.2 gait abnormality (orthopedic)

Codes:	Procedures:	Units:
97116	Gait training	1 unit (based on a 15 minute unit)
97110	Therapeutic procedure	1 unit (based on a 15 minute unit)
97112	Neuromuscular re-ed	1 unit (based on a 15 minute unit)
97010	Cold pack	1 unit (based on a 15 minute unit)

Author's Note: Non-Medicare. Although gait training was 22 minutes, as AMA CPT codes/procedures are in 15-minute increments, it only qualifies as one unit. The session qualifies for 4 units of care.

Medicare. Under Medicare coding guidelines, cold packs cannot be charged as individual procedures. Although they must be included in the documentation, they are not separately reimbursable as they are considered "bundled." Additionally, from a time perspective, as Medicare unit ranges from 8 to 22 minutes, each procedure qualifies for 1 unit, for a total of 3 units. For billing of services in SNFs, the terms limited assist and extensive assist are recommended by CMS with %s, for what were previously minimal assist and maximal assist. Regardless of the terminology used, however, the % of assist needed or % of patient/client dependence, must be included as well as a description of the behavior or dysfunction that characterizes the assistance needed.

Narrative Daily Note – Out-patient

Grant Stern
Drives I to visits, ambulatory with FWRW.

11/06/11
1:00 – 2:15 pm: Patient s/p L femur fracture, I ambulator with FWRW PWB to PT for:
97116 Gait training: 3 trials each, contact guard with axillary crutches 4 point pattern,
PWB LLE 50% on even surface x 50 feet, grass, carpet, training stairs; 5 up and down.
Contact guard and verbal cues for correct pattern and crutch placement. Short stance on
L, initial contact L with whole foot.
97110 Therapeutic procedure: in standing, active, for L hip abduction, L hip adduction,
flexion, extension, circumduction x 10 reps each, rest in between, holding handrail.
Supine: Active L knee extension hamstring stretch x2, 30 sec hold, quad sets/glut sets
bilaterally: x5 reps, 20 sec hold. Strength: L hip flexion 3+/5; abduction 3+/5.
97112 Neuromuscular re-education: Balance training without crutches: single leg stance
on R, eyes open minimal assist 10% (or limited assist 10%) for balance. Balance loss to
the left, after 10 secs, 10 reps. Assist required to right self.
97010 Cold pack L hip x 15 minutes, patient in R sidelying, pillow between knees for
comfort following gait and exercise. Reported pain level at 6/10 prior to CP and 3/10
following. Skin intact before and after with mild hyperemia after.
Pt. stated that he's able to sleep up to 6 hours per night now.
Instructed to use axillary crutches at home, instead of FWRW, on indoor surfaces only at
present for safety and to continue with home exercises as previously instructed.
Demonstrating steady improvement as evidenced by progression from FWRW to
crutches. Will continue with OP PT x 3/week for gait training, progressive ther ex,
neuromuscular re-ed and cold pack. Plan to add resistance for ther ex next visit, 2#s.

Signature: *Lynn Robert*, PT 0001234

Flowsheet Example 1

Pt: Grant Stern

Please indicate # of units as applicable for each procedure (or a check ✓ if units are non-billable) and initials of individual treating

Procedure	11/06/11									
Gait training 97116	1 *LR*									
Ther procedure 97110	1 *LR*									
Neuro-muscular re-ed 97112	1 *LR*									
Cold pack 97010	1 *LR*									
Home Instruction	✓ *LR*									

Supplemental entries by date:

11/06/11:
Progressed from FWRW to axillary crutches: CG & VC: ascend and descend 5 steps, grass, carpet, even surface 50', x 3 reps each. Ther ex, active in standing L hip: in all planes, 10 reps, single leg stance R, 10 secs with balance loss to L. CP L hip in sidelying at end of session x 15 mins. Pain ▾ from 6/10 to 3/10 following CP. Add 2# resistance next visit, cont 3x/week. *Lynn Robert* , PT 0001234

Flowsheet Example 2

Pt: Grant Stern

Please indicate # of units as applicable for each procedure (or a check ✓ if units are non-billable) and initials of individual treating

Procedure	11/06/11									
Gait training 97116	1 *LR*									
FWRW										
crutches	✓									
even	✓									
carpet	✓									
stairs	✓									
curbs										
grass	✓									
Ther procedure 97110	1 *LR*									
Active	✓									
Standing	✓									
Supine										
Sidelying										
Prone										
Resistive										
Standing										
Supine										
Sidelying										
Prone										
Neuro-muscular re-ed 97112	1 *LR*									
Balance	✓									
Cold pack 97010	1 *LR*									
Home Instruction	✓ *LR*									

Supplemental entries by date:

11/06/11:

Progressed from FWRW to axillary crutches: CG & VC: ascend and descend 5 steps, grass, carpet, even surface 50', x 3 reps each. Ther ex, active in standing L hip: in all planes, 10 reps, single leg stance R, 10 secs with balance loss to L. CP L hip in sidelying at end of session x 15 mins. Pain ▾ from 6/10 to 3/10 following CP. Add 2# resistance next visit, cont 3x/week. *Lynn Robert*, PT 0001234

Clinical Pathway Example

Medical Diagnosis:

820.9 fracture of neck of femur, unspecified, open L

PT Diagnosis:

781.2 gait abnormality (orthopedic)

Weight bearing status: FWB RLE   **PWB 50%** LLE

PT: Name: Print Jennifer Allan   **Signature:** *Jennifer Allan*   **Initials:** *JA*, DPT

PT: Name: Print: Lynn Robert   **Signature:** *Lynn Robert*   **Initials:** *LR* PT

PT: Name: Print: _____ **Signature**_____**Initials:** _____

	Gait training 97116	Gait training	Gait training	Gait training	Ther procedure 97110	Ther procedure	Ther procedure	Instructions
Date	**I crutches even surface**	**I crutches carpet**	**I crutches grass/ outdoor**	**I crutches stairs**	**3/5 strength L hip:** ✓, **abd**	**3+/5 strength L hip:** ✓, **abd**	**4-/5 strength L hip:** ✓, **abd**	**I HEP**
11/02/11					✓ *JA*			✓ *JA*
11/06/11	✓ *LR*					✓ *LR*		✓ *LR*

Discharge status:

Interim supplemental entries as indicated:

11/02/11:

Progressed from FWRW to axillary crutches 4 point gait: CG & VC: even surface 50', x 3 reps. Ther ex, active on mat in antigravity positions: L hip: in all planes, 10 reps, single leg stance R, 5 secs with balance loss to L. Able to sleep 4 hours uninterrupted by pain. Progress to ther ex in standing next visit, cont 3x/week. *Jennifer Allan*, **DPT 0002234**

11/06/11:

Progressed from FWRW to axillary crutches: CG & VC: ascend and descend 5 steps, grass, carpet, even surface 50', x 3 reps each. Ther ex, active in standing L hip: in all planes, 10 reps, single leg stance R, 10 secs with balance loss to L. CP L hip in sidelying at end of session x 15 mins. Pain ▼ from 6/10 to 3/10 following CP. Able to sleep up to 6 hours now. Add 2# resistance next visit, cont 3x/week. *Lynn Robert*,
PT 0001234

INDEX

Page numbers followed by the letters "*f*" and "*t*" indicate figures and tables, respectively.